GLEANINGS FROM VEDIC TO PURANIC AGE

Collected Papers of

Dr. Sadashiv A. Dange

(With a Biographical Sketch and a Bibliography of his writings)

GLEANINGS FROM VEDIC TO PURANIC AGE

Collected Papers of

Dr. Sadashiv A. Dange

(With a Biographical Sketch and a Bibliography of his Writings)

Edited by

Dr. (Mrs.) Sindhu S. Dange

Ex-R.G. Bhandarkar Professor and Head, Deptt. of Sanskrit, Mumbai University

ARYAN BOOKS INTERNATIONAL

NEW DELHI

GLEANINGS FROM VEDIC TO PURANIC AGE

ISBN-81-7305-237-9

First Published in **2002** by
ARYAN BOOKS INTERNATIONAL
Pooja Apartments, 4B, Ansari Road, Darya Ganj
New Delhi-110002 (INDIA)
Tel.: 3287589, 3255799; Fax: 91-11-3270385
E-mail: aryanbooks@vsnl.com

Computer Typeset at ABI Prints & Publishing Co., New Delhi
Printed in India at B.B.N. Printers, New Delhi

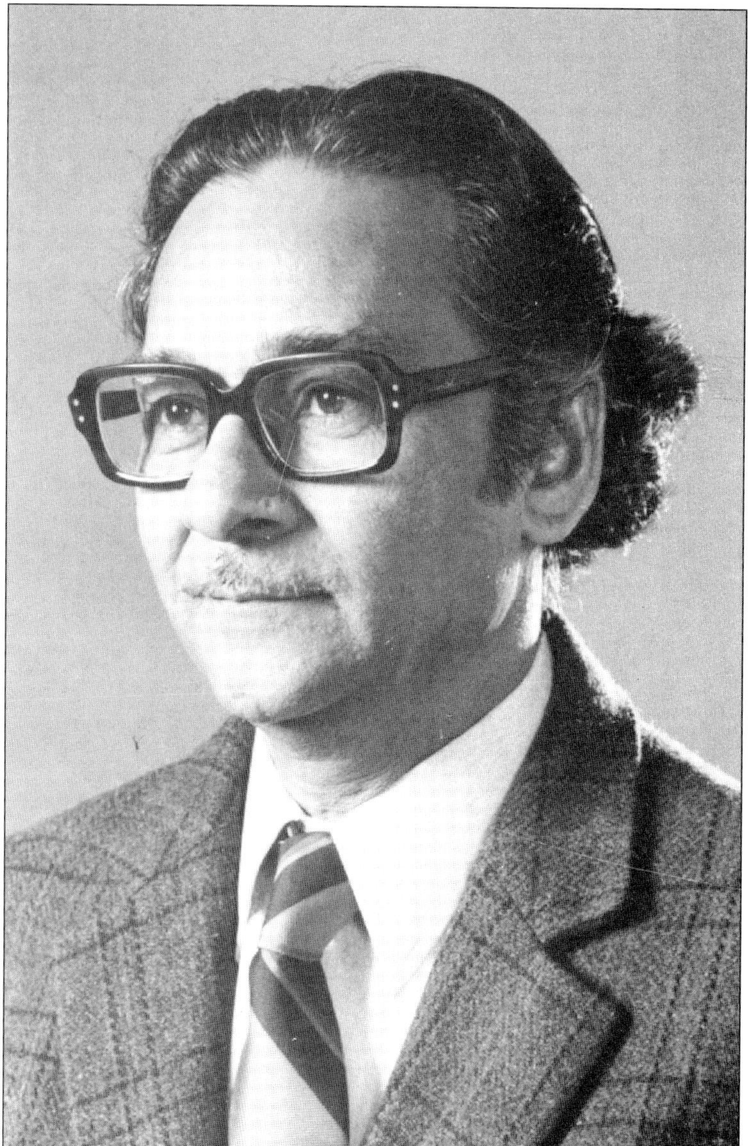

(late) Dr. Sadashiv Ambadas Dange

To
Our Daughters
Dr. (Mrs.) Varsha, Ph.D.
Dr. (Mrs.) Vinata, Ph.D.
Dr. (Mrs.) Vasumati, Ph.D.

Preface

I am presenting to the scholarly world in book-form, twenty-three papers of (late) Dr. Sadashiv A. Dange, Ex–R.G. Bhandarkar Professor and Head, Deptt. of Sanskrit, University of Mumbai, dealing with mythical concepts, poetic interpretations, rituals and 'spoken' aspect of the Sanskrit language with a focus on grammar.

These papers excepting three, were already published in reputed research journals. The details of these, are noted in the book at the end of these papers. I thank the editors and concerned authorities of these Journals for allowing me to include these papers in this book. At some places, I have made certain omissions and at some others, additions, taking into account the later researches of Dr. S.A. Dange.

As Part II of the book, I have given a bibliography of the writings of Dr. Dange, on the insistence of our students and scholars. Together with the bibliography is given a short biographical sketch of Dr. Dange, who giving a tough fight to his serious illness, could complete his projects, little before he left for the heavenly abode.

This book is a gift to our daughters. Dr. Dange always wished and was fortunate to see them in the field of research in the respective branches of their study.

I entrusted the publication of this book to Shri Vikas Arya (Aryan Books International, New Delhi). He has been publishing our books since 1994, with a sense of belonging. He has brought out this book also with the same feeling.

My thanks are to Mrs. Vidya Joshi, Lecturer in Art, J.J. School of Art, Mumbai, for the jacket-design with the picture.

19th May, 2002

Dr. (Mrs.) Sindhu S. Dange
Ex–R.G. Bhandarkar Professor and
Head, Department of Sanskrit,
University of Mumbai

Contents

Part - II

Part - I

Introduction

The *Ṛgveda* enjoys a place of prime importance for tracing any later concept whatsoever in the fields of mythology, rituals and spoken Sanskrit. The composition of the later Purāṇas practically coincides with the earlier phase of the classical Sanskrit literature, when the earlier concepts with additions in some cases did assume a final form. A detailed study of some such concepts in the field of mythology as well as in the field of rituals was undertaken by Dr. Dange in his earlier books.

The sphere of Sanskrit grammar, with its rules followed in the 'spoken' aspect of the Sanskrit language invited his attention on certain problems.

This volume presents some concepts explained and certain problems touched and solved by Dr. Dange through his papers, written from 1969 onwards, which were published in reputed research journals.

An attempt has been made here to take a bird's-eye view of these "Gleanings from Vedic to Puranic Age".

The chapter "Axis Mundi and the Vedic Yūpa" deals with the Vedic belief in *axis mundi*, which is a column or a pole that stands at the centre of the cosmos and connects the heaven and earth. The celestial tree connecting the two worlds and the sacrificial post (*yūpa*) had the same concept associated with them. In the "Visions of the Ṛgvedic Ṛṣi-kavi-s", the basic concept of '*kāvya*' is discussed as seen in the *ṚV* where it means a wonderful activity and not merely the composition called 'poetry' as we have in the later times. Here we are reminded of the *mantra* from the *AV*, which eulogises the '*kāvya*' of the (Great) God by saying that it never died (and would not die!) nor would it become worn out, i.e. old (*AV* X.8.32b). These *ṛṣi-kavi*-s of the *ṚV* are different from the *kavi-kāru*-s (no doubt, the gifted composers), the latter signifying a conscious effort on their part for poetic compositions. These *ṛṣi-kavi*-s are not only 'auto-vert',[1] but they have 'auto-vision'. This 'auto-vision' is somewhat different from simple "vision". Though basically steeped in the sacrificial set-up on the terrestrial region, the visions of these *ṛṣi-kavi*-s, crossing the mid-region embrace the farthest heaven in their supra-sensorial flights. One such *ṛṣi-kavi* is Dīrghatamas, whose visions display some of the finest images.

In line with this paper dealing with images of the *ṛṣi-kavi*-s, can be taken the following one into account, discussing the viewpoint of the *ācārya*-poetician of very late date. "Sanskrit Poetics and Semiotics" takes a note of Śaṅkuka's interpretation of the *rasa-sūtra* of Bharata. Dr. Dange points out that while advancing the imagery of the horse and its picture (*citra-turaga*), Śaṅkuka subtly introduces the principle of imagery, which glides into the realm of Semiotics. Any creative writer, while describing his experiences from the real, mixes his own imagination with them. The '*a-laukika*' (not 'other worldly' but 'of a different world') bliss experienced by the reader (spectator) from poetry is of this 'a-real' world of poetic images, created by the poet.

"Dream (Svapna) in the Vedic Concept" deals with the 'subconscious' aspect of man—a topic elaborately discussed further on a wider and comparative basis by Dr. Dange under the title "Dream, Myth and the Hindu Context."[2] Dream being a product of mind's unsettled condition, is called the sin of the mind (*manaspāpa*) and *anṛtasya prayotā*. The Greek concept of dream-making

Somnus (the god of sleep) a resident of the underworld together with his brother Death, gives him the authority of sending dreams, the 'underworld' obviously meaning the 'subconscious' in the individual. Modern age observation of Jung makes dream close to the 'dark side' of the psyche, which is the unconscious. This is verily the 'womb of *asura*', in which lies the mine of dreams, pointed out long back by the Vedic texts.

It is worthy of taking a note that the concept of dream is made to enter the realm of philosophy, while trying to know the 'ultimate'. The *Māṇḍūkya Up.* takes a note of dream as one of the four states, while explaining the concept of *ātman* (I.4). These four states are — that of being awake; of dream; of deep sleep, i.e. slumber; and of knowing the *ātman* principle (*Māṇḍ. Up.* I.2-7). In the philosophy of the Vijñānavādin Buddhists, the concept of dream can be explained by that of *parikalpita vijñāna* (which is a purely imagined knowledge),[3] as against the *pariniṣpanna-vijñāna* (i.e. pure knowledge of the ultimate).

"Act and Retribution in the Ṛgveda and the Atharvaveda" conclusively states that the theory of retribution is reflected in the *ṚV* and *AV* in the formation stage, though it developed later with its varieties.

The study of the deity Vāstoṣpati in "Vāstoṣpati, Rudra and Cyavana" results in pointing out that the deity is a mixture of concepts and beliefs. A definite presiding deity of the dwelling has already set in by the Ṛgvedic times. Though Tvaṣṭṛ and Rudra are said to be Vāstoṣpati, in the post-Ṛgvedic times, Rudra came to be closely associated with the *yajña-vāstu* (the sacrificial place) — was Vāstavya — and thus the Vāstoṣpati. Initially terrible by nature, he becomes benevolent when propitiated. The Vāstupuruṣa of the *Agni. P.* in later times, seen as a demon in appearance could be traced to this concept of the Vāstoṣpati Rudra. The sage Cyavana figuring in the account of the *Śat. Br.* and the *Jaim. Br.* is seen to know the ritual of *vāstupa* and has the behaviour and appearance of Vāstoṣpati and Rudra. Cyavana can stand as a representative of wayward sages, he himself being seen as an alter ego of the Vāstoṣpati.

The opinion of Asko Parpola that the myth of Mahiṣāsuramardinī and the later tradition of the buffalo-sacrifice offered to her is seen in the Vedic tradition itself under the influence of the Vrātyas, is taken into account in "Ṛgveda and the Buffalo-sacrifice?." It could be conclusively proved that the buffalo-sacrifice is never indicated in the Vedic texts. In fact, every trace of it has been wiped out by the Brāhmaṇa-texts as the buffalo was associated with the enemies of the Vedic people.

In "Therianthropomorphism and the Multiple-Head Motifs in Ancient India and the Middle-East", the two motifs (mentioned in the title) are dealt with from ancient India and the Middle East, cultural contacts between which have been an established fact. Though similarity in myths and art-motifs of distant lands can be explained on the basis of either independent origin or borrowing, here the point of comparison is given primary importance. The details from the Egyptian as well as the Greek mythology are therefore found fruitful.

To turn to the epics. "The Abduction of Sītā", the incident in the *Rām.* is discussed taking into account versions of the same incident in other works.

The point of the birth as also that of the marriage of the Pāṇḍavas in the *Mb.* has been discussed by scholars. Several works including even a Prakrit work have dealt with this problem. In "Birth and Marriage of the Pāṇḍavas — A Riddle?", the first problem, i.e. birth is discussed in the light of the Dharmaśāstra tradition and the second, i.e. their polyandrous marriage — a still more difficult problem — is dealt with viewing the exact situation through historical perspective. The peculiar circumstances of the Pāṇḍavas, making it difficult for them to have matrimonial relations in royal families, Drupada wishing to have political alliance with the Pāṇḍavas through Draupadī who was his (adopted!) daughter, Yudhiṣṭhira's helplessness in accepting Draupadī in a polyandric marriage as there was no other way left—all these make this peculiar marriage a politically planned affair.

Two different passages in the *Mb.* speaking of the death and subsequent cremation of Pāṇḍu and Mādrī, the latter following her husband on the same pyre, are discussed in "The 'Bodies' of Pāṇḍu and Mādrī and the Funeral Rites". These two passages appear to have contradiction, while there is none, for the two "bodies" which were brought to Hastināpura were the two jars containing the burnt 'bones' of Pāṇḍu and Mādrī. This explanation is given by Dr. Dange on the basis of the whole Śrauta tradition and also Nīlakaṇṭha, the commentator of the *Mb.* The discussion on this point has become necessary in the light of Prof. Mehendale's writings in this respect.

In "Stūpa—Vedic and Buddhistic", it is shown how the concept and practice of *stūpa* in the Buddhist tradition and *caitya* in the Jaina tradition have their origin in the Vedic practice and concept.

The Purāṇas contain several types of accounts such as those concerning creation, deluge, history of dynasties, etc. Some of these appear to be framed following the principle of 'typology' and hence need not detain us for consideration. But many other accounts are definitely challenging. To understand the implication of such mythical accounts in the Purāṇas, a transpuranic and transcultural study is indispensable. "Purāṇa and Śāstra" points out that to study the Purāṇas as a *Śāstra*, the study has to take the help from ancient Hindu law-books and has to proceed on socio-anthropological lines with material from many ancient mythologies, and has to take into account the approaches such as functionalism, structuralism and so on.

"The King with two faces" deals with a story from the Jaina text *Uttarajjhayaṇa-sutta* (*Uttarādhyayana-sūtra*), of Jaya, the king of Kāmpilya, who got the appellative name Domuha ("having two faces") after he placed the 'Great Crown' on his head. This crown he obtained when the ground was being dug up by his workers for building a *cittasabhā* (*citrasabhā,* i.e. a gallery with fascinating objects). Dr. Dange points out that the idea of two faces of the king was suggested from some such myth as that of the Roman god Janus imagined to have two faces, the god being joined with the end of the earlier year and to the beginning of the new year and also having a temple. This god (Janus) gave the name January to the month, which is at the beginning of the new year and comes immediately after the end of the earlier year. It is not improbable that Roman contacts with India from the first cent. A.D. to the fourth cent. A.D. gave rise to some such mythical accounts and beliefs. Even prior to this, the motif of the double-headed god can be traced to ancient Egyptian and Sumerian mythologies.

To turn to the points raised from the sphere of Mīmāṁsa. The Mīmāṁsā-rule "*dvayoḥ praṇayanti*" is applied by Vijñāneśvara, while deciding the woman's (wife's) share in her husband's property. It is seen that the Vedic data if strictly followed does not warrant this example.

"Moral Value and the Pūrvamīmāṁsā" points out how in the Vedic tradition, Dharma, Ṛta, Satya and Brahman were more important than even the gods, for the gods had to abide by the values indicated by these concepts. Brahman in the Pūrvamīmāṁsā context was something to be performed. The concept of *apūrva* is a definite contribution of the Pūrvamīmāṁsā to the Indian philosophical thought, a faint indication of which can be traced to *ṚV* X. 90.16, where it is said that the powers (*mahimānaḥ*) produced from the sacrifice reached the heaven. In spite of the actual sacrificial performance being perishable, there is the *adṛṣṭa* or *apūrva* produced from it, which is stored, in the name of the sacrificer. This paved the way for the further development of the doctrine of *karman,* which was earlier rooted, in the *ṚV*, because the ritual performance does not give fruit immediately but only after the death of a person (about which life he is at present completely blank). The concept of *niṣkāma karman* in its germinal form can be marked in this. Again the twin principle of *kratvartha* and *puruṣārtha* is a contribution of the Mīmāṁsā school.

To turn to the matters concerning the 'Spoken' aspect of the Sanskrit language.— "Root-Germinants in the Sanskrit Language (√*Ghas* : √AD)" points out that some (old) roots already lost some of their forms and had to be adjusted with other roots showing the remaining forms of their own. The meaning being the same, the principle of *ādeśa* came to help in this process, however, certainly showing that the roots in these cases were quite different from one another. At times a new root with a slight phonetic change is created. We can point out to the roots √*khād* as well as *kṣad* (*ṚV*) which are a combination of the roots √*ghas* and √*ad*. Thus apparently different roots are cognates and are formed from the same arch-root, if with the sound-nucleus the meaning of all is conceptually the same. As Dr. Dange has pointed out, it is interesting to see the 'history' of thought through some of the roots, which are formed on the principle of onomatopoeia. Thus √*ad* denotes simple movement of the jaws while eating; √*ghas* shows attacking prior to the actual devouring and not simply eating. Even √*khād* and √*kṣad* also run on the same lines as of √*ghas*. The roots √*grah*, √*gras* and √*ghas* show the crude hunting period of the human civilization.

The same line of thought is taken up in "Prākritization and the Germinant of the Roots of Vision". Thus in the roots of "vision", the most original root was √*khyā* — 'seeing' (Vedic) or 'telling'. The eye is the one which first 'tells' us about the object. Hence the words *cakṣu* (Skt.), *cakkhu* (Pkt) for the eye (which 'sees', i.e. 'tells'). The root √*khyā* is retained in the Prakrit language with the idea of 'telling'. As the Prakrit language shows the *kha* sound as in the normal speech of the common people, the roots of "vision" with the *kṣ* sound were reflected roots from the germinant √*khyā* or √*khyā-kṣa*.

The principle of reduplication works in the Sanskrit language when the sense is of the Desiderative, Frequentative (Intensive), in the case of the Perfect and a type of Aorist. But the point to be noted is that here the sense is changed with reduplication. The roots of the third conjugation show reduplication in actual use. In "Root-Germination and Reduplicated Roots in Sanskrit", the roots taken into account are those that have come down as reduplicated roots (*abhyasta*). These roots are seven in number, including √*jakṣ* (*Pāṇ.* VI.1.6 — *jakṣityādayaḥ ṣaṭ*). These roots do not have further reduplicated forms, √*śās,* however, having *śaśāsa* (*ṚV* II.29.5). The root √*śās* thus seems to be factually not a reduplicated root. But in the case of other six roots, the principle of root-germination seems working and a probe in the primary roots is made here.

To come to the word-study, which is taken up here. The words taken up for scrutiny are: (i) *kanyā* and *kānīna* and (ii) *dampatī* and *patnī*. In "Kanyā and Kānīna", the original word in *kanyā* and *kānīna* pointed out is '*kanī*' and with the addition of *ā* to it (*kanī* + *ā* = *kanyā*), we get the word *kanyā*. *Kanīnā* was a young maiden and *kānīna* (Masc.) was the one, born of a *kanīnā*.

In "Dampatī and Patnī", it is pointed out that the root underlying the words *sapatna, sapatnī* and even *patnī* is √*pat* in the sense 'to control' or 'to lord over', the sense 'to protect' being secondary. The root √*pat* gives the word *pati* (with the suffix *i*) (Masc. and Fem.). The same root √*pat* with *na* gives the word *patna* (Masc.) and *patnā* or *patnī* (Fem.).

"Vowel-shortening and the Sanskrit Sandhi" takes up a point, which is a matter of experience even in the modern speech. The final long vowel of the preceding word as a rule, gets shortened before the next vowel, unless it is retained with special care. In the Sanskrit *sandhi* also the long vowel becomes a shortened vowel and the latter has at once to adjust with the next one, itself taking the semi-vowel as a balancing element. Even in the case of the internal *sandhi* between a word and its suffix, this tendency cannot be overlooked. Dr. Dange was pursuing this topic right from 1969 as seen from this paper and has written two more papers on this topic in later years.[4]

Dr. Dange's hypothesis stated elaborately in his latest paper (pub. in 2001)[5] can help us to understand, as pointed out by Dr. Dange, the view of Fr. A. Esteller that *ṚV*-Saṁhitā was a palimpsest and certain changes in the *ṚV-mantra-s* of the *ṛṣi-kavi*-s did certainly take place in the times of the Saṁhitākāra.[6]

"Some Peculiarities of the Eastern Dialect according to Pāṇini" takes into account the main distinction, which prevailed between the Udīcyas and the Prācyas in the times anterior and posterior to Pāṇini. Udīcya-the northern quarter - was famous for the chaste language, while the language of the Easterners did show the deviation in the sphere of the Sanskrit and Prakrit languages. Such a deviation is noticed with respect to place-names, forms suggesting kinship, feminine forms and other stylistic peculiarities.

These papers dealing with the Sanskrit grammar take into account mainly the 'spoken' aspect of the Sanskrit language.

"Gleanings from Vedic to Puranic age" deal with varied topics. Beginning with the '*axis mundi*' and the 'visions' of the *ṛṣi-kavi*-s, which take us to the transcendental experience, we ultimately come to the terrestrial region — the sphere of the 'spoken' aspect of Sanskrit language — where, the ancient people once moved, later on making the generations to come, heirs of this great treasure — the SANSKRIT LANGUAGE.

Dr. (Mrs.) Sindhu S. Dange
Ex-R.G.Bhandarkar Professor
and Head, Dept. of Sanskrit
University of Mumbai

NOTES AND REFERENCES

1. (Mrs.) S.S. Dange, "Autovertism from the Ṛgveda", *Vishveshvaranand Indological Journal*, Panjab University, Hoshiarpur, Vo.XIV, Pt. I, March 1976 pp.7-16.
2. Sadashiv A. Dange, "Dream, Myth and the Hindu Context", *Annals of the Bhandarkar Oriental Research Institute,* Vol. LXXIX (1998), Pune, 1999, pp.61-82.
3. The Vijñānavāda Buddhist philosophy speaks of three types of knowledge *viz. parikalpita-vijñāna, paratantra-vijñāna* and *pariniṣpanna-vijñāna* the last being the pure knowledge of the ultimate. For the *parikalpita-vijñāna* see *Encyclopaedia of Religion and Ethics,* Vol.IX, p.850 a; *Laṅkāvatāra*, pub. by Buddhist Text Society, Calcutta (Kolkata), 1902, p.73; *Madhyamakāvatāra,* VI.93; *Sūtrālaṅkāra,* X.40.
4. See Sadashiv A. Dange, "Vowel-shortening in Sanskrit", *Vidyā-vratin* (Prof. A.M. Ghatge Fel. Vol.), Sri Satguru Publications (A Division of Indian Books Centre), Delhi, 1992, pp.95-100; also by the same author "Sandhi, Śākalya, Pāṇini VI.1. 127-128 And the Vedic Evidence", *Traividyam* (Vedic Studies in Memory of Durgamohan Bhattacharyya), Subarnarekha Pubn., Kolkata, 2001, pp.63-77.
5. See note 4 *supra.*
6. The view-point of Fr. Esteller was severely criticized by Prof. M.A. Mehendale, vide his Presidential Address of the Vedic Section, *Proceedings* of the All India Oriental Conference, XVII session (Kurukshetra), 1974, pub. by the Bhandarkar Oriental Research Institute, Poona, 1976, pp.39-60. Dr. Dange in his Presidential Address of the Vedic Section of the All India Oriental Conference, XXX Session (Vishva Bharati University, Santiniketan), 1980, *Proceedings*, pub. by the BORI, Poona, 1982, pp.23-34, has reviewed the contribution of Fr. A. Esteller, in view of the criticism of Prof. Mehendale of the former's views vide *Ibid.,* pp.30-34.

Chapter 1

Axis Mundi and the Vedic *Yūpa*

Though it is difficult to say that all of science that is known to us to-day was known to the Vedic people, and, for that matter, to the *Ṛgveda* and the Śrauta literature, it cannot be denied, that every clan and people have their own reasoning about the working of the cosmos and the relationship between Heaven and Earth. And time does not gainsay it. What is science to-day was not entirely fiction in the hoary past. Even to-day's anthropologists, in this advanced age of a scientific approach, believe that the ancient man had his own knowledge which could be attested as science. Among those who are to the fore and maintain this opinion are Joseph Campbell, Claude Lévi-Strauss and David Suzuki. These scholars base their proposition on the fact that the faculty of reasoning and of intellect is the same in man, and that whom we might wrongly call 'savages' and 'aboriginals' often show more marked penetration into the working of the cosmos, their instrument being close observation of Nature and the application of their keen intellect to the phenomena.[1] As this is not a speciality of any one chosen people, it is not surprising that common symptoms of observation and explaining this observation are noticed among people from lands separated by vast expanses of land and oceans. People with such keen sense, as noted above, are called, by the so-called advanced scientists, with the appellation 'shaman', 'witch-doctor' and what not. But, the Vedic tradition has a more respectable name for such knowledgeable persons. It is *brahma-vid*, and, in the later period, it is *āpta*. The *brahmavid* is 'one who knows the *brahman!*'. And what is *brahman*? Who knows? It is as good as asking, "What is Life? Is eating 'life'; is walking 'life'?" 'No' is the answer; and also, 'Yes' is the answer. In the same way, "What is *brahman*?" The etymologists and the ritualists have said, that Brahman is something that is 'Great' (*parivṛḍham bhavati*, to refer to Yāskācārya; and for Sāyaṇācārya, it was both a prayer and ritual).[2] However, the Upaniṣadic philosophers, or we may name them, now, '*brahma-vid*', even after continued deliberations, have said about 'Brahman', '*neti neti*'. And yet, we have very often heard the term "Brahmāṇḍa", as if Brahma actually produced the cosmic egg that is visible in the form of the circle of Heaven together with the Earth. If *vijñāna* is the comprehension of something beyond the seen world (*viśiṣṭam jñānam*), the very concept of Brahmāṇḍa is a phase of *vijñāna*, at that hoary period; because it is the reflection of a step to go beyond this mundane existence and touch the source of creation with our intellect. Likewise, the *brahma-vid* at the *Śat.Br.* says, "*dvayam vā-idam; na tṛtīyam asti; ārdram caiva śuṣkam ca; yac chuṣkam tad āgneyam yad ārdram tat saumyam*" ('There is only the twofold; no third exists; the moist and the dry; what is 'dry' that pertains to the fire-god; what is 'moist' that pertains to Soma, the sacred juice', *Śat.Br.* I.6.3.23). This statement, which stands at the basis of the whole Vedic sacrificial context and, particularly, the offerings, has to be seen as a scientific Truth (*vaijñānika tattva*); for, all offerings are not only moist, but, in the Vedic Śrauta tradition, they are all, conceptually aspects of Soma, which has the status of a gene for them; and various myths have explained the same principle, not to speak of the three cosmic strata: the sun with waters in its orb, the mid-region *vaidyuta-agni* with its lightning fire and the rain-waters, and the terrestrial fire at the sacrificial altar with its moist offerings. It is an easy extension to the modern experience of electricity being generated from energy commissioned from the waterfalls. Bereft of the association of the water-fire, or 'dry-moist' syndrome, the principle that emerges from such '*darśana*' (supra-mundane conception, which is 'Philosophy' according to the Western thinkers) is, that the three strata (Heaven, Mid-region and Earth) are strewn in the same system, which, on the ritual plane gave the concept of the Mahāvīra *pātra* (in the ritual of the Pravargya); and, on the cosmic plane, reflects the basic concept of the Cosmic arrangement of layers appearing as a column or as a pole, which, in modern terminology, is familiar to us in the *axis mundi*. What is *axis mundi*? Well! The word *axis* is understood in a twofold way: (i) a line about which a body rotates; and (ii) about which a figure is conceived to revolve (These are the meanings from the *Chambers Twentieth Century Dictionary*). The word *mundi* is of the Latin origin; *mundanus*, or *mundus*, has given the English word 'mundane', which has not only the sense of 'earthly' or 'worldly', but also of 'Cosmic'. Thus, *axis mundi* presents a conceptual image of a column or a pole that stands at the centre of the cosmos, around which the latter moves; or, in secular and ritual symbolism, it is the pole that stands firm as the support for Heaven and Earth. The *Jaiminīya Upaniṣad-Brāhmaṇa* (I.20.10) has very illuminating observations about the *axis mundi*. It says, that Heaven and Earth are firmly fixed at two ends by atmosphere, as are two wheels by an axle. This would reflect the belief that the atmosphere (*antarikṣa*) acts as the axle; but, if one visualizes this image in the actual position, this 'axle' would not be horizontal, but perpendicular (i.e. upright), where the circle of the sky (*dyo*, which means also 'heaven') is at the top, while the circle of the earth is at the lower end. The circular shape of the earth is attested by the Vedic tradition in the expression *parimaṇḍalā vai bhūḥ*; but, the circular shape of the sky is not quite attestable from actual observation. The circle of the earth is seen at the horizon; but, though the sky meets the earth at the horizon, it is actually half-circular and dome-like in observation. What is circular in the sky, and permanently so, is the orb of the sun. The moon is circular only on a very few days adjacent to the full-moon day; never permanently, like the sun. The axle conceived by the *Jaim.-Up.Br.* (noted above) need not be taken as having two wheels of equal size; it does not say so. It is a peculiar axle, where at the top the wheel is smaller in observation, while the earth-wheel is not so, as far as observation (*darśana*) is concerned!. In essence, in imagination, the cosmic axle joins the sun at the upper end and holds it, while at the lower end, it holds the earth. The Mahāvīra in Pravargya stands for three fires in the three worlds. The axle (Sanskrit, *akṣa*) is not the whole atmosphere; it is the conceptual column that is fixed in the orb of the sun at the upper end, while it has the earth at its lower visible end. The image to this effect obtains in the *Ṛgveda*, in the *stūpa* of Varuṇa, in a verse (*ṚV* I.24.7).

The message from the verse is: (i) King Varuṇa holds the column of a unique 'tree' in the bottomless space; (ii) its root is up; but, its filaments shoot downwards; and (iii) the rays from these filaments enter us and lie concealed within us. The exact expression about the 'tree' and the column is *vanasya stūpam*. While the *stūpa* is 'column', the word *vana* has at least three meanings in the *Ṛgveda* for the school of Sāyaṇa: (i) Tree, which is seen in the sacrificial pole (*yūpa*) being called *vanaspati* (*ṚV* III.8. 11 *vanaspate śatavalśo viroha*); (ii) Soma, as the 'lord of *vana,* vegetation' (*ṚV* IX.5.10 *vanaspatim.... sahasra-valśam;* also IX.12.7 *nityastotro vanaspatiḥ*); and (iii) in the present case, for Sāyaṇa, *vana* is *vananīya,* 'desirable'; but, further, this *vana* is 'lustre' (*vanasya, vananīyasya tejasaḥ*). This would give the concept of *stūpa* in the present context as being a 'Tree-of-light', from which filaments of lustre shoot forth. And, as they are said to enter us, they are conceived as 'rays of life' that sustain the bodies on the earth; they, in themselves do not get extinguished. When the bodies die, the light-life-filaments revert to the circular source, which is the orb of the sun. The description of the *stūpa* in this context could have no other meaning than that of a column of light. This will be clear from another, and the only instance of the word *stūpa* occurring in the *Ṛgveda*, where it relates to Agni. Agni is said to touch the top of heaven with its *stūpa*-s (VIII.2.1), where Sāyaṇa very precisely renders the word *stūpaiḥ* as *taptaiḥ raśmibhiḥ* ("with hot rays"). Though the word *taptaiḥ* in the commentary of Sāyaṇa shows two variations, as *tanvaiḥ* and *tvadīyaiḥ,* there is hardly any change in the concept; because, *tanvaiḥ* would mean "of the body" (of Agni), and *tvadīyaiḥ* would mean "of your own" (i.e. Agni's own, as the verse is addressed to Agni). In all cases, the image remains the same, 'rays of the body of the fire in the sacrifice', or 'the rays of the body of the fire in the altar'. The whole expression is illuminating, both verbally and conceptually. It says, "Accept with appreciation our *samidh*, O Agni! to-day; shine forth, releasing the profuse sacred sacrificial smoke. Touch closely the heavenly top, with your *stūpa*-s. Spread up and mix with the rays of the sun" (*upa spṛśa divyam sānu stūpaiḥ sam raśmibhis tatanaḥ sūryasya*).

The concept behind the expression is that the freshly flared fire in the altar casts away the volume of smoke and rises up in clear flames to mix with the rays of the sun, rising to the top of heaven. This top of heaven in actual observation, is nothing but the orb of the sun. This concept is based on the belief that the flames of fire, together with the rays shooting from the solar orb, form a column of light, around which the whole cosmos moves. This is an image from the *Maṇḍala* of the Vasiṣṭhas (VII.2), an earlier book of the *Ṛgveda*, in comparison with the image of the *stūpa* of Varuṇa from the hymn of Śunaḥśepa. The Varuṇa-*stūpa* image is from the first Maṇḍala, while the Agni-*stūpa* image is from the seventh

Maṇḍala (which, according to scholars, is earlier than the first, on the basis of language). This would mean, that the image of the *stūpa* with its base in the sacrificial altar is older than that of the *stūpa* with its source up in the sun and having no bottom. In any case, we have here the conceptual image along with its ritual representation. Both were familiar to the Vedic seers. Originally, the concept was of the column of light, that joins the flames of the fire with the orb of the sun. A more fashioned concept was of the tree of light and life, as Śunaḥśepa (I.24.7) uses a doubly symbolic word *vanasya,* which strikes at both the concepts. From the 'tree-light' image of Śunaḥśepa, we have further images: (i) the ancient Aśvattha with shoots growing downwards, which is the Brahman itself; and (ii) the Aśvattha, whose shoots grow downwards, having the leaves of the metres and whose shoots get associated with the *guṇa*-s of the mortals. The first is from the *Kaṭha-upaniṣad* (II.2.1); and the other from the *Bhagavadgītā* (XV.1). The image further developed into the *jyotirliṅga* ('column of lustre') under the influence of Śaivism, which also gave the myth of the *liṅga* (generative organ) of Śiva being cut asunder and later erected in a jar, in the episode of the sages of Dāruvana.[3] Another phase of the same ancient Vedic concept of the column of light, but far changed, is that of the mountain Mandara, the churning staff in the creation myth concerning the Amṛtamanthana, where light and flames do not form the column apparently; but, the principle of lustre is implied in the various 'gems' being created, including the Kaustubha; and fire and smoke are quite prominent in the process of churning. It is said, that from the mouth of the serpent Vāsuki, used as the churning rope, smoke and fire began gushing out. Further, that from the contact of the churn-staff, in the form of the mountain Mandara and the salty water of the (primeval) ocean, fire erupted and blazed fiercely (*Mahābhārata*, Ādi 18). Even if the churning motif for creation occurs elsewhere (cf. the Japanese myth of

Izanagi and Izanami), without the fire, fire and churning in the myth of Amṛtamanthana has the pattern of the churning of the fire from the two *araṇi*-s, as was the usual practice with the Vedic people. We have referred to the image from the Vasiṣṭha hymn above. Here is another expression from a hymn of Viśvāmitra, where Agni is called *aruṣa-stūpa* ('having a reddish tawny column'). There are only two places where the word *stūpa* occurs as a second member of a compound. This is one, the other one being (X.149.5) Hiraṇya-stūpa. Hiraṇyastūpa was the name of the seer from the family of the Aṅgiras-es, and he is mentioned even later. The name only shows that the concept of *stūpa* was quite familiar and was sought to be extended to individual mortals. The epithet *aruṣa-stūpa*, like the *stūpa*-s of fire noted above, occurs in the context of the kindling of the fire. The following expression is to be noted:

O (Adhvaryu)!, wise as you are, place (the kindling rod that churns the fire) on the (lower *araṇi*), spread to position (for the purpose). Lo! She has just conceived and (yet, at once) has generated the Vṛṣan (powerful Agni). He has formed into a reddish tawny *stūpa*; his lustre is reddish saffron. The son of Iḷā (offering) is born in the sacrificial rite (*vayune*) (*ṚV* III 29.3).

This will also show the belief in a column connecting the earth and the sun, through the solar fire and the fire in the altar; or we may say, the column (*stūpa*) from the eternal holy fire in the dwelling was as well set even in ritual as in the mind of the Vedic people. Along with this, there seems to have been developing the concept of the celestial tree, which was only an aspect of the concept of the axle, or, better, axis that connected the worlds.

Before we go to take some examples to show that this concept of the axis between the worlds was not restricted to the Vedic religion, we shall see how the *yūpa*, or the sacrificial pole, had the same concept associated with it. It is very well known, that the *yūpa* is required in the Soma sacrifices, or, rather, in animal sacrifices (cf. Nirūḍhapaśubandha). The *yūpa* is described as being the emblem of the sacrifice (*ṚV* III. 8.8 *yajñasya ketu)*. Though it is fixed on the terrestrial plane at the sacrifice, it is expected to reach the path of the gods. Thus, about the many sacrificial poles (fixed in the Paśubandha, or at the Horse-sacrifice) it is said that they actually provide the path for reaching the gods (*ib.*, 9 *devānām api yanti pāthaḥ*). They are invoked to carry the offerings to the gods (*ib.*, 7 *te no vyantu vāryam devatrā*), which is the prerogative of the fire-god who is acclaimed as 'messenger' (*dūta;* cf. *ṚV* I.12.1 *agrim dūtam vṛṇīmahe*). In what way is the *yūpa* expected to carry the chosen offering to the gods? It is when the victim is tied to the sacrificial pole. The parallelism between the sacrificial fire and the *yūpa* is clear. The fire carries it through the smoke and flames; the *yūpa* is believed to carry it before that, when the victim is tied to it, as its upper end is believed to touch heaven. A more vivid picture obtains at the Vājapeya. Here the *yūpa* is eight-angled,[4] corresponding to the eight quarters. The one *yūpa* is conceived as touching three worlds: Heaven, Earth and the nether subterranean. The portion that is above the *caṣāla* (ring) made of wheat-dough (cf. *Śat.Br*. V.2.1.6 *gaudhūmam caṣālam bhavati*) represents Heaven. This is clear from the rite of ascending to the *caṣāla*, made of wheat-dough, in the Vājapeya sacrifice. The sacrificer ascends to it with the help of a ladder (*niśrayaṇī*); and, while doing so, calls upon his wife, "Wife, come; let us ascend to Heaven". As soon as he ascends and touches the *caṣāla*, he utters, "We have reached Heaven, O gods" (*ib.*, 12). According to Sāyaṇa on the *Taitt.Sam* (I.7.9.1), the sacrificer stretches his hands upwards when he reaches the *caṣāla* and says, "We have reached the gods that stay in heaven" (*udgṛhītābhyam bāhubhyām*). Even out of the context of the Vājapeya, when the *yūpa* is erected (say, in the Paśubandha), it is addressed, "For the earth you, for the mid-region you, for heaven you (do we hoist you)

(*Taitt.Sam.* I.3.6. 1-3; cf. *Śat.Br.* III '.7.1.5-6). The chiselled portion of the *yūpa* is above the earth. So, from the earth to heaven, through the mid-region the *yūpa* represents the three regions. The un-chiselled portion of the *yūpa* is fixed in the pit (*avaṭa*); and the *avaṭa*, which represents the subterranean regions, is the region of the ancestors (*ib.*4). The *yūpa*, thus, is the *axis mundi*. In any religion, when there is a concept suggested to the mind of the thinker (the shaman, or the *brahma-vid* or the *āpta* in the Vedic-Hindu tradition), it often develops into a myth in the oral tradition as one phase; as another phase, it develops a ritual around it. In the case of the Vedic tradition, the *axis mundi* was suggested in the concept of the fire-column of flames that reaches the orb of the sun, on the basis of the principle of heat. Then, it gave rise to various myths, one of them being that of the *stūpa* of Varuṇa, developing further into the Aśvattha tree, which is nothing but a symbol of a tree standing with roots in the sun conceived as the horse (*aśva-stha* = *aśvattha*), a symbol obtaining at various places in the Hindu tradition. It further developed into the myth of the churning staff of the mountain (Amṛta-manthana);[5] and yet further, into the myth of Vasu Uparicara, whom Indra is said to have given his *yaṣṭi* (*Mb.* Ādi, 63.12-19). This myth of the *yaṣṭi* was perpetuated in the ritual of the Indra-dhvaja in the secular practice,[6] while in the Śrauta practice the original concept of the *axis mundi* was transformed into the *yūpa* that reached all regions, including the under-earth. There is another important angle to the *yūpa*. As the *axis mundi* it stands erect to the east of the Uttaravedi and indicates the upward move to heaven. This position is unique. If one takes into account the position of the Gārhapatya and the Āhavanīya fireplaces, it gets clear that the march is from the earth to heaven; because, the Gārhapatya is associated with this earth and it is the household fire (cf. *gṛhā vai gārhapatyaḥ*, a very common saying in the ritual-texts); and the seat of the sacrificer's wife is just near it, along with the wives of the gods, conceptually. From this fire a portion is led to the east, in the quarter of the rising sun (which is in tune with such expressions as *prāñcam yajñam pra ṇayatā sakhāyaḥ*, *ṚV* X.101.2); where the Āhavanīya fireplace is structured. As the offerings for the gods are cast in the Āhavanīya, this fire is the very gate of heaven. And, here stands the *yūpa* to its east taking a rise heavenwards. This is, by far, the upward rise. But, on the horizontal plane, the *yūpa* is posted half-inside, half-outside the altar. The reason is, that thereby it controls the sacred region and also the secular, i.e. both heaven and earth, a belief attested by the ritual texts.[7]

It has been said earlier, that the concept of the *axis mundi* obtains even outside the Hindu belief. A few examples would suffice. One of the most popular instances is that of the Titan, Atlas, of the Greek mythology. He is believed to have known the depths of oceans (thus, the nether world) and is in charge of the columns that support the sky. The columns are a later addition to the earlier phase of the belief wherein Atlas is himself the bearer of the burden of the world and heaven. Another phase of the belief is that the Titan, Atlas, got transformed into Mt. Atlas in Morocco, adjacent to the Mediterranean Sea, which was supposed to be at the centre of the Old World (prior to the discovery of America). Atlantes, another word closely associated with the concept of Atlas, signifies the figure of a man serving as a column supporting a building. It is a name given also to the vertebra supporting the skull.[8] In the Hindu concept it is the *meru-daṇda*, which is the line of backbones on the macrocosmic plane, in the Homo erectus or the Homo sapiens, while on the microcosmic it is the support of the whole world, the Mt. Meru, believed by the Hindus to be in the centre of the world. In the same way the Djed column, placed upright for the soul of Osiris to reach heaven, in the ancient Egyptian mythology, was the *axis mundi*; *djed* in that language meant 'stable'. Ancient Japanese texts speak of the 'Ame-no-tama-boko' ("Celestial Spear") with which

Izanagi and Izanami (the first brother-sister couple) churned the ocean to create islands and stabilise the islands of Japan. This spear was used by the gods to come down to the earth, where they stayed in an 'Eight-fathomed house' at the centre of which was a celestial pillar. Even today, in the Shinto shrine such a pillar is found; it is named 'Nago-no-mibasira'. At marriage it is customary for the newly-wed to go round this pillar. Ancient Egyptian temples had a central pillar which was identified with Osiris; and, in the myth of Anpu-Bata (the two brothers) Bata's soul is said to have entered a tree-trunk, which is identified with this pillar. Bata was a form of Osiris. This should be enough to understand that the concept of the *axis mundi*, which is seen in the Vedic-Hindu context as the *yūpa*, light-column or the down-growing solar tree is not isolated. Another aspect of the same concept is the separating column, that keeps heaven and earth apart. When important gods like Indra perform such a feat, they precisely act as the *axis mundi*.

NOTES AND REFERENCES

1. Betty Sue Flowers, *The Power of Myth* (Ed.; Interview of Joseph Campbell with Bill Moyers), Doubleday, New York, 1988, p.27, where exposition of the Seal of Solomon occurs; Claude Lévi–Strauss, *Myth and Meaning,* Routledge and Kegan Paul, London, 1980, p.16f; David Suzuki and Peter Kundston, *Widsom of the Elders*, Bantam Books, New York, No year, Intrn.
2. Sadashiv A. Dange, *Divine Hymns and Ancient Thought*, Navrang, New Delhi, 1992, p.39; 139, where Sāyaṇa and others are referred to.
3. Sadashiv A. Dange, *Ency. P.B. & P.*, Vol.III, Navrang, New Delhi, 1987, p.938.
4. *Śat.Br.* V.2.1.5 - *aṣṭāśrir yūpo bhavati*; the reason given is that the metre Gāyatrī has eight letters in one foot; not applicable here, as it is just hackneyed. At *Taitt. Sam.* I. 7.9.1, in this context a four-angled *yūpa* is prescribed. Sāyaṇa has no comment there.

5. For full study, see Sadashiv A. Dange, *Legends in the Mahābhārata*, Motilal Banarsidass, Delhi, 1969, pp.241-280; also by the same author, *Myths from the Mahābhārata,* Vol.1, *Quest for Immortality*, Aryan Books International, New Delhi, 1997, pp.231-273.
6. *Bṛhatsaṁhitā,* Chapter XLII.
7. *Taitt. Sam.* VI. 6.4.1; *Mait.Sam.* III.9.4.
8. Richard Cavendish, *Legends of the World,* Barnes and Nobles, New York, 1974, p.263f; *Chambers Twentieth Century Dictionary*, under 'Atlas'/Atlantes. The concept of Igdrasil Tree in the Scandinavian belief is to be compared.
9. Donald Mackenzie, *Myths of China and Japan*, G. Gresham Publishing Co., London, No year, p.350f.

Chapter 2

Visions of the Ṛgvedic *Ṛṣi-Kavis*

There are three terms in the *Ṛgveda* by which the poet is indicated, the general term being '*kavi*'. They are as follows:

1. *kavi,* which is very popular throughout the Indian literature;
2. *ṛṣi*, which could also be termed *ṛṣi-kavi*; and
3. *kāru,* which occurs exclusively in the *ṚV*.

It is very important to mark the difference that lies under these categories. While *kavi* is generally taken as a wise man, or even as a poet, he is also understood as a 'praiser' (cf. III 3.4 *purupriyo bhandate dhāmabhiḥ kaviḥ).* The word *bhandanā* is understood by Yāska as 'praise' (*Nir.* V 1.2 *bhandanā bhandateḥ stutikarmaṇaḥ).* Both *kavi* and *ṛṣi* are said to be able to see beyond the normal (*Nir.* II. 3.12 *ṛṣir darśanāt*; and XII. 2.13 *kaviḥ krānta-darśano bhavati).* But, while *bhandanā* (or *stuti*) enters the expression side of poetry, the faculty of seeing beyond the normal (*krānta-darśitva*) is closely associated with the experience side of poetry. Unlike in the post-Vedic popular context, *kāvya* in *ṚV* is some wonderful activity, not merely the composition of the so-called 'poetry' of later times. The word *kavi,* as far as the Vedic context is concerned, combines wisdom with activity; the latter may include the expression in vocal sound or some wonderful act. This is why Agni is called *kavi*; and, when Brahmaṇaspati is referred to as *'kavim kavīnām'*, his *kavitva* includes the release of the ray-cows and killing of the enemies (II.23.3f). One of the most striking examples of the aspect of activity in the concept of *kavi* is where the sun is said to show his *kāvya* (X.55.5). Though the same person may be a *ṛṣi* and also a *kavi*, these capacities may be mutually independent. A *ṛṣi* could even be mute (a *maunī)*, unlike the *kavi* who is expected to express his experience or musings. The concept in *kāru* is that of a 'fashioner'. It is that faculty of the poet which helps trim the expression. This is reflected in such expressions as *vācam akrata* (X.71.2), as if purifying speech like the malt *(saktum iva)*. This faculty of *kārutva* in a poet, or a composer, has to be taken as the basis of the later concept of *Rīti*, or *vakratā*. A *ṛṣi* need not expect an audience, while a *kavi* expects and desires it for the appreciation of his experience *(darśana)*, which he desires to express. Yāska explains the word *kāru* as 'composer of lauds' (*Nir.* VI. 2.6 *kartā stomānām*),[1] which hints at his faculty of giving tunes to the already existing, or newly composed, *ṛk*-s. Such expressions as *vidatheṣu kāru* indicate, even at the Ṛgvedic period, the activity of employing suitable *mantra*-s at the sacrifice, as also the capacity to present combinations of *ṛk*-s, known later as *sampad.*[2] It is not for nothing that the later tradition bracketed the word *kāru* (out of the poetic context) with *śilpin*. It is to be noted that even in the Vedic ritual context such combinations had the name *śilpa.*[3] That even at the Ṛgvedic period, the *kāru* faculty was considered subservient to that of the *ṛṣi-kavi* is clear from the passage where the *kāru* is said to be the son of a physician *(bhiṣaj)*, while his mother is said to be 'the grinder of parched grain' (IX.112.3).

The subtle difference in these three aspects of a poet was totally lost in post-Vedic times. The *kāvi* came to be more or less a gifted composer — in the words of the ancient *ṛṣi-kavis,* just a *kavi-kāru*; and more a *kāru* than a *kavi,* especially if we have the *citra-kāvya* in view. Even in the case of the higher type of *kāvya,* the faculty of *darśana* gave place to that of *rocana,* the sparkle being in the surrounding. This renders the poet just a tool in the chest of nature, unlike the Vedic *ṛṣi,* who has the faculty to penetrate beyond the seen nature, into the realm we call vision. The basic difference of the Vedic poet's vision from that of the composition of the latter poet can be understood by the opinion of the *Agni P.*[4] mentioned by Ānandavardhana, according to which the poet is the *Prajāpati*; but, he is conditioned by the faculty of *rocana* and *parivartana (yadasmai rocate viśvam tathedam parivartate).* The stage of *rocana* is that of experience, where the nature or a situation shines before his eyes. It is the same as *pratibhāna* where the imagerial intellect of the poet interacts with his surroundings. The stage of *parivartana (cf. parivartate)* is in the expression of the *pratibhāna*, which involves rearrangement of the experience in suitable words and phrases. It is difficult to be sure if the Vedic seers called their experience *pratibhāna;* but, there is no reference to *pratibhāna*, or *pratibhā* in the *Ṛgveda*; and *darśana* is not *pratibhāna.* However, there is no way to ascertain if this *darśana* entailed Truth, or if it was only metaphoric imagination on the part of the seers. Yet, the basis to believe, that it was not mere imagination on the part of the Vedic seers, when they gave vent to their vision, is in their avowance: "I HAVE SEEN". The main difference between metaphorization and vision is, that in the latter there is no contrivance or a conscious effort for superimposition (*adhyāropa),* which is the basis of a metaphor (*rūpaka).* This process is also different from 'autovertism'.[5] We might term it as 'autovision', and might differentiate it from the general term 'vision'. The difference between autovision and vision is very thin, and here we would name it just vision. In the former the seer particularises himself as 'I': 'I have seen' or 'I see', or 'I saw'. And, there should be no reason why we should not take him by his expression, which, after all, may be to himself! Once uttered to himself, it gained the status of a magical charm, and came to be repeated with the expectation of a particular effect that the images in it were believed to bring about! We take such expressions, with an open mind, not with the pre-notion that, "the hymns are meant to puzzle, surprise, to trouble the mind".[6] The puzzle, surprise and the trouble come when one does not get familiar with the images the seers appear to fling. As noted above, in a vision, there is nothing of art, like a pure myth.[7] The seer enters the vision, which appears before him, with his mental compromise (if we could put it that way). Here are the examples:

(1) III.38.6:

> O you, two lustrous ones! you protect all three (and) various
> places, being at the sacrifice *(vidatha);*
> Reaching here with my mind
> I beheld the Gandharvas — even them
> With their hair fluttering in the air;
> In the *Vrata.*

The two lustrous ones are the gods Indra and Varuṇa, from the context. There is no definite mention in *ṚV* of the three places *(sadāṁsi)* being the three fireplaces that figure in the later ritual. The three places, here, are the three worlds: Heaven, Mid-region and Earth. The thought of the seer centres round the sacrificial altar, and leads him to believe that the presence of the two gods at the sacrifice activates the three worlds. The expression 'Gandharvas with fluttering hair' with the word *vāyu* reflects the image of the Mid-region, of which Vāyu is the deity in the Vedic tradition. This, with the flames of the sacrificial fire, which together present the vision to the poet, it is clear that here there is a mixture of the mid-region and the flames of the sacrificial fire before the mental eye of the seer. In other words, the vision lifts the flames to the mid-region and the sacrifice gets to be supra-terrestrial. The word *urate* does not have the idea of law which holds the Gandharvas in the command of the two gods, as is generally understood.[8] *Vrata,* in this context, stands for the sacrifice itself through the medium of which the vision appears before the seer.

(2) V.2.1-3:
Here we have the vision of the seer Jana, or Vṛṣa, of the family of the Atris. The seer says:

1. The young mother conceals the child, fully grown;
   She gives it not to the 'Father;'
   His scorching face the people see not;
   Though laid in front, it is hidden
   In a place, uncozy.

What is the seer up to? He indicates that the face of the unborn one is visualised by him, though others do not see it. He also knows that it is scorching, though dormant.

He further asks:

2. Why, O lady, do you withhold the child?
   Cruel are you, though conceived and great;
   For many an autumn the foetus grew;
   As the mother delivered, I saw.

And, suddenly he says:

3. I saw him from afar
   Coming out of the *kṣetra*
   With golden teeth and lustrous form, wielding weapons;
   All-sustaining nectar do I give unto him;
   What will they do to me—
   They, who are devoid of Indra
   And offer no praise?

Further the seer says:

I saw him as swiftly did he move, by himself
From the *kṣetra* (birthplace)
Shining profusely;

Those ladies - they held him not for support,
As by himself he got born, indeed;
Young again did the old ladies become. (V.2.4)

Sāyaṇa mentions here a legend from the *Śāṭyāyana Br.*, but, as he finally says, the whole image is of the fire that is kindled from the kindling apparatus (the *araṇi-mantha*), where the lower *araṇi* is called the *kṣetra,* a word that became symbolic of a woman and the womb, getting further developed in the concept of the *kṣetraja* son. On the other hand, Agni coming out of the *araṇi-*s at the ritual at the sacrifice is a common image in the Veda; but, that he is seen as wielding his weapons as he emerges from his 'birthplace' (*the araṇi-*s) serves as the basis of such mythical accounts of birth, where the hero is seen as being born from the altar to indicate his divine birth, or he is said to be born fully grown and wielding his weapons to punish the evil-doers.[9] In the vision in question, others do not see the fire-god as he is dormant in the apparatus; but, the seer indicates that he has seen his lustrous face. The lower *araṇi* hides her foetus for a long time, which serves as the source of myths which speak of delayed births.[10] The interrelationship of later myths and the Vedic visions, a subject of interesting research (which the present author has worked on), becomes clear at many places like this. The flames act as the mothers, after the birth of the fire as if they support him. When they diminish, they are seen as pale white, their radiance exhausted; they are seen as old. The 'Father,' or, in fact, 'protector', is the sacrificer or the priest who pours offerings. The moment he offers an oblation of clarified butter in the fire, the flames regain their youth. The whole vision centres round the fire and the sacrifice, as did others mentioned earlier.

Another set of visions, with the "I saw" pattern, starts from the sun, mixing various images. In one the seer says,

The steadfast *Ṛta* that concealed by *Ṛta* itself
Where the horses of the sun get unyoked;

Ten hundred, they stand together;
Among the gods with wondrous forms,
I saw the One, lustrous! the Highest! (V.62.1)

The *Ṛta* that conceals is the orb of the sun; the other *Ṛta,* that is beyond this one, is the potent force of the cosmos. Both are *ṛta*, as they are constantly active (√*ṛ*). The horses, where these two aspects of *Ṛta* meet, are the rays of the sun which get unyoked and released from the orb to descend to the world of the mortals. The image of the concealed and non-concealed *Ṛta* developed later on in the image of "Truth with its face covered by the golden container" (*Iśāvāsya-Up.* 15). Another seer says that he 'saw' by his penance those places which were created by the wise when they conducted the sacrifice. These places do not appear to be the fireplace at the sacrifice, but, are the result of sacrifice. But, which? (VIII. 59.6[cd]). In spite of varied interpretations, 'the *drapsa* at the depth of the river Aṁśumatī' which the seer says he 'saw' remains a mystery.[11] If it is a 'drop' (disk) in the bed of the river of rays (*aṁśumatī),* which could it be? (VIII.96.14). Another seer proclaims, "I have seen the god Narāśaṁsa, spacious and well-formed, residing in the home of light like heaven (with its stars)" (I.18.9). It is impossible to take it just to be the description of the fire in the altar, or the sun. Though Narāśaṁsa is, generally, taken to be fire, this god who sits in his home of light is beyond the normal experience.

Some of the finest images obtain from the visions of Dīrghatamas. He sees the sacrificial horse sacrificed; he assumes it to be going to the heavenly world (I.162.21), but the form of the beast changes in his vision. It has the wings of the hawk and front-legs of a deer. He sees Yama giving it to Trita who makes it ready for Indra who is to mount it, the first to do so. He says, that is fashioned by the Vasus from the sun (I.163.1), which imagery is based on the traditional identification of the horse with the sun even at his time. Though the wings for the horse here may be the influence of the sun being seen as the bird, the 'front legs' (*bāhū*) of a deer do not fit in the Vedic solar imagery. In spite of this mixed image in his vision, it reverts to the sun; and he says:

> [O horse!]
> These your auspicious reins of *ṛta*
> These that guard you,
> I have seen here.
> With my mind have I recognised your form,
> The 'bird' moving in heaven and hereward.
> Your winged head have I seen flying
> On dustless paths, easy to move along
> (I.163.5-6).

The head of the horse seen in the sun has its counterpart in the myth of *Dadhīca* and the lost head of the horse.[12] But, the vision continues, and the seer says,

> (O horse!) Your form—the very best
> Gliding towards the footprint of the Cow (Bull),
> Which is nourishment (incarnate)
> I have seen here (*atra*) (I.163.7).

The foot-print of the cow (goṣpada) occurs in the myth of Indra and the Vālakhilyas, where it is said to be filled with water; and the thumbkin Vālakhilyas get almost drowned in it.[13] The 'footprint of the cow', both in the myth and the vision mentioned here, is the sun. The seer sees the horse entering it and getting merged in it. This is a rearrangement of the known symbols. But, for the seer here, Dīrghatamas, the one horse gives place to a row of horses,

> With their tail-ends speeding alike
> Their mid-bodies evenly aligned
> These divine horses speed on
> Like swans in lines, they fly
> Along the divine path, they cover (v 10).

He addresses them,

> The hairs of your manes,
> Perched variously all over,
> Flutter freely on the forest-trees (v 11).

The description takes the horse from its own frame to a larger entity, as its hairs are seen as the leaves on the trees in the forest. The description may be taken as just a poetic imagination like "bow to trees having green hairs" (*namo vṛkṣebhyo hari-keśebhyaḥ Taitt. Sam.* IV. 5.2.9), that occurs even in a ritual context. But, very probably, it passes the realm of mere poetry. Earlier, at the very start of the long hymn, known as '*Asyavāmīya*,' the seer starts with the image of three fires: the sun in the heavenly region, the mid-region fire (lightning, or Vāyu traditionally) and the altar-fire on the terrestrial level. He describes them as brothers of each other; but, suddenly says,

> Here have I seen the lord of all,
> The One that has seven sons. (I. 164.1).

This shows a constant flight from the sacrificial level to the cosmic, which is noticed also in other seers. At a later stage in the same hymn, he avows,

> I have seen the *gopāḥ*, who tires not
> Moving hereward and far, along many paths;
> Lustrous in his garb,
> As he moves, now herewards now afar
> And traverses many worlds (v 31).

The *gopāḥ* is, apparently, the sun (as attestable from *Taitt. Ār.* V.6.4); but the thought of the seer does not stop only here. He visualizes a 'Cow', from whom oozes the 'un-oozing' (*tataḥ kṣarati-akṣaram,* v 42). It is right that *akṣara*, here, indicates a twofold image: (i) the supreme point whence waters (rains) ooze out; and (ii) the expression of Speech.[14] Yet, the 'Cow' at the source gives a new flank to the imagery. This has to be taken as vision;

for, just later the seer says,

> I saw the smoke up there,
> Far away from this smoke that is near;
> The skilled activators (*vīrāḥ; vi-īrāḥ*) cooked the bull
> That was variegated;
> Those were the rites of yore (v 43)

The seer starts with the sacrificial smoke and flies to cosmic height, where there is another smoke. His mental eye joins him with the source of all nourishing waters and that of the very first symbol of Speech; the latter he calls *akṣara* in the sphere of audible speech. The imagery already gets the status of a vision, when the seer has said, earlier, that he has become macrocosmic — a son of suprahuman parents,

> Heaven is my Father, the generator;
> My navel is here, the binding force;
> This great Earth is my mother (v 33).

He says:

> This altar is the farthest end of the earth
> This Sacrifice is the navel of the universe (v 35)

He is candid in admitting:

> I know not if I be this all (universe);
> (But) Well-equipped do I traverse, in secret,
> With my mind (v 37)

The thought of Dīrghatamas, that the altar is the farthest end of the earth, is unique; and obtains at various texts later on, where the ritualists say, "The earth is only as far as is the altar" (*yāvatī vedis tāvatī).*[15] This may be symbolic in the precincts of the ritual. However, with the seer it is the vision. It is this visionary expression that guided the rituals.

Another seer, whose name is not exactly known (and, hence, who is named Pataṅga due to the word occurring in the hymn),[16] says:

> The wise, with their mind and heart,
> See the *pataṅga* (bird);
> The seer-poets visualise
> In the interior of the ocean,
> The *pada* (='foot', source) of the rays;
> They desire THAT. (X.177.1)

And even this seer avowedly says:

> I have seen the *gopā* never tiring,
> Moving along the paths, near and far (v 3)

Here, again, it has been usual to understand the *gopā* as the sun. But, let us take the vision of Vasukra (X. 27). After experiencing many and varied images, he says:

> With each other the cows mixed
> And have 'eaten the barley'[17] of the lord,
> As they wandered with their *gopā*;
> I have seen them. (X. 27.8)

Even if we may take these images as suggested from the sun, often the mind of the seer pierces the appearance and flies into vision—which are the cows? Rays? But, is that all? Even with the parallel of the 'honey-eating birds' (I.164.22), the image cannot rest only at the solar orb. There can hardly be any doubt about the fact, that the *gopā* in all such experiences is the Protector of the universe. In such cases, the normal experience (about the sacrificial fire or about the sun) catapults the seer in the *a-laukika*. It has to be remembered, that the *a-laukika* is never entirely different from the *laukika*.[18] It has its source in the experiences from this world; but, these experiences are rearranged by the mind of the seer in such a way, and in such relationships, that they assume the status of the *a-laukika* (or, better, *atilaukika*). The ordinary poet does the same thing. But, while in the case of the ordinary poet the effort is conscious, as noted already, for the *ṛṣi*, it is supra-sensorial; and without effort. That is why, probably, the seer Sadhri of the family of Virūpa says:

> The Suparṇa; he entered the ocean;
> The whole world does he look over;
> Him did I see near me
> With my mind 'filled'.
> He licks his mother, (and lo?)
> His mother licks him (X.114.4).

And Dīrghatamas is confident, when he says:

> The *gopā* of this whole - He, the lord
> He, the Wise One
> Has entered me, here
> Me — whose mind (now) is 'full'.

The mind is said to be *pāka,* a word which has a unique sense. It is indicative of 'fullness', clarity and purity. There is a strong reason to believe, that it is this concept of the *gopā* (cowherd, as *go* + √*pā*, "to protect") and the supreme protector (√*gup,* "to protect") that stands at the basis of the 'Cowherd god' in the later devotional poetry, howsoever unnoticed the process was.

The *ṛṣi*, with his *pāka* mind, visualizes images which are wonderful. Why not believe in him when he says. "I am the Firstborn of *ṚTA*" (X.61.19)?

NOTES AND REFERENCES

1. This basic difference between *kavi* and *kāru,* as also between *ṛṣi* and *kāru* has not been marked by Gonda in his *Epithets from the Ṛgveda*, Mouton and Co., Gravenhage, 1959, p.153. He connects *kāru* with *gṛṇat* ('praising'), but does not touch the basic concept behind the *kāru*. Prof. H.D. Velankar (in his paper "Kavi and Kāvya in the Ṛgveda", published in the *Proceedings* of the All India Oriental Conference, Twenty-third Session, Poona, 1969, held at Aligarh, 1966, pp. 253-258), rightly says that *kavi* is 'visionary'; but he leaves *kāru*; see also T.G. Mainkar, *Some Poetical Aspects of Ṛgvedic Repetitions,* University,

of Poona, Poona, 1966, and earlier, *Mysticism in the Ṛgveda,* Popular Book Depot, Bombay, 1961. He also leaves away this difference, and, in the latter, he uses the term 'mystic songs' rather than 'mystic poetry'. According to L. Renou, *kavi* is a worker at sacrifice, both manual and oral, *Journal Asiatique,* Vol. 241, 1953, pp. 180 ff.

2. Sadashiv A. Dange, "Ritual Variations and the Principle of Sampad", *Brahmavidyā* (Golden Jubilee Vol.), Madras, 1986, pp. 498-511; for a detailed study see (Mrs.) Sindhu S. Dange, *Aspects of Speech iṇ Vedic Ritual,* Aryan Books International, New Delhi, 1996, pp.182-205.
3. *Ait. Br.* VI.27 (=30.1) *śilpāni śaṁsati, devaśilpāni*; for the application of this, see, S.A. Dange, *Sexual Symbolism from the Vedic Ritual,* Ajanta Publications, Delhi, 1979, pp.68f; 127 ff.
4. *Agni, P.* 339.10.
5. (Mrs.) S.S. Dange, "Autovertism in the Ṛgveda", *Vishveshvaranand Indological Journal,* Panjab University, Hoshiarpur, XIV, pt. I, March, 1976, pp.7-16.
6. Wendy Doniger O'Flaherty, *Anthology from the Ṛgveda,* Penguin, 1981, from Frits Stall, *Agni* (The Vedic Ritual of the Fire-altar), Motilal Banarsidass, Delhi, 1983, p.xxix.
7. Sadashiv A. Dange, On vision and pure myth, and the various types of myth, *Towards Understanding Hindu Myths,* Aryan Books International, New Delhi, 1996, pp.xxiv ff, p.10.
8. Geldner, *Der Rigveda*, I, p.380, "*(eurem) Dienste*"; H.D Velankar, *Ṛgveda Maṇḍala* III, University of Bombay, Bombay 1968, p.94, "your law". There is no word here for "your" *(eurem).* In the ritual-texts *vrata* has the sense of a drink in vow, generally milk. The sacrificer (or, seer who might be a sacrificer) actually got weakened in the course of the sacrifice. And, in the Ṛgvedic period, when Soma was the available drink, it might cause the drinker glide into a vision.
9. Cf. The birth of Dhṛṣṭadyumna, *Mb.,* Ādi 166.136-139; see Sadashiv A. Dange, *Ency. P.B. & P.,* I, Navrang, New Delhi, 1986, 136 ff; also see Dange, *Myths from the Mahābhārata,* Vol.2, Aryan Books Internạtional, New Delhi, 2001, Chapter II "Supranormal Birth", birth from sacrificial altar, pp.162-170.

10. Indra's birth, *ṚV* IV. 18.1-5; *Mb.* Ādi, 176.46 f.
11. Sāyaṇa, referring to an *itihāsa,* says that Kṛṣṇa was an Ausra, hidden in water; was found out by Indra with the help of Bṛhaspati. He also states a varying account, according to which *Drapsa* was a drop of water (*udaka-kaṇaḥ)*, being only a form of Soma. The allusion, according to this account, is to Soma, who had run away, being afraid of Vṛtra and had taken resort to the river Aṁśumatī *(Bṛhaddevatā* VI, 109-115). This latter account amounts to be a pseudo-myth formed from the account of *ṚV* itself. See Geldner, *op.cit.,* II, p.422, note to his tr., for other opinions.
12. For a detailed study of this myth, see Sadashiv A. Dange, *Towards Understanding Hindu Myths,* pp.242-251.
13. Sadashiv A. Dange, *Legends in the Mahābhārata*, Motilal Banarsidass, Delhi, 1969, pp. 131-134; also Dange, *Myths from the Mahābhārata*, Vol.1, Aryan Books International, New Delhi, 1997, p.9; p.10ff; pp.103-105.
14. See Sadashiv A. Dange, *Images from Vedic Hymns and Rituals*, Aryan Books International, New Delhi, 2000, Chapter II: "The Thunder and the Akṣara", pp.25-59.
15. *Taitt. Sam.*, III.6.4.13; *Śat.Br.,* I.2.5.7; III.7.2.1.
16. The general maxim is, *yasya vākyam sa ṛṣiḥ (Anukramaṇī* II.4), which has to be taken as modified here. Though Pataṅga does not speak here, "he holds speech in his mind" — v 2.
17. 'Barely-eating' indicates good health and satisfaction; cf. X.27.9 *yad vayam yavasādo janānām aham yavādaḥ.* Later, 'eating of barely' occurs in a figurative sense of sexual satisfaction leading to conception, *yad hariṇo yavam atti na puṣṭam paśum manyate;* for subtle meaning of this expression, Sadashiv A. Dange, *Vedic Concept of 'Field' and the Divine Fructification,* Bombay University, Bombay, 1971, p.36, and n.15 where he examines, and differs from other scholars.
18. As the present author has proposed in a previous Seminar at the Asiatic Society of Bombay, "Sanskrit Poetics and Semiotics", 1995, the same paper later on published. See Journal of the *Asiatic Society of Bombay*, Bombay, Vol.71 (for 1996), 1997, pp.47-57. It is this sense of the *alaukika* that applies to all types of creative art. For the context of myth, see, *Towards Understanding Hindu Myths,* p.2f;

p.31, n. 6; also *Purākathñcā Artha-Vāda āṇi Vivecana* (Marathi), Continental Prakashan, Pune, 1993-94, p.2.

* Included here from the *Journal of the Oriental Institute,* M.S. University of Baroda, Baroda, Vol.45, Nos.3-4, March-June, 1996.

Chapter 3

Sanskrit Poetics and Semiotics

In the sphere of Sanskrit Poetics, the contribution of the three *ācārya*-s, viz. Lollaṭa, Śaṅkuka and Bhaṭṭa Nāyaka is too well known to require any detailed comment. The author of *Dhvanyāloka,* Ānandavardhana, goes a step further in his exposition of Dhvani, the propriety of which has been acclaimed and questioned by other *ācārya*-s. Apart from whether *rasa*-realization is *pratīti* or *pratipatti,*[1] it could be observed that the first three *ācārya*-s fall into one group, while Ānandavardhana and his eminent commentator Abhinavagupta fall into another. This division is obvious in view of the fact that the first group has elaborated its exposition with the *nāyaka* (character) as the starting point ending with the spectator; and the second group has extended the start to an earlier point, i.e. the *kavi*. Though Bhaṭṭa Nāyaka initiated the principle of *sādhāraṇīkaraṇa,* the frame of *rasa*-activity remained the same: character (*nāyaka*) → *pātra* → (actor) → *sāmājika,* or *sahṛdaya* (=spectator). The frame for the *rasa*-activity contemplated by the latter class is: *kavi* (poet, dramatist, or creative writer) → *nāyaka* → *naṭa* → *sāmājika*. In this scheme Śaṅkuka's contribution, though somewhat obscured under the showers of the *rasa-dhvani* eulogium by the posteriors, it has to be stressed, not only from the Semiotic approach but also from the independent observations regarding poetic appreciation available in the writings of poets and writers.

Śaṅkuka who advances the imagery of the horse and its picture *(citra-turaga)* subtly introduces the principle of imagery, which glides into the realm of Semiotics. According to Śaṅkuka the spectator oscillates between accepting the reality of the actor being Rāma (the character, or actual Rāma) or otherwise, finally accepting him as Rāma (character, or the original person). Śaṅkuka's observation has two parts: (i) *Rati* is not present, according to the first observation of the spectators, in the actor, as it is in the character. But, it is inferred to be so in the actor (= dancer) due to his imitation, which is artificial. Though artificial, this imitation, aided by the stage-arrangement, leads the spectators to believe that the *rati* (about Sītā, or the female actor) is the *sthāyi-bhāva* (inherent emotion) even in the case of the actor. This inference of the spectators is based upon the active perception of the spectators. (ii) This activity is called *carvaṇā* of the *vāsanā.*

To take up the first point: It is very clear, that the actor serves as the human symbol (the term is used as a general class-name for the character) because, like a symbol, or sign, he is artificial and counterfeit. Another point, apart from *rasa*-realization, in the observation attributed to Śaṅkuka is that there is hesitation in the mind of the spectators regarding the presentational ability of the actor, though it is not expressed in clear words. Otherwise, knowing that they are witnessing a dramatic presentation, they should be taken as being pretty sure that the actor is not Rāma (or the character)! Another reflection in the observation is, that actors are likely to misrepresent the character originally contemplated by the dramatist - especially if the dramatist is not alive, or is long dead. It is almost impossible to find, in the sphere of Sanskrit Poetics, such a suggestive statement regarding the basic difference between the actor and the original character being made by any *ācārya*. This reminds one of the statements by Charles Lamb about David Garric, the famous Shakespearean actor, after seeing the epitaph on the actor's tomb. The epitaph said (rather boastfully), that:

> Though sunk in death the forms the poet drew
> The actor's genius bade them breathe anew.

The comments of Lamb are, that it is impossible for an actor to possess "*a mind congenial with the poet's.*" He says, "Of the motives and grounds of the passion (with which the poet, or dramatist drew his characters) the actor can give no more idea by his face or gesture than the eye can speak or the muscles utter intelligible sound." (From his essay, "On the Tragedies of Shakespeare", 1811). This is about a very renowned actor. Yet, the difference between the artificial (actor's acting) and the original (character contemplated by the poet/dramatist) is clear. It is also true that, in spite of this difference, the spectators enjoy the drama. Will the spectators enjoy it if the drama is presented with the help of cartoons? Yes! In the case of the imagery suggested by Śaṅkuka, the picture of the horse may be in any style. As long as there is some resemblance, it would be taken as the horse. This would mean, that the original can have more than one images within a set sphere and yet the cognition would not suffer. This is a step towards symbolization which does not concern us at the moment.

The second point: This does not concern Semiotics so much as *rasa*-realization. However, the Semiotic value of *vāsanā* is to be noted. Now, *carvaṇā* is repeated chewing. In the present context, it is a repeated but effortless activity of the mind to cognize the various actions of the actor, or of the character depicted by the author in case one is reading a piece of poetry or drama. This *carvaṇā* is conditioned by the *vāsanā,* which is the impression of anything remaining in the subconscious (fr. √*vas*, "to stay"). It should be noted, that *vāsanā* spoken of here is that of the *sāmājika*-s (spectators).[2] But, it is not restricted to them. It is equally inherent in the reader and also in the dramatist (or poet) himself if he witnesses his own drama, whereby he becomes one of the *sāmājika*-s. The *vāsanā* acts as the conductor common for all the *sthāyi-bhāvas,* inherent in the spectators (readers), who get stirred on viewing a respective situation concerning the real/original (character) or concerning even the counterfeit (actor). To put it slightly differently, *vāsanā* is the psychic faculty which, not only causes the release for relish (taste; *rasana*[3]) in the *sthāyi-bhāva* complex but also, subtly categorizes it into various components. These various components are, hence, categories inherent in the *sthāyi*-complex.[4] We might explain the phenomenon as follows. While remaining dormant in the *sthāyi*-complex, the various categories are unclear and unnamed. With the conduction through the *vāsanā*, the impressions, gathered by the outer senses, in the form of the acting and dialogue of the actor together with the environmental situation on the stage, the *sthāyi*-complex gets activated. This is the stage of the *rasyamānatva* of the *sthāyi*-complex, which immediately serves to jettison the process of categorization resulting into a particular emotion to surface corresponding to the impression that percolated through the *vāsanā*. This stirred-up and surfaced emotion is *rasa,* given a name suiting to the impression. With an addition to the already known impressions, a corresponding name to the added type of *rasa* becomes necessary. This is clear from the case of the Śānta *rasa* and also the Vatsala. This also explains the dispute regarding Śānta *rasa*. We could, now, classify the whole experience as: (i) Psychophysical; and (ii) Purely psychical. The first, is that which precedes the conduction of the impressions by the *vāsanā* to the dormant *sthāyi*-complex; the latter is that which follows it leading to the *rasana* (stir). Though we have analysed it in these details, the process of the transmission of impressions by the *vāsanā* faculty is continuous (we might say, *a-saṁlakṣya-krama)*. The same is the case with *rasa*-realization throughout the dramatic performance. This, obviously, means that there is a constant shifting of the *rasa*-s during the whole duration of the drama (and while reading), till the finale, which determines the main *rasa* in it. And, it is here that one speaks in terms of the Main *rasa*[5] and the associate *rasa*-s. Viewed from the Semiotics angle, the relationship between the *sthāyi*-complex and the individual *rasa*-s is that of an undefined unit and the defined categories that comprise it. But, yet it is not Semiotics. However, if the *sthāyi*-complex is given a new technical name indicative of this relationship without actually using the original names of the *rasa*-s from the said complex, it would very much come under Semiotics. An example from the metalingual method of Pāṇini would indicate this. The *pratyāhāra* method is one such example, where *ac* stands as a symbol for the vowels.[6] In the context of Poetics such terms as *Dhvani* has a Semiotic value. This is a juncture at which Semiotics and Poetics could be viewed more closely. We have said earlier, that in the *citra-turaga* relationship the *citra* is the symbol of the horse, or it gets the status of a symbol. Flatly speaking, a symbol is something which stands for the thing it indicates or suggests; but it is not the thing itself. In the case of the horse and its picture, the latter is like the objective, but it is not the object. We could say that it is a weak symbol; but it is not just a sign. It is a weak symbol, as in this case the picture is not different from the horse in appearance though there is difference in contour and size. As Śaṅkuka's comments were in the sphere of dramas, the *citra-turaga* exactly suits the *naṭa-nāyaka* relationship. However, the example is not entirely exhausted in this relationship alone; because, the *naṭa* (actor) indicates the *nāyaka* (character) who is only the image contemplated by the dramatist. Actually, for the *sāmājika*, the *naṭa* stands for the original person, not the *nāyaka*, who is real only in the drama, or a novel. So, the position is: the *naṭa* is the *citra*. To put it to graph:

Real person (Rāma) (life-stage)

- *citra* (*nāyaka*) (poetic stage–drama) → *citra* (*naṭa*) (dramatic stage) → *sāmājika*
- *citra* (*nāyaka*) (poetic stage–novel, long poem) → *pāṭhaka* (*pāṭhaka*)[7]

The weakness of the symbol in the *citra-turaga* example does not lie in the symbol being a concrete object. It lies in the visible non-difference between the symbol and the symbolised. The same is the case with the *naṭa*. However, the *rasa-niṣpatti* is not restricted to drama or dance. When the *kavi,* as distinct from the dramatist, was brought into the discussion on Poetics[8] we could say, from the modern point of view, that Semiotics gained more scope. Applied to shorter forms of poetic expressions, it would help stride over such disputes as to whether for *rasa*-realization, or for appreciating *camatkāra* in a particular poetic expression, we have to resort to inference (*anumāna*), *dhvani (vyañjanā)* or the *liṅga-liṅgī* relationship.[9] Let us take some famous examples:

To turn to the first—

O wayfarer! There is no bedspread (*srastara*) here, whatsoever, in this village that is strewn with stone-slabs. (However) seeing the *unnata-payodhara,* if you (desire to) stay, then stay!) (*Kāvyaprakāśa* IV. verse 58).

This is taken as an example of *vastu-dhvani.* The very fact that *dhvani* is categorized here as *vastu* (*niṣṭha*) as different from *rasa-dhvani* indicates that, for the Dhvanyāloka-kāra, *rasa* and *dhvani* do not always go together. But, could we say that this is an example of a *nīrasa-kāvya?* While writing about *citra-kāvya* he says, that a poet should not attempt a piece of poetry that is devoid of *rasa*, etc. (*rasādi-tātparyam anapekṣya)*. Whether he includes *vastu-dhvani* in *adi (rasādi)* is not clear, but it could be taken as implied (to speak in his favour). Apart from the fact that Ānandavardhana was not followed whole-heartedly, and by all, the influence of the concept of *dhvani* is clear even in casual use when somebody says, "Well, it is *dhvanita* in a particular expression", and so on. The actual position about the example mentioned above is that the poet presents an expression which at once throws two images:

Payodhara	breast	(1) fully developed	*un-nata*
	cloud	(2) poised above	

which are activated by the double meaning of the word *payas* (= i. water; and ii. milk), the fusion of this double meaning well rooted in the mind of the *rasika*-s, as in that of the poet. There is a further aid in the expression itself in the word *srastara*, which subtly serves as an *uddīpana*. This, without any elaboration, serves to render the verse striking. Here the word *payodhara* stands not only as a symbol for the objects, viz. the cloud and the breast, but for enjoyment. The Semiotic principle involved here is that experience leads to direct cognition at the same time, without any intermediary process. This would relieve the cognition of the aid of any *dhvani* or *vyaṅgya*, or *liṅga* and *liṅgin* and the disputable discussion accompanying these views.

Another example may be that where the *viṭa* (sex-agent/or a paramour) desires to know the time of meeting and the woman signals him with her eyes, smiles a little, and closes the lotus in her hand.[10] The closure of the lotus is indicative of the evening time; because the lotus is the *padma,* which is the sun-symbol and the sunset is suggested by its closure. For any other woman this action would have been just a mute one. Here the woman is said to be *vidagdhā* which means she is cultured in such symbolic communication. In fact, she is a courtesan of accomplished sense. Though here we may see *śābdī-vyañjanā* or *vakrokti,* which cannot be denied, the understanding of the symbol is an important factor.[11] In such pithy expressions there is no scope to *carvaṇā;* but one cannot deny the potentiality of *rasa.* It will be seen that in both the examples, what strikes us is the quick and apt imagery which is the very essence of Semiotics. In another example, where Pārvatī is described as standing at the back of her father as the sages broach the topic of her marriage, her instantaneous action of the head tilting down and hand fondling the petals of the lotus it held,[12] suddenly gives the image of a coy girl drenched in shyness. Though in both the examples the actions of the *vidagdhā* and the *mugdhā* (skilled and the coy) may be termed technically *vyabhicārin* what strikes the reader is the perfect image. The same is the case with the expression *na yayau na tasthau,*[13] which suggests the psychic condition oscillating between the strong desire to stay due to love, at the same time pricked by a feeble impulse of modesty (like the *ardham antarvedi ardham bahirvedi*[14] position). These are the poetic images based on the observation of the poet from actual life. When they are repeatedly employed, they tend to become symbolic for all such emotions; and, then, they come to be mechanically followed in creative art, whether it is drama or picture or sculpture. Semiotics and Poetics, thus, become complementary to each other. Examples can be multiplied; but we take one more from the *Rāmāyaṇa,* where Rāma asks Lakṣmaṇa to identify the ornaments of Sītā. The latter says, "I know not the *keyūra*-s (bracelets on the upper arm), nor do I know the *kuṇḍala*-s (in the ears). I know only the *nūpura*-s (anklets) - due to always bowing down at the feet" (*Rām.* Kiṣkindhā 6.22).[15] Here, the image of Lakṣmaṇa never looking intently at the face of the wife of his elder brother is created by the poet.

But, the strikingness in it is due to the norms of behaviour prevalent in a particular society. It is the impression of this image that serves as a stimulus to appreciate the inner emotion of the character (if dramatised), or the real younger brother contemplated by the poet. One feels, however, that, to do more justice to Lakṣmaṇa, the statement of this younger brother should have ended with, "I know only the *nūpura*-s", the portion *nityam pādābhivandanāt* being uttered by Rāma himself with a nod of his head. That would have rid Lakṣmaṇa of the thin tint of virtue-consciousness and heightened the effect of the imagery. Dramatization of the situation with this split at the last quarter of the verse, put in the mouth of Rāma with an appreciative gesture, even in that condition of grief, would make all the difference. Of course, the poet is helpless by the natural limits of poetry.

From what has been said above, it would be clear that for the experiencing of poetic beauty, or enjoyment of *rasa,* the formation of imagery, sometimes leading to the formation of symbols, is necessary. This formation of symbols starts with the poet (dramatist included), who tries to transmit them to the reader (spectator included) through the medium of words and expressions and through the actor. Bhaṭṭa Tauta implies this when he says, *nāyakasya kaveḥ śrotuḥ samāno anubhavaḥ.* But, the word *samānaḥ* does not mean 'same'; because, the images created by the poet (or, for that matter, any of the creative writers including the dramatist) and transmitted, are not the same for the reader. The creative writer does not describe his experiences from the real world as he gets them directly, in which case he would lose his claim to creativity. He mixes his own imagination with them and floats them for the readers (spectators). The reader fits them in his own experience. In the words of Wordsworth, who was himself a renowned poet, and examined the process of poetic composition, "However exalted a notion we could wish to cherish of the character of a poet, it is obvious that, while he describes and imitates the passions, his employment is in some degree mechanical". According to him, the poet should consider himself "as in the situation of a translator who does not scruple to substitute excellencies of another kind for those which are unattainable hy him; and endeavours occasionally to surpass his original". (From "Poetry and Poetic Diction", being Preface to the second Ed. of his *Lyrical Ballads*, 1800). The pertinent point is that the poet, or dramatist, is an artist who has to impress the reader or the spectator. The last sentence, that he endeavours occasionally to surpass the original, is true of the actor also, and more so, as he constantly has the spectators before him whom he wants to win over. We are now at a stage to mark the difference between the poet (dramatist) and the actor on the one hand, and the reader and the spectator on the other. Both the poet (dramatist) and the actor are artists; their effort is artificial. In between the poet (dramatist) and the actor, the former (or any literary creative artist) takes real impressions and situations from nature, rearranges them and then presents them for the reader or spectator. So, the artistic presentation is not real. We might say, that, in a way it assumes the status of the myth[16] with some difference.[17] What a myth expresses is real within its own sphere and period. Likewise, the incidents in a novel or a long poem or a drama, even if based on real incidents or historical facts, appear real for the duration of the reading or dramatic session. The poet or the creative artist has a double role (1) as a manipulative artist (we may term him *bhāvayitṛ*): and (2) as a proto-spectator (proto-reader). The spectator (reader) has a single role, that of a *bhāvuka* from the beginning, and at the end *bhāvita* (or, *prabhāvita*). Both are *sa-hṛdaya* to each other. It is not only the *sāmājika*, or the reader, who is the *sa-hṛdaya*. but, while the poet-dramatist is an 'artisan'[18] of poetic (dramatic) situation, the spectator (reader) does not require any art to enjoy the performance. The former creates imaginative situations and tries to transfer them to the other, who is to be impressed to believe them as real. For both, however, the situations are 'a-real'; not real! Semiotically speaking, the former re-arranges his experiences and even creates symbolic situations, or forwards already known symbols, while the latter does no such thing. In this scheme the actor has to be un-creative imitator, more or less. In a diagram it could be as in the Table (see p.51).

As has been said earlier, formation of images is the very first step in Semiotics. The second aspect of Semiotics is of a synchronic nature, which is seen in the formulation of groups of categories. In other words, it is visible in the various codes. A faint idea of this was indicated in the relationship between *vāsanā* and the *sthāyi-bhāvas,* though in Sanskrit Poetics such a relationship, as the *vāsanā* and the *sthāyi-bhāva* was not further developed. But, as the single semblance of a tree on the Shakespearean stage was a synchronic symbol for the garden or orchard, the whole arrangement on the stage stipulated by Bharata (*Nāṭyaśāstra* 1.39ff) was synchronic in essence. The Jarjara symbolized order, being the *axis mundi;*[19] it also symbolized the destruction of evils (v 65 *jarjarastv abhisaṁpūjyaḥ syāt tato vighna-jarjaraḥ*); it was the symbol of the thunderbolt of Indra (*ib*.58) and at its joints were believed to be settled various gods *(ib.)*. The same is the Semiotic value of the jar filled with water. Another important aspect of Semiotics is non-taxonomicism, which serves as a base for codification. (Taxis fr. Greek *tasseim*, 'to arrange') means 'split-category' arrangement; non-taxonomy indicates arrangement into groups forming codes. This is seen in the various formations of the hands indicating various emotions. For example, the *patākā* type of hand-formation (*Nāṭyaśāstra* IX.17), in which fingers of both the hands are spread and the thumbs are a bit curved, forms a code to express lightning-fall (*prahāra-pāta*, torrents of rain or fire, and even the shower of flowers (*ib*.19). Though it is not specifically mentioned, we could name it as 'shower-code'. Another example is of the codification of colours;

Creative Plane			Receptive Plane	
I	**II**	**III**	**IV**	**V**
Poet	**Character**	**Actor**	**Spectator**	**Reader**
(dramatist) Re-arranges; imagines (i.e. creates images etc.)	Image; 'a-real'; symbol.	Image of the Image; 'a-real'; human symbol.	modified by his own experience ↑	
i. Proto-actor	i. Poet's alter ego;	i. un-real as		
ii.Proto-reader	ii. Real during the presentation;	= character;		
iii.Creative artist ↓	iii. Unreal as compared to factual; imitative artist.	ii. Real as common man		
→ Impressions and Images ——→		Similar		

for example, the same colour indicates a different group of categories.

(vi)	Soft Black — Śṛṅgāra	(xxi)	Ghosts, demons, etc. -Black
	White — Hāsya		Varuṇa, Soma, etc. -White
	Red — Raudra		Aṅgāraka — Red
	Deep Dark — Bhayānaka		—
	Blue — Bībhatsa		
	Yellow — Adbhuta		Budha, Agni

Thus (and so on) is also the case with non-divinities; but here we have only a twofold codification; *Vidyādharas* - like heated gold; the same with the *Pitṛ*-s. Among the humans, the southerners are to be shown as dark, while the northerners and the westerners as fair (ib. XXI. 76-88). Even a particular type and shape of the beard symbolized the difference in the categories:

> *śuddha* (white): Liṅgin, Amātya, Purodhas (i.e. a religious student, minister, priest)
> *vicitra* (variegated): Divya (divine being), Vidyādhara, Pārthiva (king), Śṛṅgārin, *yauvanamada (-yukta)*
> *śyāma* (black): *tapasvin* (ascetic), *duḥkhita, vyasana-abhihata* (i.e. all dejected persons)
> *romaśa* (woolly, shaggy): *vaira-baddha* (hostile)
> Likewise and so forth.

Semiotically, one of the most pertinent concepts in Poetics is that *rasa* is the 'womb-mate' of 'Bliss-of-Brahman' (*brahmānanda-sahodara*). It has to be noted, that all *śāstra*-s in the Hindu tradition show Brahman as their source, or, in any case, a divine source. This is a fact of faith, which is not to be doubted and need not be proved! It is equally doubtful if all the founders of the Śāstras had actually known what Brahman is. Yet, realization of Brahman is taken as giving unsurpassable Bliss. This is not to doubt the reality of Brahman, but to show how it had a normative value; and, to express this value in plain words it would be 'The Excellence in every sphere'. This value is not the *abhidhā* potential of Brahman.[20] We may call this value by any name, But, plainly, it is symbolic. In other words, Brahman in Poetics (like other Śāstras) has a Semiotic value. In the same way, what is said to be *a-laukika* is not 'other-worldly', meaning heavenly! It means 'of a different world'. And, that world is of Poetic images, which is 'real' only in the sphere of Poetics; not actually real. In other words, it is 'a-real', i.e. non-real but similar to real (*laukika-sadṛśa*);[21] and the '*a-laukika*' bliss is due to the creation of this 'a-real' world, which is more fascinating than the stark real - as Māyā is!

NOTES AND REFERENCES

1. Bhaṭṭa Lollaṭa, *pratīyamānaḥ, pratītiyogyaḥ; pratipattyā* rendered as *pratītyā* at Bālabodhinī on *Kāvya-Prakāśa,* IV.28.
2. *Ibid. sāmājikānām vāsanayā carvyamāṇo rasaḥ.*
3. Rudraṭa, *Kāvyālaṁkāra,* XII. 4 *rasanād rasatvam eṣām.*
4. Cf. Bharata, *Nāṭyaśāstra,* VI. 37-38 *evam bhāvā rasāścaiva bhāvayanti parasparam*(37) and *tathā mūlam rasaḥ sarve tato bhāvā vyavasthitāḥ* (38). The word *vyavasthitāḥ* is to be marked.
5. Cf. Bhavabhūti, *Uttararāmacarita,* III.47.
6. Pāṇini, Māheśvara-sūtras, and *Aṣṭādhyāyī* I. 1.71.
7. Bālabodhinī, *loc.cit. nartake iti upalakṣaṇam kāvya-pāṭhake'pi.*
8. Bhaṭṭa-Tauta in Abhinavagupta's Locana, *nāyakasya kaveḥ śrotuḥ, samāno'nubhavas tataḥ.*
9. According to Mahimabhaṭṭa, *Vyaktiviveka;* see P.V. Kane, Ed. *Sāhityadarpaṇa,* which includes his *The History of Sanskrit Poetics,* Bombay, 1951 (Third Ed.,), p.238 for a brief discussion and the anticipation of this theory by *Dhvanyāloka*.
10. The verse is: *saṅketa-kāla-manasam viṭam jñātvā vidagdhayā hasannetrārpitākūtam līlāpadmam nimīlitam.*
11. There is an interesting point. The *viṭa* is a companion of a courtesan and also a paramour. Here he appears to be

a paramour. If he is a companion of the courtesan in the present context, the subdued symbolic communication would indicate, that the woman (courtesan, in that case) is having another customer at the moment, whom she would not like to embarass!

12. *Kumārasaṁbhava* VI.84-
evamvādini devarṣau pārśve pituradhomukhī
līlākamalapatrāṇi gaṇayāmāsa pārvatī
It is hardly surprising that the *nāyika* here and at note 10 *supra* have a lotus in their hand, though they are socially different. The lotus had clearly become symbolic with women and for soft emotions, among other things.
13. *Ibid.,* v.85.
14. *Śat.Br.* III. 6.1.24; of course, this is the position of the pandal called Havirdhāna.
15. *Rām.* Kiṣkindhā 6.22.
nāham jānāmi keyūre nāham jānāmi kuṇḍale
nūpure tveva jānāmi nityam pādābhivandanāt.
16. For example, if one has not seen the place being described by the writer (say, London), the city that gets figured up in one's own experience (say, Mumbai. If he is a resident of Mumbai, it would be different from Mumbai; it may be any foreign city seen in a film or so).
17. On this see Sadashiv A. Dange, *Purākathāñcā Artha-vāda āṇi Vivecana* (Marathi) Continental, Pune, 1994. The difference between a myth and creative literary work is that while the former is not artificial, the latter is a work of art; see p.27ff.
18. The word *kāru* used by the *Ṛgveda* for a poet is very perfect; 1.11.6; II, 43.1 and at a number of places.
19. See Sindhu S. Dange, "The Stage of Bharata: Some Symbolic Rites", *Ṛtam, Baburaṁ Saksena Fel. Vol.,* Lucknow, 1983, pp. 119-124.
20. The concept of *Brahman* was not the same originally as in its later absorption in the Upaniṣadic philosophical context. The ritual concept was of *karman*, as it was viewed against the backdrop of *karma-kāṇḍa*. As against the subtle principle it got evolved into in later times, originally it was tinted even with the idea of grossness (cf. *parivṛdham sarvataḥ, Nirukta* 1.9; *karmāṇi* XII.36; concurring only with the later idea of *mahato mahīyān;*

not with *aṇor aṇīyān).* The concept of *rasa* in the philosophic context occurs first in the *Taittirīya Upaniṣad* (II.7), where it is identified with the *sat* principle, with the comment that *sukṛta* (good deed) is itself *sat* and also *rasa*, but further with a new tint; that *sat* created itself on its own; hence it is called *sukṛta* (*ātmānaṁ svayam akuruta, tasmāt sukṛtam ucyate)* thus fusing the older idea of *karman* and the subtle *sat,* which, though known to the *Ṛgveda* (X.72.2.3) as the creative force, gained new dimensions in the Upaniṣadic period, Śaṅkara understands *rasa* (Comm. on *Taitt Up.*) as the *jīvātman,* which may not quite fit with the real expression *raso vai. saḥ*; but it would fit in the concept of Poetic *rasa*, as being the subtle element in the body, closely associated with the *vāsanā,* or the *sthāyibhāva* concept of Bharata. Later theoreticians just gathered it and stuffed their argument with it, without paying heed to its symbolic value and development. See also Dange, *Divine Hymns and Ancient Thought,* Vol. II, New Delhi, 1995, Intr. and p.357ff.

21. *a (nañ)* has the sense of *sādṛśya* also among its other five senses, *ct tat-sādṛśyam abhāvaśca,* etc.

* Included here from the *Journal of the Asiatic Society of Bombay*, Bombay, Vol. 71 for 1996 (New Series) pub. in 1997).

Chapter 4

Dream *(Svapna)* in the Vedic Concept

The subconscious in the humans has been an absorbing and striking subject for speculations.[1] The subconscious expresses itself most picturesquely in a dream, on which the dreamer has no control. That is why, a dream is dreaded, and in the case of a bad dream measures are stated to avert its probable influence. Information on this topic is scant in the Veda, but, there are illuminating suggestions. One of the most instructive references is from *Ṛgveda* where Vasiṣṭha is afraid of the wrath of Varuṇa due to a probable sin he committed in dream and he pleads before Varuṇa that on certain things one has no control. Among them he includes *svapna*. The word has a double meaning: (i) sleep, and (ii) dream. In the present case, it is 'dream'. He says, "Well, indeed, a dream is a mixer (*prayotā*, it may also be understood as 'contriver') of *anṛta*". *Anṛta* is opposite of *ṛta*, the order of things including the behaviour normalised by a society. Sāyaṇa explains the word *prayotā as "prakarṣeṇa miśrayitā"* and glosses, that a dream is a medium through which a sin, or untoward behaviour, is mixed up with a dreamer in his state of dreaming, though in actual life he might be pious (*ṚV* VII. 86.6).[2] In such a case, the dreamer is not at fault. The word *prayotā* (*fr. pra* + $\sqrt{}$*yu*), though it occurs only here, is very suggestive in the context of dream; it has the sense of uncontrollable rearrangement of events from actual life in the subconscious, which cannot be taken at its face value. At another place the seer Kakṣīvant, laments that he gets depressed by a dream, which has to be taken as a bad dream (*ṚV* I. 120. 12, *adha svapnasya nirvide*); and this verse has been a charm against bad dreams (*duḥsvapna-nāśinī*). In the event of delivery, or pregnancy, there was the belief that an evil power might snare the woman through *svapna* or *tamas* (= dream or sleep, X. 162.6 *svapnena tamasā*, which Sāyaṇa, rightly, takes to mean *svapnāvasthayā* and *nidrayā*). There is also the probability that a friend and a relative in real life may appear in dream as an enemy and cause worry (II.28.10),[3] the worry, after the dream, being that the dream may turn out to be portentous. Actually, such a dream may indicate strain due to conflicting situations in real life, one being good and the other bad. Here (as at VII.86.6) Varuṇa is invoked to protect, if such a situation does arise in real life. Indra is said to have resorted to the trick of involving the demons Cumuri and Dhuni in *svapna* (II. 15.9 *svapnenābhyupya)*. Vṛṣākapi is said to be *svapnanaṁśana* (X.86.21). Yāska (*Nir.*XII.28) and, later, Sāyaṇa render this word as "destroyer of dreams", i.e. bad dreams.

The *Atharvaveda* provides some more details regarding the beliefs about dreams. Here, dream is levelled up to the status of a deity, who is invoked to avert bad dreams. Dream, as a deity, is conceived as both living and not-living (*AV* VI. 46, 1, *yo na jīvo' si na mṛtaḥ).* This is based on the belief that the dream-reality is different from actual reality. For a person the dream is not unreal, as long as he is in dream. He realizes the dream to be unreal only when he gets up and faces stark reality. Dream (*svapna*) is said to be the 'son' of the sisters of the god[4] though his mother is said to be Varuṇānī and Yama is his father. He is also the agent (*karaṇaḥ*) of Yama, being himself the 'life-ender' and death. Dream's (other) name is Araru (*ib.*1-2).[5] The dream is called 'sin-of-the mind' (*AV* VI.45.1, *manasaspāpa*). Though at this particular verse the word *svapna* does not occur, it is enjoined as a charm against bad dream (*Kauśika-Sūtra* 46.9), which is admonished for portending inauspicious things (*ib. kim aśastāni śaṁsasi*). At the *Atharva-Pariśiṣṭa* these two hymns (*AV* VI. 45 and 46) are termed '*Duḥsvapna-nāśana-gaṇa*' (34.8). The *Kauśika-Sūtra* (*loc. cit.*) further enjoins that a *puroḍāśa* prepared from various grains (*miśra-dhānya*) should be placed in the quarter of the enemy, if one has a bad dream. It appears that the sacrificial cake (*puroḍāśa*) of various grains is in view of the nature of the dream, which mixes up things and events. The dream is not taken to be totally unreal, as it is believed to portend future events. This is clear from the atonements for deeds done in dreams. The *AV* already hints at the practice when it prescribes atonement for food taken in the dream and which is not found in the morning, indicating that such food was from some insecure source (*AV* VII. 101).[6]

At *AV* (XIX. 56) we have some information about how a dream takes shape. It has been noted above, that dream (as a deity) is the son of Yama, the god of death. In the present place, it is stated that the dream (*svapna*) arrives from the region of Yama and that it associated the mortals with error (*ib.* 1, *pramadā martyān pra yunakṣi dhīraḥ*).[7] The suggestion is that the dream-state leads a person's mind to experience regular things in an unexpected situation or new irregular situations, causing disorder or new order of things and behaviour. Dream is said to wander in the company of the "lone one" (*ib. ekākinā saratham yāsi*). Now, who is this 'lone one' (*ekākin*) with whom dream wanders, or who is led by dream? He is the person who dreams. He is alone with dream in the state of dreaming. There is none of his relatives or friends from actual life. This deity of dreams, called dream himself, is said to wander with the dreamer in the 'womb of the *asura*' (*ib. asurasya yonau*). The womb of the *asura* is the state of hypnosis, wherein mind gets loose from reason and flows with imagination. This is how dreams get formed. The *AV* (*loc.cit.*) indicates this by saying that dream fashions the dream in this way (*svapnam mimānaḥ*). Sāyaṇa takes this to refer to the condition of a dying man, which is absolutely off the mark; and there is not the least suggestion here for such a hypothesis and for understanding *ekākin* as one who has left his relatives and is being led by dream to the region of Yama as a result of a bad dream. Dream is said to be the son of Yama, all right; but, that does not mean that a bad dream takes a dreamer to Yama's abode. The belief that is reflected in these places is just, that sleep (*svapna*) creates a state which is akin to death, but with an important difference. In sleep dream (personified) takes charge of the mind; in the 'sleep' at death, there is no such thing. As sleep and death take a person away from the realities of life, the former temporarily and the latter permanently, both are associated with the god of death. Further, as sleep is the state where dreams (*svapna*) rise up they are also believed to be related to death. It is in this sense, that Yama is said to be the father of dream, the deity of dreams, bad or good. The request to *svapna* (dream), "*O Svapna,* protect us from bad dreams" (*AV* VI. 46.2 *sa naḥ svapna duḥṣvapnyāt pāhi*) is meaningful this way. This is about the relationship of dream with death.

Dream is said to have been first visualised by the 'all collecting' *Bandha* (*AV* XIX. 56.2 *bandhas-tvā agre viśvacayā apaśyat*). The time when this happened is said to be 'the day before the night was born' (*purā rātryā janitor eke ahni*). This has, obviously, an allusion to the first ever division of day and night in the primeval time. As dreams occur, normally, in sleep at night, but are not restricted to the night-sleep, the expression appears to suggest that the birth of dream was at the joint of day and night. This would mean that they occur at the confluence of light and darkness. The events in the dream may be clear, but they arise in the darkness of sleep. There is no ground to deny that the seer of this hymn is describing the phenomenon after a close watch on the process of dreaming. We may compare the modern scientific finding, that dreams are generated in the state of Rapid Eye Movement (*REM*, as it is known) not in sound sleep. In the state of sound sleep the person is completely in the dark about the events in his subconscious. The passage has been a riddle;[8] and what exactly is the nature of *bandha,* who is said to have first ever visualised this 'birth' of dream has been a problem. The easy way Sāyaṇa seems to have thought was to understand *bandha* as *bandhu;* and this choice out of other variant readings cannot be questioned. However, his choice does not make any difference in the explanation he gives, which is applicable to both *bandha and bandhu,* "the creator (*vidhātā)* who binds the creatures due to the actions of each one". But, the point is, why the well-known *vidhātā* should be called *bandhu* here; and, moreover, the word has variations. If one takes the word as *bandha* itself, there is no room for this philosophisation. This is the reason why Whitney discarded this interpretation of Sāyaṇa as just unacceptable; also because most of the authorities have followed the reading *bandhaḥ.* We may discard the spacious explanation of Sāyaṇa and restrict to the etymological meaning of *bandha* or *bandhu,*[9] 'tie', and understand *bandha* as the force that ties the day and night together, to give rise to dream in the present context. This way, *bandha* represents the stage, which, like the twilight, ties the day to the night and the real to the un-real in the dream together. This goes well with the statement that from this visualization stage of *bandha* dream was formed (*ib. tataḥ svapna, idam adhyā babhūvitha*). As dream is the product of hazy circumstances (dark and light mixing up; also real and unreal fusing together), it is seen as hiding its true nature even from the psychiatrists (*bhiṣagbhyaḥ rūpam apagūhamānaḥ*). The statement is important. Though the post-Vedic literature shows a system of the study of dreams, their grouping and the efforts to attribute meaning to the dreams on the basis of symbols in them, there are instances of the attribution of conflicting meanings to the same symbols.[10] In the modern time even Freud and his school fell into distrust regarding the exact implication about the symbolic objects seen in dreams. Dream, being powerful and yet slippery, was considered even by the gods as superior to them. They, or the manes, did not understand the implication of dreams, though they prattled about them, says *AV*. Ultimately, they gave it to Trita Āptya, who came to be regarded as the surest resort for all such things that were either harmful or of dubious nature (*ib.*3-4).[11] In fact, this hymn from *AV* has the characteristics of a regular myth; and, a myth and a dream are of similar nature.[12]

From what has been seen up-till now, the Vedic belief regarding dream appears to be as follows. It is product of the mind's unsettled condition, due to bodily ailment or pressure. This is more so about the formation of bad and disturbing dreams. It is called the sin of the mind *(manaspāpa)*. Though there is next to nothing about good dreams, we can take that good dreams were believed to be a creation of pious thoughts, as mind could also hold such thoughts. It was believed, that a dream was produced from a mixture of clarity and haziness, which gave rise to a disorder and rearrangement of things and events. In the Vedic terminology, a dream was *anṛtasya prayotā*. The concept behind *anṛta* is not of something diagonally opposite to *ṛta*. It is not non-order; it is disorder. It is not false; it is true in its own arrangement in the case of the dreamer.[13] It is produced from the mind of a person who is 'being heated' (*ib.* 5. *tapyamānasya manaso' dhijajñiṣe*). This state of the mind is not of actual heat; it is of persistent thoughts, either good or bad, a state of emotional fervour.

A comparison with ancient mythical ideas about dream from the Greek mythology will be interesting. According to the Greek mythology, Hypnos was the god of sleep; and the name is the Greek version of the Vedic *svapna* (dream), who is the god of dreams, as we have noted. Another name of Hypnos is Somnus, which also tallies with *svapna*. As in the Vedic beliefs about *svapna*, who controls dreams, Somnus has a close relationship with death, or the god of death. Somnus is the brother of death. Both Somnus and death stay in the lower world,[14] which is a mythical way of saying that sleep which generates dreams is but another aspect of death. The idea is the same as Yama being the father of dream (*svapna*). Staying in the lower world along with his brother death, Somnus (the god of sleep) sends dreams, that rise up. As dreams are restricted to individuals, sleep (Somnus) and death have to be understood as microcosmically staying in the individual. Hence, the 'underworld' for the individual is his subconscious. This is exactly the case with the *asurasya yoni* of the *AV*. *Svapna*, in his aspect of the god of dreams, leads the lonely dreamer through this 'womb', situated in the dreamer himself, fashioning dreams. The Vedic *svapna* has a twofold aspect, as noted above: (i) god of sleep who controls dreams; this is his and generalised aspect; and (ii) an individual dream, which is the particular aspect. In the Greek mythology there is a further nicety. The god of dreams, who actually sends dreams, or is dream himself, is called Morpheus, who can assume any form[15] and is endowed with wings. This is just the personification of a dream and its nature. The Vedic *(AV)* detail of the creation of dreams at day before the oncome of the night is a way to suggest that dreams assume a mixture of light and dark, as we have noted above. This rough belief may be compared with a modern scientific observation. Jung, for example, says that a dream represents the *terra intermedia* between moral and pathological psychology. He says that a dream is close to the dark side of the psyche, which is the unconscious.[16] This modern day observation, together with the Greek myth about the formation of dreams, appears to be already suggested in the concept of the womb of the *asura* in which lies the mine of dreams.

NOTES AND REFERENCES

1. Sigmund Freud, *Interpretation of Dreams,* 1900: 1953; *On Dreams,* 1954; 1968 (Basic Books, London); *Collected Papers,* London, 1925; Karl Abraham, *Dreams and Myths,* 1909; also Ann Faraday, *Dream Power and The Dream Game;* Calvin S. Halls, *The Meaning of Dreams and so on.*
2. The passage is *svapnaś cana-it-anṛtasya prayotā*. Geldner, *Der Rigveda (HOS., 34)* Cambridge, Massachusetts, 2nd Printing, 1978, p.257, renders it as meaning that sleep (or dream) "is not the diverter" of *anṛta*. The root *yu* has both the meanings of joining and separating, however, *prayotā* has to be contrasted with *viyotāraḥ* (IV.55.2) and *viyoṣat* (IV.16.20).
3. *yo me rājan yujyo vā sakhā vā svapne bhayam bhīrave mahyam āha.*
4. *AV* VI.46.1cd *varuṇānī te mātā yamaḥ pitā-ararur nāmāsi.* At XIX. 57.3 we have *devānām patnīnām garbha yamasya kara.*
5. Araru occurs in *ṚV* twice, I. 12.3 and X.99.11. At the first place it is rendered by Sāyaṇa as *araṇasīla* ('moving'); at the other he is said to be *catuṣpāt.* The idea is that he is a demon, with four feet.
6. *yat svapne annam aśnāmi na prātar adhigamyate / sarvam tad astu me śivam nahi tad dṛśyate divā / /.*
7. Whitney renders *pramadā* as "with mirth (?)", with a question mark. In that case we expect the reading *pramudā.* There is no variant for *pramadā.*
8. And there are variations, *budhnastvāgre viśvavyacā; bandhustvāgre viśvacayā: bandhastvāgre,* etc.
9. In the same hymn *svarmadasi parameṇa bandhunā* occurs at v.5 below.
10. See, Sadashiv A. Dange, *Ency. P.B. & P.,* Vol.II, Navrang, New Delhi, 1987, pp.445-451.
11. See A.A. Macdonell, *Vedic Mythology* (Hindi Tr. by Ramkumar Rai), Chowkhamba, Varanasi, 1961, p.128; cf. *ṚV* VIII. 47.13 *trite tad viśvam āptye,* 14-17. These five verses are enjoined by the *Āśvalāyana Gṛhya-Sūtra* to be recited after seeing a bad dream. The last one occurs in *AV* (VI.46.3; and XIX. 57.1) with a slight variation. *ṚV yathā kalām...yatha ṛṇam saṁnayāmasi / evā duḥṣvapnyam*

sarvam āptye saṁ nayāmasi / / (v.17); *AV* VI. 46.3[b] = XIX.57.1[b]. *yatharṇam saṁnayanti;* and *dviṣate saṁ nayāmasi at* VI.46.3[d], while *apriye saṁ nayāmasi* at XIX. 57.1[d].

12. For discussion on this point, see Dange, *Towards Understanding Hindu Myths,* Aryan Books International, New Delhi, 1996, p.175*ff.*
13. In this case the particle *an* in *anṛta* has to be taken as meaning 'like' or 'little less than'; cf. *tatsādṛśyam abhāvaś ca tadanyatvam tadalpatā,* etc., the famous line from *Vaiyākaraṇabhūṣaṇasāra.*
14. Edith Hamilton, *Mythology,* Little Brown and Co., Boston, 1942, pp.44 and 143.
15. Morpheus connects with morphia which causes drowsiness; and, on the other hand, with the Greek word *morphe,* meaning 'form'. Morpheus, as dream, has both these traits.
16. C.G. Jung, *The Archetypes and the Collective Unconscious* in *The Collected Works of C.G. Jung,* Vol. IX, pt.I (tr. in English by R.F.C. Hull), Bollingen Series XX, Princeton University Press, Princeton, 1990 (1968), p.152.

    In the *Chāndogya-Upaniṣad* (VIII.10) we have an illustration of the self through the experience of the dream, where also the dream self is said to be different from the normal self.

* Included here from the *Vishvesharanand Indological Journal,* Panjab University, Hoshiarpur, Vol.XXX, pts.i-ii, June-Dec., 1992, pub. in 1997

* For a detailed discussion on the topic of 'Dreams' on a comparative basis, see Sadashiv A. Dange, "Dream, Myth and the Hindu Context", *Annals of the Bhandarkar Oriental Research Institute,* Vol. LXXIX (1998), Pune, 1999, pp.61-82 (being the R.G Bhandarkar Anniversary Address delivered at the Bhandarkar Oriental Research Institute, Pune, on Ṛṣipañcamī, Sunday, 7th Sept. 1997).

Chapter 5

Act and Retribution in the Ṛgveda and the Atharvaveda

It has been stated that a clear statement about the prevalence of *karman* and its *phala* is absent in the *Ṛgveda.*[1] The same is believed to be the position regarding the *Atharvaveda,* more or less. This is in spite of the fact that the concept of the 'world of the performers of good acts' *(sukṛtām loka)* was quite well settled in the *ṚV.* It has been said, that the concept of 'deed' and its fruit (*karman* and its retribution) is an afterthought, influenced by the concept of Hell and Heaven, in the history of Vedic thought. While commenting on the passages from *ṚV* which say, that persons bereft of Ṛta and Satya create a deep pit for themselves (*ṚV* IV.5.5), and where the gods are invoked to strike down the evil-doers into the bottomless darkness (VII.104.9), Kane says that here we have the glimpses of the concept of hell, as in the *sukṛtām loka* the glimpses of heaven. He opines, that "Later on, when the doctrine of *karman* and *punarjanma* (deed and rebirth) came to be universally believed, in India, the theory of heaven and hell came to be modified by holding that the author of sins was born again and again as an animal or a tree or human being suffering from disease and defects".[2] This and such opinions need re-examination. Apart from the fact whether the belief in rebirth is attested by *ṚV* and *AV*, a question needs to be answered. Who is supposed to reach heaven and who the hell, according to the belief in *ṚV*, as reflected very clearly from its statements. For whom is the *sukṛtām loka?* The answer lies in the very expression itself. It is for those who are *sukṛt,* i.e. 'The performers of good deeds'. Who are desired to go to the bottomless pit of darkness? The word for such persons is just the opposite of *sukṛt;* it is *duṣkṛtaḥ*. So, it is the evil-doers that are desired to go to the dark pits. Such persons are called *pāpāsaḥ* (cf. IV. 5.5 *pāpāsaḥ santaḥ-anṛtā asatyā idam padam ajanata gabhīram)*. The thought is very clear: The persons who are sinful, not steadfast in their promises, and are against Ṛta, create (*ajanata*), for themselves the deep place. They are termed *duṣkṛtaḥ,* and for them is the bottomless dark abode (cf. VII.104.11). The reference to the *duṣkṛtaḥ* occurs at many other places. What is pertinent to note is, that such people are said, as noted above, to create for themselves the dark pit. Thus, the action lies with them; and they have to bear the responsibility.

It is true that there is no one-to-one correspondence between a particular act and its fruit in these texts. The reason is that they are not treatises on Dharmaśāstra. However, one cannot deny the very presence of the concept of act and its retribution here. The belief and concept of heaven is closely associated with merit in this world. The later maxim and injunction: *svargakāmo yajeta:* which stresses the need to sacrifice, has its origin in the belief that if one desires to achieve heaven, after death, one has to sacrifice here, which, in plain words, is 'heaven is the fruit of the act of sacrifice'. The basis of this belief lies in such expressions as, "Those who reached heaven by their penance" (*ṚV* X.154.2 *tapasā ye svar yayuḥ*). The point is that heaven was believed to be a place of joy and, hence, desirable. The way to attain it was *tapas*, which involved sacrifice and good deed. This is closely associated with the concept of *iṣṭāpūrta.*[3] *Iṣṭa* includes the daily duties and sacrificial rites, while *pūrta* is the fulfilment of the vows—which may be in the context of a sacrifice or the social behaviour according to recognized norms, and also performance of deeds useful for general good. The *ṚV* records the belief that by *iṣṭāpūrta* a person establishes himself among his ancestors, after death, and also that he reaches the highest heaven thereby. With *iṣṭāpūrta* he is able to discard whatever sin that contaminated him in this world; and, that, finally he obtains a new body to come back home in this world for performing further meritorious deeds (*ṚV* X.14.8).[4] In the social context, about merit through donation, *AV* says, that such a donor attains heaven, and that (interestingly) he is not obliged to give any bribe to a higher-ranking person. *AV* clarifies, in this context, that the assessors in the assembly of Yama (the god of death) take the sixteenth part of the *iṣṭāpūrta* of the person, which might stand for the smallest portion of demerit, if any, in the mass of merit. This small portion might turn against the person in the abode of the dead. So, to nullify even this probability a white-footed male goat is to be given in one's lifetime (*AV* III.29.1).[5] The concept behind *iṣṭāpūrta* is, hence, that of storing merit with good acts in this world for the final settlement of accounts before the judges of Yama. Care has to be taken to remove even a speck of demerit that might cling to the bundle of merits, lest it should counteract the good actions, which implies the fruit of those actions, though it is not specifically stated in so many words. There is no mention of heaven and hell here. The gain of heaven would come after the judgement. If rebirth happens it is not arbitrary; it is not even through Fate. It is due to one's own accrual of merit or demerit. If one scrutinizes the thought in *ṚV* and *AV* carefully, one would see a gradual evolution of the concept of *karman*—from a mere deed or exploit to action that has the power to turn into merit or demerit. And, probably, herein lies the difference between *apas* and *karman*. We have to understand *apas* to be just a 'deed' or just a mere act or exploit, without any retributive or merit-involving power. It is restricted and has a limited application. On the other hand, *karman* had gained, at the period of the *Ṛgveda* itself, the status of a capsule with far-reaching complex results. Thus, it came to be believed that *karman* was consolidated with *apas* (*ṚV* 1.31.8 *ṛdhyāma karma apasā navena*).[6] The family-books already indicate the progress in the concept of *karman* from just an exploit (*ṚV* III.30.13;-32.8; see also - 12.6) to a meritorious and sacrificial act. It is said, "Manifold bondages set him free, who abodes with Indra through his *karman* (*ṚV* VII.32.13 *pūrvīś cana prasitayas taranti tam ya indre karmaṇā bhuvat*). Here *karman* has the sense of a sacrificial deed, involving merit. The same is the case when the juices of Soma are said to invigorate Indra with their *karman*-s (IX.46.3 *indram vardhanti karmabhiḥ*). Flatly, the juices can hardly be said to 'act' like a sentient person. Their *karman,* hence, has to be understood as 'power' to promote action (the flat sense of action, or exploit) in Indra. Such passages give clue to the evolution of the meaning of *karman,* which, now, involve the power to cause a result, in the *karmin* (performer). On the level of the sacrifice, *karman* assumes the sense of a rite, or a group of rites in a larger ritual. The rite and the larger group of rites get into the relationship of part and a whole. In technical language, they have the *aṅga-aṅgin* relationship. With this stage of evolution, the sacrificer or any wonder-worker came to be called *sukṛt (su-kṛt).* The next step is heaven being called *sukṛtām loka* and the precincts of the sacrifice *sukṛtasya yoni,*[7] where demerit has no place. On the other hand, whatever is done in the context of the sacrifice, howsoever unusual it might look, is nothing but *sukṛta* (auspicious).

As against the *sukṛt ṚV* speaks about the undesirable persons, *duṣkṛt (duṣkṛtaḥ*; plural) at many places. The *duṣkṛtaḥ* (evil-doers) are desired to be punished or thrown into the dark pits and so on (V.83.2; 9;VII.104.3 and so on). By far, the most suggestive is the invocation about the personal evil, or sin (*duṣkṛta*). It is said, "Whatever *duṣkṛta* we have committed with greed, while awake or in sleep, may Agni cast it away" (X.164.3); or, "Whatever sin, concealed or in open, did we commit (*yad āvir yad apīcyam asti duṣkṛtam*), O Gods! Separate it from us. May it be tacked on to Trita Āptya" (*ṚV* VIII.47.3).[8] Any sin committed even in dream, let alone while awake, under the influence of wine, or in anger, or at dice-playing and while being not in senses, is sought to be avoided (*ṚV* VII.86.6). Why should the seers be so afraid of an evil deed, which is termed *pāpa*? Why should *AV* lay down hymns for freeing oneself from sin (*pāpa-mocana;* cf. IV.23-25; VI.45-46, etc.)? The obvious implication is that, as meritorious acts (*iṣṭāpūrta*) are recorded to be judged in the life after death, as noted above (*AV* III.29.3 *yad rājāno vibhajanta iṣṭāpūrtasya ṣoḍaśan)*, so does the sinful acts get recorded, though it is not seen, and it might harm the doer some time in this very life, or after death—may be in the next life. This would show that, though there is no direct enumeration of retribution, the belief is obvious. It is this belief that is at the base of the doctrine of 'Apūrva' and 'Adṛṣṭa' of the Pūrvamīmāṁsakas of later years, the *karmakāṇḍin*-s who evolved a regular philosophy of *karman.* Every rite, according to this doctrine, creates some thing new; but, it is not immediately seen or witnessed. It accrues to the doer or performer. The rite is a part of a larger performance, which is the complete sacrifice. As the single rite, or action in the sacrifice, is the *aṅga*, the *adṛṣṭa-apūrva* of that part is called *aṅgāpūrva.* The sum-total of all such *aṅgāpūrva*-s join together at the end of the whole of the sacrifice, which is the *aṅgin.* The *apūrva* of this *aṅgin* accures to the sacrificer and reserves for him place in heaven. Care is taken that each rite is clear of any blemish, lest the future deposit of total virtue should get contaminated by it. Such specks of blemish are sought to be wiped off by expiations at various places, should they happen.

Retribution, in the true and expressed sense of the

term obtains in certain places in *AV*. For example, it was believed that a sterile cow belonged to the gods. If any one, promising to donate such a cow, goes back on his words he would be afflicted with manifold calamities (*AV* XII.4). It is said that one who usurps a brahmin's cow moves away from the heavenly region of Yama to evil worlds far away (*ib*.XII.5.64). This is a clear indication of the belief, that the cow stealer transmigrates, after death, away from the assembly of Yama, where he is first led, to other worlds. As against this, the donor of a cow enjoys all desires in the heaven of Yama. And, read with *ṚV* X.14.8 (noted above), a person who performed meritorious or virtuous acts in his life-time could be back in this world with a new unblemished body, having washed his blemish, if any, in the region of the fathers above, after getting judged by the assessors of Yama's assembly! For, one who committed sin and gained only demerit is sure to be withheld in the 'Naraka-loka' as if he himself asked for it (*AV* XII.4.36 *athāhur narakam lokam nirundhānasya yācitam)*. The point is, nobody forces his stay in heaven or pushes him to lower worlds. It is his own *karman* that does it. Though the concept of Naraka does not obtain in *ṚV* proper, *ṚV-Khila* has it (X.106.1),[9] where it is said that, by offerings in the sacrifice some attain heaven directly from here; but, that, if crookedness sets in us, we are sure to fall in Naraka. The concept of Naraka, as explained by Yāska, who quotes the verse with accents, is "that which leads down and down" (*Nirukta* I.11 *ni-arakam; nīcair gamanam)*. Probably, this indicates lower and lower birth in a chain. This gets support from *ṚV,* which reflects the belief that a person who is set in the cycle of births enters Nirṛti (I.164.32 *bahuprajā nirṛtim āviveśa)*. The word *bahuprajāḥ* (with the accent on the last syllable, indicating the compound to be Tatpuruṣa) has to be particularly noted. Sāyaṇa renders it as "one who undergoes many births" (*bahujanma-bhāk*).[10] This is further supported by the preceding expression, "mother's womb" (*mātur yonau*). Nirṛti is the deity associated with sin (*pāpābhimāninī devatā*).[11] She is associated also with Yama (*AV* VI.29.3, where, earlier, her messengers are said to be the pigeon and the owl; cf. *ṚV* X.165.1;4). Hence, Nirṛti, like *anṛta,* is a hindrance—a sin—which causes instability and trouble, as against *Ṛta* and merit, which generate virtue with its good results. This is the basic principle of the theory of retribution. The *Ṛgveda* and the *Atharvaveda* reflect it in the formation stage, though it developed later with its varieties.

NOTES AND REFERENCES

1. P.V. Kane, *History of Dharmaśāstra,* Vol.V, pt. II, Second Ed., Poona, 1970, p.1536.
2. *ib.* Vol.IV, Second Ed., 1973, p.158.
3. For this concept, cf. *Kauṣītaki Br.* VII.4; *Jai. Br.*. II.53; *iṣṭa* at the former, *iṣṭāpūrta* at the latter; both are non-perishable. The expressions are, respectively, *iṣṭasya akṣiti*, and *iṣṭāpūrtasya akṣiti.*
4. Kane, *op.cit.*, p.156, says that with *iṣṭāpūrta* he stays in the company of the manes in heaven. He does not take the sense of rebirth here. Obviously, he *ignores punar astam ehi.* Keith, A.B., gets the point and understands fresh birth here; see *The Religion and Philosophy of the Veda and Upanishads,* (Part II, reprint), Motilal Banarsidass, Delhi, 1989 (HOS, Vol.32, 1925), p.478. For a critical assessment of Kane's criticism of Ranade and Karandikar, see Dange, *Images from Vedic Hymns and Rituals,* Aryan Books International, New Delhi, 2000, p.266f.
5. *AV* III.29.3.
6. Sāyaṇa renders *apasā* as *putreṇa* ("with the son"), which is off the mark. Geldner, "neue Machwerk" (new work), and at the bottom-note "Das neue Lied" (i.e., a new song), out of which the former is more to the point.
7. *ṚV* III.29.8. Agni is asked to take his seat in the *sukṛtasya yoni*, which is his own region (*sva loka*). Cf. X.61.6 and 85.24 *ṛtasya yonau sukṛtasya loke.*
8. Trita Āptya is conceived as taking upon himself the sins

and bad omens or bad dreams, cf. *Ṛ̣V* VIII.47.14-17; *AV* VI.46.3.

9. *Vaidika Sam. Mandala* ed., Vol. IV, Poona in *sūci* (Index), p.956. However, here no accents occur. But, cf. *Nirukta* I.11.
10. See Dange, *Images from Vedic Hymns and Rituals,* p.269, for a full discussion.
11. *Iriṇa* occurs as the form of Nirṛti. It is said, this *iriṇa* should be self-formed. Now, *iriṇa* is a hollow pit in the earth. It is also said, that the *iriṇa* is the earth itself, *Taitt. Br.* I.6.1.1-3; *Śat, Br.*V.2.3.2-3. The combined image of Nirṛti will be of the 'womb of the earth'. At the Ṛgvedic and the later Vedic period, it is mixed with 'falling in hell'. The place of Nirṛti was to be at the south of the southern fire (Dakṣiṇāgni). Later, this quarter came to be associated with Death. These references are from the context of the Rājasūya, where, at the start itself, Nirṛti is to be pacified. For another ritual, at a sudden hollow *(iriṇa)* appearing, for pacification, cf. *Kauśikasūtra* XIII. 28, where *mantra-s* from *AV* (XII.1, 19-21) are enjoined.

Chapter 6

Vāstoṣpati, Rudra and Cyavana

The deity Vāstoṣpati presents a rather interesting mixture of concepts and beliefs. He is first mentioned in the *Ṛgveda* and has maintained his importance through ages to the Puranic period (A.D. 200-1000 or later). The *vāstu-s (vāstūni)* of Viṣṇu are spoken of in the *ṚV* (I.154.6); but Viṣṇu's association with these *vāstu*-s is not as being their 'lord'. He is not the special deity of the *vāstu-s*. The idea is that he owns the vā*stu-s* and stays in them, as Mitra and Varuṇa stay in their *vāstu-s*, that are full of riches (*ṚV*. VIII.25.5). It is also observed that the meaning of the term *vāstu* shows variation as it was used in various periods and contexts, as is shown by Ram Gopal.[1] In the present article, the idea is to examine the status of the deities (mentioned in the title), as also to see a phase of the personality of Cyavana, a point that has been unnoticed by scholars. That *vāstu,* in one of its connotations, was a dwelling is already noted by the *ṚV* in a hymn to Vāstoṣpati (*ṚV*. VII.54 and cf. also 55). This deity was invoked at the building of a dwelling, as Sāyaṇa says referring to the *Āśvalāyana-gṛhyasūtra* (II.9.9). This would clearly show that a definite presiding deity of the dwelling was already set at the period of the *ṚV* (cf. also VIII.17.14). However, there are two other gods who are said to be Vāstoṣpati, irrespective of the implication of the term Vāstoṣpati (whether *yajña-vāstu* 'place of sacrifice', or the dwelling or any other place). One is Tvaṣṭṛ (V.41.8: *(aham) vāstoṣpatim tvaṣṭāram rarāṇaḥ)*;[2] and the other, more frequently, is Rudra. He appears to be more so in the context of the *yajña-vāstu,* as we shall see. Rudra, as Vāstoṣpati, is clearer in the post-Ṛgvedic texts. In this capacity he is also called *vāstavya* (*Śat.Br.* 1.7.3.1; 7). According to a myth at the *Śat.Br.,* the gods went to heaven by means of a sacrifice; but, the 'god of the cattle' (Rudra) was left behind in the *vāstu*. This would mean that Rudra is the master of the sacrificial site after the sacrifice is over, and, when the main offerings were cast into the fire. The text specifically mentions that whatever remains (of the offerings and of the place of sacrifice) is the *vāstu*. Rudra, being its lord, is Vāstavya. The myth further says that when the gods had almost left, Rudra followed them (like a sentinel?) and appeared in the north with his weapon held high. He told them to set apart some portion for him. The gods instructed the Adhvaryu priest to replenish the portions and, from a share of each god, to form a whole share for Rudra. The Adhvaryu did it. This new share was the *vāstu*. Rudra was the Vāstavya on this account also,[3] as this new share belonged to him. It has to be noted, however, that this offering, as such, is not called *raudra* ('meant for Rudra'). It is also to be noted, that in the *ṚV* in one hymn by the seer Dīrghatamas, where the birth of Vāstoṣpati is described, the act is called *raudram brahma* (X.61.1). In the present context, the offering is called *sviṣṭakṛt,* and even the god is named Sviṣṭakṛt. The point is, why the god is Agni Sviṣṭakṛt, when the offering is made for Rudra? Another point is, that the *sviṣṭakṛt* offering is always the last — or, more correctly, an additional one when the main gods have been offered to. The idea is twofold. Rudra is to be kept away from the main offerings; and, at the same time, his inclusion is arranged by proxy. Rudra is acclaimed, even here, as the 'lord of cattle'; and yet, he is to be kept at a distance. This has been his trait in rituals.[4] Even so, he has to be satisfied. This was done with this *sviṣṭakṛt*. The proxy in this case is that he is not mentioned as Rudra, but as Agni. The proxy, however, is very thin here. If we see the various names of Agni Sviṣṭakṛt here it would be clear that they are the names of Rudra. It is said, that 'Agni' is called Śarva by the eastern people; 'Bhava' by the Bāhīkas; he is also called 'lord of cattle' (*paśūnām pati;* cf. the name of Rudra in the myth just referred to above); he is also Rudra. The point is that Rudra is here suppressed by the concept of Agni; and even elsewhere Agni and Rudra are fused, as is seen in the context of the birth of Kumāra.[5]

Being the controller of the *vāstu* in the double sense of the term, Rudra gets to be called Vāstoṣpati. It is seen that he not only is the 'lord' of the sacrificial place (*yajña-vāstu),* after once the sacrifice is over, and of the offering made after the main offerings are offered, but he is the deity of the household, in which capacity he equals Vāstoṣpati (known to the *ṚV.* VII.54) mentioned above. This is clear from a ritual. When a householder went on a journey he was advised to invoke Vāstoṣpati with the hymn from the *ṚV* mentioned above (VII.54); and it is said that, if he did not do so, Vāstoṣpati would harm him and the dwelling (*Taitt. Sam.* III.4.10.1-3). The same hymn is prescribed when a new dwelling is constructed and it is to be entered for the first time. The *brāhmaṇa-s,* who are to be fed at this entry, would utter: *śivam vāstu* ('auspicious be the dwelling'), thus handing over the new dwelling to the owner with the propitiation of Vāstoṣpati (*Āśvalāyana G.S* II.9.9). The Vedic people had a clear idea of the difference between the status of Vāstoṣpati and Gṛhapati, though both were seen as aspects of Agni. Gṛhapati was the visible form of Agni, who is also termed Damūnas. The aspect of Vāstoṣpati was invisible and lying under the visible 'lord of the dwelling'. In essence, he was the god of the basement and the whole structure, if any, above the main. The structure above the main is termed by the *Manusmṛti:* 'Pṛṣṭha-vāstu' (III.91; Kullūka, *gṛhasyopari yad gṛham).* At the daily worship a *bali* was to be offered in the centre of the main house (*ibid.* 89 *vāstu-madhye)* to Brahmā and also to Vāstoṣpati, separately. The mention of Brahmā is as, by that period, he was considered to be the lord of the cosmic space with also the Vedic ritualist concept of Brahman (ritual and prayer) and the altar being at the centre.[6] The fusion of Vāstoṣpati and Agni (the unseen and the seen aspects) is seen in the fact that, if Vāstoṣpati is not propitiated by the householder while going on a journey, Agni would burn the dwelling; but, here we have a further identification, "Rudra, indeed, is Vāstoṣpati". If he goes away without offering the share to Vāstoṣpati (*vāstoṣpatīyam)*, "Agni would kill him becoming Rudra". Thus, Agni, Rudra and Vāstoṣpati are identified. According to a famous myth, Manu, the father of Nābhānediṣṭha, divided his wealth among his sons. At that time, Nābhānediṣṭha was in his preceptor's house practising the vow of a *brahmacārin* (and was learning the *Vedas*). When he returned, and seeing that the division was already made leaving him, he asked his father what happened to his share. Manu said that, now, he should go to the sacrifice of the Aṅgirases. The Aṅgirases are leaving for the heavenly world; but, they cannot proceed, as they get confused each time when they come to the sixth day. Manu tells Nābhānediṣṭha that he should go there and get them recite two hymns (*ṚV* X.61 and 62) on the sixth day.[7] Their impediment being cleared, they would give him whatever they had collected for the sacrifice. Nābhānediṣṭha did it; and the Aṅgirases gave him saying the thousand (cows, that are remaining), now, belong to him. As he was about to gather the thousand, a man wearing black (soiled) garment approached him suddenly from the north and said that the thousand, that is the remainder in the *vāstu (vāstuham),* belonged to him and that Nābhānediṣṭha should not take it away *(Ai.Br.=* V.14 22.9; *Taitt. Sam.*III. 1.9.3ff). The man in the soiled garments is Rudra; and the 'remainder' in the *vāstu* (here, *yajña-vāstu*, place of the sacrifice) belonged to him. Hence, he is the 'lord of the *vāstu*', Vāstoṣpati (cf. also *Taitt. Sam.* 3: *rudraḥ khalu vai vāstoṣpatiḥ; and* III.1.9.5: *yajñavāstau rudra āgacchat*). Comparing the two myths regarding Rudra certain points come to the fore: (i) in both Rudra is said to be Vāstoṣpati; (ii) Rudra, as Vāstoṣpati, has a double nature. Propitiated, he is benevolent. Even in the second myth, it is further said, that he eventually granted the thousand cows to Nābhānediṣṭha; this would show him to be kind. But, he is also cruel; because he, as Agni, would kill the householder, if not propitiated before the start of his journey; he wields his weapon against the gods; and (iii) Rudra's quarter is the north. This would show that the basic concept behind Vāstoṣpati was of a mixture of good and evil. This brings us to the association of Vāstoṣpati with Cyavana (Cyavāna).

Apart from the two myths regarding Vāstoṣpati mentioned above, there is an important reference to Cyavāna and Vāstoṣpati, together. In the second myth mentioned above, Nābhānediṣṭha figures; and he is successful in winning over Rudra = Vāstoṣpati. Now, the hymn in which Vāstoṣpati is mentioned is the *ṚV*. X.61. This one, along with X.62, is enjoined to be recited, according to the myth, to clear the Aṅgirases from getting confused and make their ascent to heaven sure. This means that the myth presupposes the hymn. According to the hymn (X.61) it is Cyavāna who readies the altar (v.1: *amimīta vedim*). The ritual is called Raudra *brahma* (*ibid.*) as we have noted earlier. Later in the hymn, it is said that the gods fashioned Vāstoṣpati (*ibid.* v.7: *vāstoṣpatim vratapām atakṣam*). Sāyaṇa (on v.1) does not say so in many words; but, he is reminded of the myth and jots down a sentence from it relating to the confusion of the Aṅgirases. The manner in which Vāstoṣpati was fashioned is to be noted. It is said, that this was when the father united with daughter; and this daughter is said to be Kṣmā, which is earth (*ibid.* v.7: *kṣmayā sam jagmānaḥ*).[8] This makes Vāstoṣpati an autochthon, i.e. a being born from the earth. There is a minute suggestion that, as soon as he was born from the earth, Vāstoṣpati was held and fashioned by the gods. This detail, with his nature of being cruel, is the basis of the Puranic myth which tells that, as soon as Vāstoṣpati (or Vāstupuruṣa) was born from the earth, he was seized by the gods and other powers and was pinned down to the earth. The Purāṇas further say that, the gods and the other powers (including the evil ones) are to be shown and propitiated in and around the area where the building is to be structured. According to the Purāṇas, the Vāstupuruṣa (Vāstoṣpati of the *Vedas*) was terrible to look at and was deformed (like a dwarf). It is also said that the Vāstupuruṣa, called also Vāstu, was like a demon in appearance (*Agni P.* 93.3: *asurākṛtim*).[9] The mixed nature - benevolent and cruel — of Vāstupuruṣa makes him of unpredictable nature. Cyavāna's mention in the hymn of Nābhānediṣṭha, which also speaks of the fashioning of Vāstoṣpati, has to be taken note of in viewing Cyavāna's personality in the Brāhmana texts.

First of all, the good-evil (cruel) syndrome is seen in the case of Cyavāna (Cyavana). This is clear in the account of king Śaryāta and his daughter. Undisturbed, Cyavana is not harmful; but, being disturbed, he spreads confusion in the people of the king. Later, being propitiated by the king by giving his daughter to him, he officiates at the king's sacrifice. The *Śat. Br.* (IV. 1.5.1ff) and the *Jai.Br.* which has about the same account (III.120-128), give some more details about his nature. It is said that, when the Bhṛgus or the Aṅgirases went to the heavenly world, Cyavana was left behind; he was ghostlike in appearance (*Śat. Br., op.cit.* 1). The motif of the others going to heaven and someone left behind is seen also in the myth of Nābhānediṣṭha noted above. The *vāstuha*, in that myth, of which Rudra is said to be the lord and which very much tallies with the concept behind Vāstoṣpati, and also tallies with the expression *jahe* (*ibid. kṛtyārūpo jahe* 'he was left, of evil form as he was'). The word *vāstuha* would mean *vāstau hīnam* ('left in the *vāstu'*). Though the expression is about any object that is left, it also reflects the position of Rudra - Vāstoṣpati, who is separated from the other gods. He is 'left' away; and he is the lord of what is left away. According to the *Jai.Br.* (III.120) he asks his sons to leave him near the pool of the Sarasvatī. So, he is *vāstau hīnaḥ*. Not only that, he knows the technique, or ritual, of *vāstupa* (*ibid.*). The appearance and the behaviour of Cyavana reflects those of Vāstoṣpati and Rudra. In the *Mahābhārata* we meet a person very much of this type, and also named Cyavana, who tests the king Kuśika and his wife very torturingly.[10] It is clear that he could not be the same Cyavana as we have in the Vedic context. But, Cyavana seems to have become a type, the other such being Durvāsas;[11] and myths came to be woven round them. In all such myths, and legendary accounts, about these persons the common trait is the same. The person is endowed with suprernatural power; he is a mixture of good-evil; he acts waywardly. Another such one is the 'sage' known as Aitaśa,[12] who asks his sons to leave him away in the uninhabited place and prattles like a mad man. However, the oldest and the earliest is Cyavāna, who appears to be a veritable alter ego of the Vāstoṣpati, and also knows the science of the Vāstupa. It is not improbable, that, as being the very embodiment of the deity or the lord of the *vāstu,* he chose to appear like the Vāstoṣpati. And, the norm for Vāstoṣpati was Rudra.

NOTES AND REFERENCES

1. Ram Gopal, "Vedic Vāstu and its Derivatives", *Bhāratīya Vidyā,* Vols. XLV-XLVII (Mm. Prof. J.H. Dave Fel. Vol.), Bombay, 1987, pp.37-42.
2. Geldner, 'Vāstoṣpati (und) Tvaṣṭṛ'. *Ca* is found in a variant commentary. The *Saṁhitā* does not warrant it. Hence it is not in the regular commentary of Sāyaṇa.
3. Vishva Bandhu, in his *Vaidika-Padānukrama-Kośa,* p.2828, suggests *vāstu* to be 'ashes, rubbish', etc., and

vāstavya to be 'one covered with ashes'. This may suit the later appearance of Rudra. Ram Gopal rightly rejects this suggestion; *ibid.,* p.38f.

4. Cf. the rite at the 'Tryambaka-*havis*' at the Sākamedha, where Rudra is requested to go beyond the Mūjavat mountain, *Śat.Br.* II.6.2.17.
5. *Śat.Br.* VI.1.3.9ff. Here the boy Kumāra, said to be an aspect of Agni is said to have various forms - Śarva, Paśupati, Ugra, Bhava, Mahādeva and so on — which characterize Śiva-Rudra. On this see Sadashiv A. Dange, 'Kumāra, Kārttikeya and the Peacock', *Journal of the Asiatic Society of Bombay,* Vol.74(for 1999) (New Series), 2000, pp.39-53.
6. *Nāṭyaśāstra,* 1.48 for the places of different deities and powers; *Matsya P.,* 235.39-46.
7. The sixth day was important. It indicated full birth or a change in the state of the foetus; cf. the birth of Kārttikeya, *Mb.,* Vana. 229.52. On the sixth day in the twelve- day sacrifice, the Śukra cup of Soma is taken up, with the identification of Śukra and the sun, both being the givers of life. Cf. also the belief in *ṣaṣṭha kāla* for meals, *Mb.*, Āśvamedhika, 57.18; also 90.26-27; cf. also other beliefs regarding the sixth day at Dange, *Ency. P.B.* & P., Navrang, New Delhi, Vol. V, 1990, pp.1543, 1549.
8. On a detailed discussion on this point and the meaning of the myth, see Dange, *Sexual Symbolism from the Vedic Ritual,* Ajanta Publications, Delhi, 1979, pp.141-160.
9. See Dange, *Ency. P.B. & P.,* Vol.V, p.1502f., where a figure is also given. See also, by the same author, "Vāstupuruṣa", in *Purāṇa-Itihāsa-Vimarśa* (Essays in Honour of Prof. S.G. Kantawala), Bharatiya Vidya Prakashan, Delhi, 1998, pp.46-51.
10. Here he comes into his place any time, goes out any time; but, he has to be attended to by the king and the queen. He yokes them to a chariot and asks them to pull it. Ultimately, he gives them boons, being pleased with their sincerity. See *Mb.,* Anuśāsana, Chs. 52-55. For the whole legendary account, see Sadashiv A. Dange, *Myths from the Mahābhārata*, Vol.2, Aryan Books International, New Delhi, 2001, Ch. "Tests", p.50f. The author has also studied here parallels from the *Mb.* and elsewhere.

11. See Dange, *Myths from the Mahābhārata*, Vol.2, Appendix A, "Durvāsas—A Pattern", pp.229-239
12. *Ait. Br.* VI.33 - 30.7.

* Included here from the *Oriental Journal,* Sri Venkateswara University, Vol.XLII, Pts.1 & 2, 1999.

Chapter 7

Ṛgveda and the Buffalo-Sacrifice?

The position of the buffalo (*mahiṣa*) in the Vedic ritual tradition is unique, in the sense that it has been recognised as the norm of strength; and, yet, it was never sacrificed to any deity. The word 'sacrificed' is to be particularly noted. An ordinary killing and eating are different from killing at a rite and partaking of the flesh of the sacrificed beast; such is not the case with the buffalo. From the point of power, important gods are compared with the buffalo. They include Agni, Soma, Indra and even Aśvins.[1] The goddess Vāc identified with the Uttaravedi is said to be both lioness and she-buffalo (*mahiṣī*). It is of some interest to note that, in Sanskrit literature — which reflects the practice current among the people — the human king is rarely denoted as *mahiṣa,* though his chief queen is termed *mahiṣī,* which has also been the Vedic practice. In a suggestive symbolism, the Uttaravedi (situated to the east) is addressed as lioness and *mahiṣī* (*Taitt. Sam.* 1.2.12.1; VI.2.7.15). In all such places the power-aspect of the *mahiṣa* is at work. As for the sacrifice of the buffalo, as is found in the case of the Devī in the post-Vedic period, the Vedic texts are silent; because, there was no such practice among the Vedic people. It is not to deny that the killing and cooking of the buffalo are not mentioned in the Vedic context.

Though it is never mentioned in the post-Ṛgvedic Vedic texts, the *Ṛgveda* alludes to this practice; but, it is only in the context of Indra's victory. Thus, after the battle with the roaring 'serpent', Vṛtra, a hundred buffaloes were cooked for Indra (*ṚV*. VI.17.11). He is also said to have eaten (or killed: *aghaḥ*)[2] a thousand (*sahasram)* buffaloes (VIII.12.8). Viṣṇu is said to have brought to Indra a hundred buffaloes and milk-cooked rice (*kṣīrapākam odanam)*, when the latter seized Emuṣa, who was his enemy. These references could hardly be taken to mean, that Indra alone devoured the multitude of buffaloes. These have to be taken as indicating a general feast after war, or a great battle; and, in this all his helpmates (read, soldiers) participated. Also, *śatam* and *sahasram* could not be taken to indicate the exact number of buffaloes killed for the feast; the words are indicative of just a 'large number'. When it comes to Indra, himself, offering a buffalo (*mahiṣam mṛgam*) and cooking it, it is only for his 'mother' and 'father' (VIII.69.15), whosoever they may be. Indra's father and mother are not clearly defined and identified. The father cannot be Tvaṣṭṛ, as is generally believed; because, he is the 'general' father of all the gods. He is, rather, Indra's mythological 'father'; but, actually, socio-historically, he is the senior adversary who has to be defeated for Indra's deification. The point is, Indra was never a god, in the real sense of the word.[3] He was god, as Rāma was (and has been, since) a god, and also as Kṛṣṇa was such. Or, as was the ancient Egyptian king Zaru, or as Alexander, the Great, would have been a god - but could never achieve godhood.[4] There is no other reference to the killing of a single buffalo. And, it is doubtful if the *mahiṣa* in this context (*mahiṣam mṛgam)* is the buffalo. It is more likely, that the main beast is indicated by the term *mṛga* while *mahiṣa* is the epithet suggestive of greatness, the whole image reverting to the power aspect. Moreover, the context shows that the whole image is of the dark waterful cloud seen as the big beast; because, in the same breath, Indra is said to have 'broken' open the moist nourishment (*odanam),* which is a typical rain-symbol in the Ṛgvedic imagery (cf. X.123.4). It is, thus, clear, that there is no reference to the killing of a single buffalo in the *Ṛgveda* - far less as a ritual act. The many buffaloes that are referred to be killed and cooked are not for a god at a regular ritual; they are in connection with the war-feast. They certainly indicate the eating of the flesh of the buffalo by the unpriestly class. But, they cannot be mistaken as at a sacred ritual. In other words, this act was never a sacrament; hence, there was no sacrificial killing of the buffalo. As such, even in the later Vedic-ritual texts the sacrifice of a buffalo is never mentioned.

The necessity of the observation, that the Vedic literature does not have, nor does it attest, the sacrifice of the buffalo, is in view of the opinion of Asko Parpola[5] that the Mahiṣāsura-mardinī myth, and the later tradition of the buffalo being sacrificed to her, is initiated in the Vedic tradition under the influence of the Vrātyas whose rituals the Vedic people incorporated. This is no place to go into all the arguments and suggestion of Parpola. (The present author has done so and has examined them elsewhere.[6]) However, it will be proper to touch the most important of the arguments which concerns the present purpose. Referring to the ritual at the Rājasūya sacrifice wherein: (i) a tiger-skin is laid on the ground; upon it a piece of lead is placed; (ii) this piece is said to be the 'head of Namuci'; and (iii) Indra kicks away the piece and, according to myth related in this context, a demon springs forth. Parpola sees here the rudiment of the detail in the later Mahiṣāsura-mardinī myth, where from the body of the buffalo, killed by the Devī, the demon Mahiṣa comes out. Parpola thinks that here there is just an inversion of the later myth ('inversion' is not the word used by Parpola; it is a rather technical term from the context of the study of myths). He feels that the king, who is a human aspect of Indra, acts as the Devī. Thus, according to him, the equation is:

Indra (= king) is the Vedic aspect of the later Devī; and Namuci, the demon, is the suggested Mahiṣa (buffalo).

There is no necessity to meet this argument. It is sufficient to say that, in myths, similar motifs do not attest sameness of the ultimate meaning; and far less the sameness of characters. The point is, that we just do not have the mention of the buffalo and its sacrifice - or, the buffalo-demon and his killing by Indra. We have already noted how the cooking of buffaloes does not prove ritual killing, or offering at a rite. Parpola cites another ritual and a myth associated with it from the *Vadhūla-Śrautasūtra*.[7] According to it, Prajāpati runs after Vāc, who wants to escape from his lustful clutches. They take various forms. Finally, Prajāpati sees that Vāc entered the mouth of the Puruṣa. Vāc sees him approaching; so, she makes the teeth of the Puruṣa her protective walls (*puraḥ*); and watches Prajāpati's move. Now, Prajāpati takes the form of the rice-porridge (*odana*). To attract Vāc he decorates himself (covers himself) in that form with melted butter (ghee). Vāc cannot control herself and swallows the ghee-smeared porridge, which is nothing but Prajāpati. In this state of Vāc, behind the *puraḥ,* Parpola sees Durgā (the deity of the mountains). And, in this ritual and in the myth, he sees the following equations:

Prajāpati = porridge; Vāc = tongue= Durgā.
Prajāpati swallowed = Mahiṣa sacrificed.

So, he suggests that Prajāpati is the earlier one whose later version is Mahiṣa; because, both are sacrificed to, and eaten by, the female deity. Here again, the difficulty about this argument is that it sees the form but not the pattern - of both the ritual and the myth. Here, and in another example (which Parpola has not taken) where a male victim is sacrificed to Sarasvatī, in her aspect of Vāc who is said to have sustained Prajāpati, one might as well say that there is a base for believing the male victim to be Mahiṣa (though here it is a goat) and Sarasvatī the Devī (*Śat.Br.* III.9.1.7). But, the pattern of the Devī myth and ritual shows that, in it the buffalo (= demon) and the Devī are not only juxtaposed in a sexual tie as a suitor (soliciting lover) and the desired female; the buffalo is on a lower level than the Devī. In the Prajāpati–Vāc relationship both are on the same divine level. Moreover, the Prajāpati-Vāc myth is only a version of the Prajāpati-Daughter myth; and the demon Mahiṣa is never said to be the father of the Devī. Further, the sacrifice in the Vedic context is never associated with the offering of the head, or blood, which are prominent features in the ritual of the Devī and the buffalo. Yet further, the motif of 'swallowing' does not indicate 'murder' as the meaning, as Parpola proposes.[8] It suggests oneness, as is clear from a number of such cases. This will show that the sacrifice of a buffalo is never indicated in the Vedic texts. Buffalo-sacrifice was a unique rite among the non-Vedic people who, later fused with the Vedic; and there is no ground to believe (as Parpola proposes variously), that it was present among the early Vedic people, but that every trace of it has been wiped out by the Brāhmaṇa texts because the buffalo was associated with the enemies of the Vedic people, and that these later texts show a deliberate discrimination, of the later conservative priests, against the buffalo.

NOTES AND REFERENCES

1. Indra I.121.2; II.22.1; III.46.2; IV.18.11; X.54.4, etc.; Agni I.95.9; I.141.3; X.8.1 etc; Soma IX.82.3; IX.86.40; IX.95.4; IX.113.3, etc. Aśvinau X.106.2; for *mahiṣa-mṛga* as a cloud see also X.123.4.
2. Sāyaṇa takes it, alternatively from √*ghas*, 'to eat'.
3. Cf. L.D. Barnett, *Hindu Gods and Heroes,* London, 1922, p.28.
4. See, for Zaru, Donald Mackenzie, *Egyptian Myth and Legend,* Gresham and Co., London. p.36; for Alexander, see Peter Green, *Alexander of Macedon*, University of

California Press, Los Angeles, Oxford, 1991, pp.164, 314.
5. Asko Parpola, "The Metamorphosis of Mahiṣa Asura and Prajāpati", in: *Ritual. State and History in South India* (Essays in honour of J.C. Heesterman), ed. A.W. van Den Hock and others, E.J. Brill, Leiden, 1992, pp. 276-295.
6. Sadashiv A. Dange, *Towards Understanding Hindu Myths,* Aryan Books International, New Delhi, 1996, pp.440-466.
7. Parpola. *op.cit.*, p. 287f.
8. Cf. Swallowing of Kaca by Śukrācārya; of Śukra by Śiva; sometimes, swallowing gives place to keeping the male in the vagina by a female power, say of Śukrācārya by the Kṛtyā; for these see Sadashiv A. Dange, *Legends in the Mahābhārata*, Motilal Banarsidass, Delhi, 1969, pp. 171ff-esp. 183ff; or his, *Myths from the Mahābhārata,* Vol.1, Aryan Books International, New Delhi, 1997, p.160ff.

* Included here from the *Oriental Journal,* Sri. Venkateswara University, Vol. XXXIX, Pts.1 & 2, 1996.

Chapter 8

Therianthropomorphism and the Multiple-Head Motifs in Ancient India and the Middle East

Cultural contact between ancient India and the Middle East has been an established fact, the reason being either trade-routes or early conquests, which facilitate migration of concepts and myths. Like the similarity in the case of myths from distant lands,[1] similarity of art-motifs may be ascribed to either independent origin or borrowing; and, it is difficult in many cases to fix the exact direction of dispersion. Especially, in the case of the topic in hand, this becomes further difficult, because, the idea of the theriomorph of a deity need not be a case of borrowing. In the same way, the one head developing into multiplicity could, very well, be a natural process, the reason being a fusion of various god-heads or concepts into one. On the Indian side the earliest literary records, in this context, go back to the *ṚV*, the period of this text being yet in dispute. The Western-oriented scholars take the period to be about 1500 B.C., which, however, is unacceptable. In the state of our present knowledge, sculptures relating to the Vedic data are hardly available beyond about the second century B.C. There has been dispute regarding the identity of the Ṛgvedic data and the finds from the Indus civilization. (The present writer has expressed his opinion that the two do not tally in most of the cases).[2] This being the case, it would be better to survey the two motifs, noted above, through the span mentioned in the title; the question of borrowing may be kept at rest, comparison being given ascendance.

The *ṚV* describes the Year (Saṁvatsara) as a bull having three heads, or faces (*ṚV* III.56.3 *vṛṣabhaḥ... tryanīkaḥ*). The fire-god is seen as being 'four-faced' (*ṚV* V.48.5 *catur-anīkaḥ)*; also, 'having four eyes' (*ibid.* I.31.13 *catur-akṣaḥ),* indicating that he has two heads. Obviously, the four faces in the case of Agni are in view of the flames of the fire being open to the four quarters. This idea gets developed, in the Puranic context, in the four faces of the god Brahmā; but, with a regular explanatory myth. According to the myth (which has its origin in the Vedic period), Brahmā sexually desired his own daughter, when she circumambulated him. To be able to fix his eyes on her, as she went round and in the four directions, he developed one head each in every quarter.[3] Traditionally, the three heads of the Year (Saṁvatsara) have been explained as the three seasons,[4] though it is not clear whether he is contemplated as a pure theriomorphic deity or a pure anthropomorphic one, or a therianthropomorphic complex deity. The case of the fire-god should not pose a problem. Yet, in the description at the places noted above, there is no clear indication of his being an anthropomorph or a theriomorph, though in *ṚV* the deities are compared or identified with such beasts as the Bull or the Horse. Some men and gods are said to have 'seven mouths' (Brahmaṇaspati, *ṚV* IV.50.4; Aṅgirases, the seers, IV.51.41). Even the cloud is seen as (a demon) having seven faces (*ibid.*, X.40.8). The first son of Tvaṣṭṛ (the older god, often believed to be father of the gods), and the elder brother of Vṛtra, is described as 'three-headed', or is named so (Triśīrsan). The *ṚV* does not mention whether the heads were theriomorphic or anthropomorphic. In the later texts he has normal (human) heads; but, from each of his heads cut by Indra various birds are said to have been created.[5] Indra is said to have impelled Trita Āptya to smite the 'three-headed' demon who wielded seven ropes, or fetters, to bind and subdue his opponents (*Ṛ̣V* X. 99.8 for Triśīrṣan; and *ibid.* 8.8 the latter). A Gandharva (semi-divine human being) is said to be of the name Triśīrṣan (*Jai. Br.* I.125). It is clear, that he did not actually have three heads. However, the very name would reflect the belief in such a being - divine or demoniac - being current at the period; and this falls in line with the Ṛgvedic belief in a demon (*asura*) having three heads. The *Avesta* also speaks of a three-headed demon, Azi Dahāka, the three-mouthed serpent (*ahi* in Sanskrit), who was killed by Thraetaona. He is described as having three jaws and three heads, and having six eyes (Yasna, IX 7-8). Here Thraetaona (=Vedic Trita) is said to be the son, or scion of Athwya in the Avesta,[6] while Trita, in the *Ṛgveda*, is himself Āptya (= Avestan Athwya); and Āptya is associated with water not only by Sāyaṇa (the commentator of the *Ṛgveda*), but also by modern scholars. However, this association should not be taken to make Āptya as identical with the god Apām Napāt. The picture of Azi Dahāka (i.e., *ahi daśaka,* 'the biting serpent') that we get from the *Avesta* is of a serpent who dwells in deep waters. The 'Three-headed demon', from the *Ṛgveda,* having six eyes, is not specifically said to be a serpent; but, he has all other traits exactly as the Azi Dahāka, which would show him as serpent. The fact that he is the elder brother of Vṛtra, the serpent of the Vedic context, would support this image of the Ṛgvedic 'Three-headed' son of Tvaṣṭṛ. In the Avestan context, later in *Shahnamah, Azi* Dahāka came to be identified with the Chaldaean enemies of the then Aryan Iran.[7] All the same, his original image of a serpent demon in the deep waters does not get diluted. Azi Dahāka is said to have offered sacrifice to the goddess of water, Ardwisūra Anāhita, in the land of Bawri, which is the early name of Babylon. According to Darmesteter the origin of the Azi myths was in the southern coast of the Caspian Sea.[8] In any case, there can hardly be any doubt that the Avestan Azi myth centred round the serpent of the deep subdued by a hero. Even in the case of the anthropomorphism of Azi in the later *Shahnamah,* his association with the serpent form is clear. There he is depicted as a man from whose shoulders, on either side, a serpent is seen as springing.[9] This image would be therianthropomorphic, like the Nāgas of the Indian context. The latter, however, do not appear much before (the B.C. era) coming in connection with Mahāvīra or the Buddha. Comparing Indra and Trita in the myth of the killing of the 'Three-headed' demon, the position of Trita appears to be more popular as it obtains both in the *Ṛgveda* and the *Avesta.* In all probability, the Trita (Thraetaona)-serpent myth is older than the Indra-'Three-headed'/Vṛtra myth; and it is certainly different from the concept and myths of Apām Napāt ('Foetus-of-Waters') who has rarely any association with the serpent in the *Ṛgveda* and the *Avesta.*

Now, while on the Indian side there is no therianthropomorphic imagery clearly associated with the serpent in the Vedic period, and even later up to the early Jaina-Buddhistic context, there is clear mention of Azi Dahāka as a therianthropomorphic being (Man-serpent) in the Middle-Eastern theatre. Though the period of Z(Jh)arathuṣṭa (Jarad-uṣṭra) is taken to be 1500 B.C.,[10] there can be no doubt about the motif of the 'Three-headed' serpent (Azi Dahāka) being far older. Therianthropomorphism can be seen even in the case of the Tiamat-Marduk myth from the Assyrian-Babylonian context. The Babylonian influence on the Avestan image of Azi Dahāka can be seen from the mention of Bawri (noted above) in the *Avesta.* In Sumerian imagery the mixture of various animals is quite frequent, and it is not restricted to the serpent motif. Thus, Nintu, an aspect of the Mother-goddess Ma, was half-serpent and half-woman; but, in addition, she had a horn on her head. She also held a babe sucking her breast.[11] The one horn may be symbolic of fertility from the pre-agricultural stage, and indicative of the hoe that was used for ploughing. This therianthropomorphic goddess was a human, serpent and also a horned beast in one, the symbolic implication apart. The Sumerian king, Ea-bani, was deified as a human goat. His legs and hooves were those of a goat.[12] Lilith, the Sumerian goddess, was depicted as a woman (nude) with a hood on her head from which two wings came down covering her back and going below her waist. At her feet, on either side, there was an owl. Her feet were those of a bird, suiting the winged hood. In between each owl and her foot, on either side, there was some wild beast, its ears erect. These depictions go back to about 2000 B.C.[13]

The point is, whence is the therianthropomorphic motif? For this, we have to turn to the ancient Egyptian records. The chief god of the Egyptian pre-dynastic period was Ptah; and the region of lower Egypt where he was worshipped came to be called 'Hiku-Ptah' or 'Het-ka-Ptah' (= 'House of Ptah'), which came to be pronounced as Egypt (Hiku-ptah > Ikupta > Egupta > Egypt), by the Greeks. He was a dwarf; but got fused with another equally ancient god, Sokar (or Seker), who was conceived as a hawk-man. In the dynastic period, especially by about the fourth dynasty (3000-2500 B.C.), just prior to the period of Chepos (Khufu), Sokar came to be the underwater god having three human heads, a serpent-body and having two mighty wings.[14] The combination of the serpent and the bird, or the fight between these creatures is almost a universal motif; but, it is more prominent in ancient Egyptian records. This is also the earliest of such records, as far as our knowledge stands at the present stage. The Vedic records do not strongly vouch a combination of a beast and a human. The position there, is of total identification with a beast or the birds like the hawk in certain descriptions. The pattern is more metaphoric, and, at the best, verging on theriomorphism rather than therianthropomorphism. This is not to say that this trend is never seen on the Indian scene. As a matter of fact, from the early centuries of the Christian era glimpses of this trend appear, and later myths show it prominently, as we shall see later. In ancient Egypt we meet a large number of gods and goddesses who are half-human, half-theriomorphic. The jackal-headed god Anubis (termed 'Finder or Opener of the Ways'), the cow-faced Hathor who is seen as frog-faced in her cruel form, Heket, and the cow-faced Isis are only some of the examples. To these may be added Bast, who was cat-headed and was regarded as a therianthropomorphic aspect of Isis.[15] According to an ancient myth, Horus (the son of Isis and Osiris) cut off the head of Isis and substituted it with the head of a cow.[16] This is corroborated by her figure having the horns of a cow between which is shown the solar disk.[17] This myth corresponds to the Hindu myth of the head of an elephant on the human body of the god Gaṇeśa, or that of Viṣṇu Hayagrīva ('Horse-headed'), in the post-Vedic period. From the Vedic period we have the myth of the head of a horse on the body of the sage Dadhīc, which is, by far, the only example of this type indicative of therianthropomorphism[18]. The tenth dynasty Egypt shows a variety of such therianthropomorphic motifs, in the case of the chief god Her-Shef who was believed to be an aspect of the solar god Re (Ra). In one depiction he is seen as having four heads; one is that of a ram, the other that of a bull, while two heads are of hawks. Thus, he had a double-hawk head and two of beasts. The older motif of the serpent, or the serpent and a hawk, is changed at this period. In another depiction this god has a ram's head and wears a white crown of plumes.[19] In both the depictions, the body is that of a man. The second depiction is worthy of note, as it presents further details. His plume-crown is surrounded by two disks representing the sun and the moon. By the side are two serpents - one on either side - with disks on their heads. In the twelfth dynasty, the new god Amon Ra came to be represented as a frog-headed man, serpent-headed man, ram-headed man and also a purely human figure.[20] The period of the twelfth and the tenth dynasties comes roughly to the twentieth to eighteenth century B.C. In the earliest phase in the Egyptian religious belief the serpent plays an important part, which is marked with other religions also. We have already seen how Sokar was a combination of the human, serpent and the hawk. However, the serpent is more prominent as 'Son of the Earth' in his name of Sito having two necks and heads, or "Creator of the Earth" in his name of Iru. He is also the "Provider of attributes",[21] like the Vedic Prajāpati; however, the latter is not seen as the serpent. The counterpart of the Egyptian Sito or Iru is the Vedic Ahirbudhnya ('Serpent of the Bottom') or the Śeṣa of the later Hinduism. The latter is said to be endowed with a thousand hoods, as he serves as the bed for Viṣṇu (*Mb.* Vana 272.38), who is the Puruṣa with equal number of heads. But this has to be taken as just extravagant description, without any indication of a definite number of hoods, like the 'thousand faces' of Puruṣa (*RV* X.90.1). Ahirbudhnya has no multiple faces, nor is he said to be a serpent in *Mb.* and later. The Egyptian primeval serpent is the creator of multiplicity in its form of Sito, the 'provider of attributes'. In one depiction this "great surviving serpent, when all mankind has reverted to slime".[22] is double-necked. According to the ancient Egyptian belief the serpent was the symbol of the cosmic ocean, and the world was enveloped by him, as he lay with his tail in his mouth. In the innermost shrine of Tutankhamen there is a strange mummy-like bearded figure. It is in the erect position, and has no hands (probably, they are covered due to its being a mummy). It is encircled by a serpent each at the head and the feet. These serpents have their tails in their mouths, while the feet of the figure are not separated, but form one whole appearing like a robust curved tail.[23] These two separate serpents, encircling one human bearded figure are a variant of the double-necked serpent noted above. In any case, it appears that the two heads, or the two separate serpents with their tails in the mouth, symbolize the beginning and end of the existence being controlled by the primeval serpent in his two aspects. Though not expressed in so many words, one suspects that there is a seed here of the motif of double/multiple heads. We do not have here a clear image of therianthropomorphism. In the double-necked serpent anthropomorph is absent; but, the other figure is suggestive of therianthropomorphism. The human figure does not have the serpents right from the shoulders; but, they are closely associated with it. A subtle instance of therianthropomorphism is seen in the 'Eye of Atum.' The Eye was worshipped in ancient Egypt as the 'most ancient female'. According to a myth Atum was alone in the primeval waters of the abyss. He created his children Shu and Thefnut; but, they got lost to him in the dark waters. So he sent his eye (presumably, he had only one eye) to search them out. When the eye came back with the children, it saw another in its place and got furious. He became a rearing cobra with swollen neck. Atum pacified the eye-cobra by tying it around his head, with its mouth to the front on the forehead, to guard his crown. This explains the custom of the crown of the Pharaohs. As the eye went on flying through the primeval dark waters, it developed wings. So it developed a double morph, serpent and the bird. This way, the eye with its lashes developed into a hairy serpent; and also into a winged creature, the hawk. This is the source of the 'uraeus' on the crown of the Pharaohs. It is the combination of the human eye (of Atum conceived as a divine human) and the serpent.[24]

We leave away such instances of theriomorphs that were believed to be representatives, or symbols, of gods without a mixture of an anthropomorph. Osiris, for example, was represented variously as a gazelle, pig, a boar, and so on; or the crocodile which came to be regarded as the god Sebek. But the Bull form of Osiris, as the Apis, has to be particularly noticed. Though he had no anthropomorphic traits, he was a combination of creatures that had a long history of sacred adoration in the ancient

Egyptian belief. He was to be carefully selected and kept in the temple at Memphis. He had to be black in colour, with a triangular white mark on the forehead (probably representative of the moon, as Osiris himself was). On his back there had to be the sign of an eagle; and under his tongue there was to be a lump resembling the beetle, called Khoprer (or Khopri, as the creature was called in later dynastical period). Khopri, the beetle, was depicted in pictures from the pyramids as pushing up the sun for rise[25] from the underworld waters through which he had to travel in the night after sunset. Independently, Khopri symbolized Atum (the Creator god), as he (in the beetle-form) was seated on the mound of soft earth that he brought up. The mound of earth visible after the flood in the Nile receded was considered to be an aspect of Atum. One more peculiarity about the Apis Bull is that he had to be the only issue of his mother-cow.[26] It is not improbable that Osiris was worshipped as a Bull-headed human-bodied god in the origin. In that case, he would be therianthropomorphic. In the Apis Bull we have another phase of theriomorphism. It is not therianthropomorphism; but multiple theriomorphism. Like the Khopri, the eagle-hawk has a long tradition. As we have noted earlier, Sokar had the wings of the hawk (together with his serpent body and human faces) in the very early layer of Egyptian belief. The solar hawk that was brought by the Horus worshippers from the east got fused with the Sokar-hawk. The Sokar-hawk had already fused with the cult of Osiris, the moon-god; and, with the advent of the solar Horus-hawk, and its fusion with the Osiris cult, the latter became the father of Horus. The Apis Bull showed this merger with the eagle on its back; with the Khoprer Atum under his tongue, there was the representation of a further merger. Already in the earliest period, that of the god Ptah, gradually a merger came about among three gods: Ptah, Tanen and Osiris. Ptah was a dwarf, as already noted; he was an autochthon for that matter. Tanen was also an earth-god; and Sokar, with his serpent body was an autochthon; but, he had the mixture of the Solar/sky-god as indicated by his hawk-wings. What exactly was the nature of the three human heads is unclear. But they appear to indicate merger of three different gods, or powers.

The influence of the mixed motif of serpent, hawk and the human appears also in some of the Greek gods, though it is difficult to say if it is from Egypt or Assyrian-Babylonian context. For example, in the cave of Phigalia, the ancient figure of the Black Demeter was made of wood, seated on a rock. She had the face of a mare. Above it there were figures of snakes and other monstrous beasts. She had a dolphin in one hand and in the other she held a dove. At another place she is shown as goat-faced and having wings. Her body is short and columnar and she wears a spreading skirt. At yet another place she is shown as an eagle-lady, with prominent breasts.[27] This is her therianthropomorph, and it may be compared with that of the Sumerian Lilith, noted earlier, with the difference that in the case of Lilith the face is of a woman and she wears a feathered hood. In the case of the Minos-bull, the Minotaur, the head is of a bull while the body is of an anthropomorphic monstrous creature. According to a myth he was born from a bull; but his mother was a human, the wife of King Minos. In the case of the Sphinx guarding the entrance to Thebes we have a multimorph. This creature has the face of a woman, the body of a lioness and has wings.[28] The Minotaur falls in the pattern of Egyptian gods, where the face is of a beast and the rest of the body is human. The Greek Sphinx does not fit in the Egyptian pattern, generally, where the head of the Sphinx is of a man. The Great Sphinx, representing the head of a man upon the body of a lion is an example. In the case of Thefnut, the wife (and sister) of Shu, the head is of a lioness and the body of a woman. Moreover, the Sphinx near the pyramid of Gizeh shows the mutilated face of a lion; it does not appear to be that of a human. In the case of the Theban Sphinx, from Greece, unlike the Great Sphinx from Egypt, the head is of a woman (not of a man as in the Egyptian pattern). Also Thefnut is a lioness in her face, and not in her body as is the case with the Greek Theban Sphinx. Even so, the motif in the Greek Sphinx should be taken as showing the influence of the Egyptian Sphinx, not without, however, that from the Babylonian lion-headed eagle form of Ningirsu. The wings of the Greek Sphinx betray the latter influence. A non-bird showing wings appears to be peculiar to the Middle East. Apart from Sokar, hardly any other Egyptian god appears as a beast with wings. On the other hand Babylonia and Assyria show it frequently. Here Shedu was the destructive bull. He would kill anybody wantonly; but, he was the protector of the temples. Another bull, but having wings, was Lamassu. He had a human head and was believed to be protector of palaces.[29] The winged bull, with a human face appears also among the Persians and is seen placed at the entrance of their fire-temples in India. This has to be taken as due to the influence of the Lamassu, through ancient Persian practices. As such, the source has to be taken as the Middle-East. The influence of Assyria on ancient Persian architecture is seen even in the vast colonnades in front of the palaces, and also inside.[30] The winged horse of the Greek mythology, Pegasus, appears to have been suggested from the winged bull of the Middle East. It may be noted that the Zeus Bull, who carries Europa on his back, is not winged. And there is no winged bull in the Egyptian mythology. The winged sandals of Hermes, together with his low-crowned hat and his winged magic wand (Greek)[31] fall in a different category. Here we have faint anthropomorphic traits, as contrasted to the Assyrian instance of the bull mentioned above; for, in Lamassu there is mixed theriomorphism. The case of Icarus is different; as his wings are not natural; they were attached to him with glue, and were artificial[32]. In the ancient Persian context, and in Zoroastrianism, therianthropomorphism is seen in the figure of the

Fravashi (sixth century B.C.) and the bearded winged figure (which is common with the bearded man-faced bulls at the entrance of the temples). Then we have the Griffins, that are winged lions with horns (fifth century B.C.). We also have the Ibex, which is a winged goat with long curved horns.[33]

If we compare the various forms of the gods mentioned above, together with the multimorphic beasts, with the data from the Vedic context, we see that in the latter the motif is not a very marked one. As we have noted above, we do have identification of gods with beasts; but, we have no sound ground to accept that gods were believed to be beasts or that a particular beast was taken to be a particular god. To believe that the various vehicles of gods were their theriomorphs is a blunt argument as there is no corroboration for it either through depiction or description. Even looking to the various victims the riddle does not get any solution; because a particular beast is not wholly reserved for a particular god. Even when it is said, for example, that a dwarf victim (goat) is to be offered to Viṣṇu (who was considered as a dwarf in the post-Ṛgvedic texts;[34] he was not so considered in *ṚV),* a dwarf beast was never treated as Viṣṇu. A horse was said to be the beast for Varuṇa; also for Prajāpati; and it also symbolized the sun, and also Prajāpati (in the context of the laying down of the sacrificial fire).[35] It may be argued that the Vedic people were not worshippers of idols, and it is difficult to find traces of pictures or depictions as are available in ancient Egypt and Babylonia and Assyria. Even granting this, we expect literary descriptions, transmitted through the oral tradition, in the *Ṛgveda* and the later Vedic texts, of concrete god-heads to match the theriomorphic or therianthropomorphic representations from the Middle East and Egypt. We have referred to the case of the 'Three-headed' demon, as a solitary case, coming in a later book (I *maṇḍala*) of *ṚV;* and we have compared it with the three-headed demon from the *Avesta* and from the earlier context of Egypt.

The *Ṛgveda* mentions Agni (the fire-god) and the sun as having seven heads (*ṚV* III.5.5 and VIII.51.4 respectively). It also speaks of the faculty of reasoning (*dhīḥ*) as having seven heads (X.67.1). Bṛhaspati is described, once, as having seven heads (or, properly, mouths), due to his manifold births by virtue of his roar (*ibid.* IV.50.4). This is due to his being the deity of hymns and songs (*sāman-s*). The same is the case with the band of divine seers, the Aṅgirases, who are believed to be having seven mouths as they have mastered the art of singing in the seven metres (*ibid.* IV.51.4). In all these cases the heads (or mouths) are metaphorical. Agni has three heads as he is seen in the form of the sun in the sky, in the form of the lightning in the cloud in the mid-region, and as the sacrificial fire on the earthly plane. This is the position in the *Ṛgveda;* and, to extend the image in the context of the later ritual, the three heads of the fire-god are: the Gārhapatya (house-hold) fire, the Dakṣiṇa (southern) fire, and the Āhavanīya fire (in which the oblations are offered with the invocations to various gods). Whether these faint presentations of the motif of multiple-heads would have influenced the pictures and images of gods having more than one head in the later Hindu tradition, as we shall see, is doubtful. The seven heads of the sun are sometimes seen as his rays, which epithet is transferred to the god Bṛhaspati (*ṚV* IV. 50.4). Even if it is granted that these instances of the motif of 'multiple-heads' might have suggested the later Hindu depiction of more heads than one in a figure, it is almost certain that the source of the therianthropomorphic figures and idols is not in the Veda. Of the mixed theriomorphic motif, the only clear example is of the horse, rising from the ocean, having the wings of a hawk and the forearms (or, fore-feet) of a deer (*ṚV* I. 163.1).

Some of the most prominent sculptural depictions on the Indian side involving the therianthropomorphic motif are: the Varāha, Hayagrīva and Nṛsiṁha from the Hindu context. All these are the forms of Viṣṇu; and in all these the face is of the beast while the lower body is of a man. These therianthropomorphic depictions are supported by literary evidence from the Purāṇa texts where some others are mentioned, though they are not associated with the cult of Viṣṇu. The fire-god is represented by a goat, or has the head of a goat and the body of a man.[36] Gaṇeśa has the head of an elephant. He is one of the *gaṇa-s* of Śiva; but there are other *gaṇa-s* having various heads with human body covered with hair. Some of the heads are those of the lion, elephant, horse, pig, goat, donkey and even of a fish.[37] Nandī, the vehicle of Śiva is generally conceived as a *gaṇa* having the head of a bull, or a bull-vehicle of Śiva. An interesting variant is that he had the head of a monkey.[38] One of the best known therianthropomorphic examples is of the head of Dakṣa Prajāpati. His human head was cut and substituted by that of a goat.[39] Apart from these examples, there are others of local female deities, such as Mṛgīmukhī ('Deer-faced'), Barkarī (who had the head of a she-goat) and Ajeśvarī or Ajāpāleśvarī (indicating that the face was that of a she-goat).[40] And to these we may add the elephant-headed and the mare-headed Lakṣmī, and also Sarasvatī who is said to have assumed the form of Gaurī and was seen in the form of a mare.[41] The motif of the beast-head is not restricted to certain gods and their attendants. Even Fever is described as such. Fever was conceived as having three eyes in (each of) his three heads, and had three legs. He was not a demon, but a deity of fevers, with sacred ashes applied to his forehead. He was sought to be pacified with a regular *mantra* in the holy Gāyatrī metre.[42] Except for his beast-heads, he was an anthropomorphic god, and a fine example of therianthropomorphism together with the motif of multiple heads. In the case of Brahmā, in addition to the four heads (mentioned above), he is said to have also the fifth head; it was that of an ass according to one account, in view of the fact that with it he told a lie. It is also said to be of a horse; because, for his daughter, he had lust. It was, hence, cut by Śiva with his nail as a punishment (or chastisement!). According to another account it was that of a tiger.[43] In both the accounts this fifth head was cut, maintaining the original four heads, which were human. The fifth head made Brahmā an example of therianthropomorphism. Examples could be added.

We may take note of the Vaikuṇṭha and the Viśvarūpa motifs. In both cases Viṣṇu is the main deity. In the first case the heads are: (1) Saumya (i.e. normal and placid or complacent); this is the main face, and it is to the east (i.e. east-facing); (2) Nārasiṁha (i.e. of the Man-lion); this is to the south; (3) Kāpila (i.e. of Kapila; it is said to be *raudra,* 'fierce'; demoniac); it is to the west: and (4) Vārāha (i.e. of the boar); it is to the north.[44] In the Pāñcarātra system these heads were adjusted as those of Vāsudeva (Kṛṣna = Viṣṇu originally, as indicated by the heads of the boar and Man-lion), which is the main head, the others being of Saṁkarṣaṇa, Pradyumna and Aniruddha. On the very face of it, it is clear that the original idea was of the *avatāra-s* of Viṣṇu. But, even earlier the heads appear to have been simply of a man and three beasts. This doubt is supported by the fact that the head said to be Nārasiṁha ('of the Man-lion') could not be really of a man with the head of a lion; because, only the head is shown and not the lower portion. Thus, it was just the head of a lion. This suggestion gets support from the same text (*Viṣṇudharmottara-purāṇa*) which, in the same chapter, later, says that it should be 'of the appearance of a lion' (*siṁha-vaktrābham),* calling it *jñāna-vaktra,* the quarter of the head being the same (south). In this place, *raudra* appears; not *kāpila,* as is the case at the first place (*ibid.,* III. 44.11 and III.44.44^{cd}-45). Generally there is the direction of the idol being prepared as showing four faces; but, the details differ in other texts. At the latter place the *Viṣṇudharmottara-purāṇa,* as noted, has the faces: (1) East-*Saumya,* the chief one; (2) South - Lionlike, which is *Jñāna-vaktra;* (3) West - *Raudra,* which is said to be indicative of overlordship (*aiśvaryam*).[45] In a sculpture at Kharar, near Chandigarh, a figure of this type shows three faces, the face at the back being unseen or not shown. The central face is of a man; and it is flanked by the face of a lion and that of a boar.[46] It is not necessary to go into other details for our purpose here. In the Viśvarūpa sculptures there are five visible heads, with a circular arrangement of nine human heads. In the five visible heads the central is that of man; it is flanked by the heads of Varāha (boar), Narasiṁha (actually, lion), Matsya (fish) and Kūrma (tortoise).[47] Without doubt, this is the *avatāra*-motif. But, the principle of therianthropomorphism is clear. The point is, where do we get the earliest mention and representation of this motif?

The idols of the Vaikuṇṭha and the Viśvarūpa types appear more frequently from the ninth century A.D. and such types can hardly go before the fifth century A.D. In one representation of the Vaikuṇṭha image, at Khajuraho, there is the head of a horse in place of the expected *Kāpila*.[48] Whatever might have been the reason for the interchange of the horse-head for the *Kāpila,* and in spite of the confusion between the Hayagrīva Viṣṇu and the demon named-Hayagrīva, one thing is sure. During the seventh and the ninth centuries A.D., the horse-head was gaining prominence. This is supported from the mention of the mare-faced goddess, said to be both Gaurī and Sarasvatī, at the Prabhāsa region. Likewise, there is a myth that once a *brāhmaṇa* girl slept on the bed of Viṣṇu, through childish curiosity and was cursed by Lakṣmī to be turned into a mare. When the *brāhmaṇa*, the girl's father, came to know of this curse, he counter-cursed Lakṣmī to have the head of an elephant (hence, she became *gaja-lakṣmī*)[49] The mare-faced goddess of this account is said to be stationed at the Hāṭaka region, which corresponds to the Prabhāsa (though Hāṭaka is variously identified). These accounts occur in the *Skanda-purāṇa*, which is dated from the seventh to the ninth centuries A.D. This will show that the underlying idea in the

Vaikuṇṭha images is dominantly of the aspects of Viṣṇu; and the adoption of it by the Pāñcarātra is a veneer. It is also clear that the multiple-heads motif here, together with that of theriomorphism or therianthropomorphism, does not go far back, as far as the present Indian sculptural evidence is concerned.

In the case of the Indus seals the case is a bit different. Though it is not quite certain if the seals were depictive of religious motifs or they were purely of commercial value, some of the figures are of interest for the point we are discussing. The most prominent is the so-called Śiva figure having three human heads with a headgear, which apparently is horned; and the horns appear to be those of a buffalo. This figure has been interpreted variously; but, there could be no difference of opinion about the point that it is the earliest of such figures in the ancient region. Other figures that show multiple beast-heads are such as a bull with two antelope-heads, elephant with bull's head and so on.[50] These may go back to 2000 B.C., but do not come near to the heads in the Vaikuṇṭha set.

In this context it will be pertinent to note the practice at the Vedic Agnicayana. The earliest clear mention of this practice occurs in the *Taittirīya Saṁhitā.* The idea behind the Agnicayana was the symbolic construction of the cosmos. In the lowest layer, out of five total layers, four heads were placed in the firepan. According to this text the following were the heads: That of a man, which was to be placed at the centre (it faced the east; however, it is not specifically so stated). To the east was placed the head of a horse; to the west was the head of a bull; also the head of a serpent was placed; but its direction is not mentioned. No head is specified for the north. Thus, in all there were four heads (*Taitt. Sam.,* V.2.9.2-4). Earlier (*ibid.* V.2.8.7) the sacrifice is said to be Viṣṇu. Though the heads were without their bodies, and dead, they were sought to be made endowed with life by pouring curds and honey over them, and stuffing them with seven chips of gold. In essence, they were the heads of Viṣṇu, the sacrifice, one anthropomorphic and the rest theriomorphic. Together they formed the therianthropomorphic multiheaded body of Viṣṇu. It is not clear why there was no head on the north. The period of the *Taitt. Sam.* has to be taken as about 2000 B.C. or even earlier. The *Śatapatha-Brāhmaṇa* prescribes five heads; but, the arrangement is different. The heads are to be in one line. The head of the man is to be at the centre. To its left side, to the north, the heads of the horse and the ram are to be placed; and to the right side of the man's head, i.e. to the south, there are to be the heads of the bull and the goat (*Śat. Br.* VI. 2.1.14). The practice must have been quite in vogue. Even to this day Agnicayana is performed[51] (though without the heads). At the early period, the Śrauta-texts continued the tradition. The memory must have continued, though the practice might have become less frequent. The myth of the *avatāra-s* of Viṣṇu, together with this practice might have served as the basis for the Pāñcarātra concept of Vaikuṇṭha and Viśvarūpa. Actually, the 'Viśvarūpa' of the *Bhagavadgītā* is far wider. It could not be taken to be the basis of the Pāñcarātra concept of Viśvarūpa,[52] which is narrow and limited to the beast-heads from the *avatāra*-s with a few more faces added. However, for the sculptural depiction of this motif one has to revert to the Middle East for comparison, though the contexts differ. It will also be good to note that the first ever concept of Viśvarūpa, when it occurs in *ṚV* for an anthropomorph, is for Indra and the son of Tvaṣṭṛ (*ṚV* III. 38.4; II, 41.3; II. 11.19). In later texts, it is only the son of Tvaṣṭṛ who is so, and has three heads as noted above.

If the four heads at the Agnicayana be taken as forming the basis of the Vaikuṇṭha and "Hayagrīva-in-the Vaikuṇṭha" motifs, it could be said that the motif of the multiple heads goes back to at least the period of the *Taittirīya Sam*, i.e. 2000 B.C. It will be of some interest to note that, by about the same period, the motif is seen in the throne of King Solomon. At its back was the figure of a bull; and on the two arms was the figure of a lion each.[53] The vision of Ezekiel showed that in the centre of a storm there were four living creatures in human form; but each had four faces and four wings. They had the hooves like those of a bull. In each, the four faces were: human in front; a lion's at the right, a bull's at the left and an eagle's at the back.[54] Ezekiel lived in the sixth century B.C. There is reason to believe that this composition of heads must have been suggested from actual experience in sculpture. Was the influence from the Indian region? Or, was the source of the motif in the Middle East? We may mention here an Orphic cosmogonic myth. According to it, at the beginning of creation, from the mass of earth and slime, first there arose a dragon with the face of a god. He had wings on either side; and to his main face (which was human), on one side there was the head of a bull; and, on the other side, there was the head of a lion.[55] The period of this myth is prior to the sixth century B.C., as both Pythagoras and Plato were influenced by the Orphic mystery.[56] It would not be wrong, from what has been said until now, that the source of the multiple-heads motif was somewhere in the region between Egypt (cf. the two-necked cobra) and the Middle East, whence it spread to Greece in the west and India in the east. This motif was an aspect of therianthropomorphism. It was used in Vedic ritual in the later Vedic period (i.e. after the Ṛgvedic and the Atharvavedic period). But in sculptures it was introduced in India not before about the fifth century A.D.

NOTES AND REFERENCES

1. For the borrowing and stratification of myths, see William Robertson, *History of America,* 1997; Hugh Miller, *Scenes and Legends,* London, 1835; Donald Mackenzie, *Myths of Pre-Columbian America,* Gresham Publishing Co., London (year not mentioned), pp.39-42; also Sadashiv A. Dange.

Towards Understanding Hindu Myths, Aryan Books International, New Delhi,1996, p.14f
2. "Indus Civilization and the Vedic Culture (Re-examination of the Problem)", *Journal of the Mythic Society,* Bangalore, Vol. LXXIV-1, Jan.-March, 1983, pp.49-82.
3. *Skanda P.*, 1.3.5. 49-62, also Dange, *Ency. P.B. & P.* Vol. I, Navrang, New Delhi, 1986, p.206 for similar accounts.
4. Commentary of Sāyaṇa, on *Ṛgveda* - IV.56.3.
5. *Taitt.Sam.*II. 5.1.1-2. He was also named Viśvarūpa; cf. also *Mb.* Śānti, 342. 32-34.
6. *athvyo... yo janat azim dahākăm thri-japhnăm thrikamărădhăm.*
7. James Darmesteter, *The Zend Avesta*, Pt.II, SBE Vol. 23, p.60 n.3. The period of the *Shahnamah* is eleventh century A.D. It is an Iranian text.
8. *Ibid.*
9. *Ibid.*, n.2.
10. Khojeste Mistree, *Zoroastrianism - An Ethnic Perspective,* Bombay, 1982, p.5.
11. Donald Mackenzie, *Myths of Babylonia and Assyria,* Gresham, London, p. 75.
12. *Ibid.*, p.135
13. The present writer is thankful to Dr. Mrs. Vidya Kamat for this information; see also Asis Sen, *Animal Motifs in Ancient Indian Art,* Firma K.L. Mukhopadhyay, Calcutta, pl.XXXVIII.
14. Donald Mackenzie, *Egyptian Myth and Legend,* Gresham, London, p.12.
15. *Ibid.*, p.73.
16. Donald Mackenzie, *Myths of Crete and Pre-Hellenic Europe,* Gresham, London, p.183.
17. H.A. Davis, *An Outline History of the World,* Oxford University Press, London, 1950 (1928), Fig. on p.35. Isis has the Horus babe supported on her left lap by her left hand; cf. Nintu above.
18. *ṚV* I. 84.13-14. For a full description, see Dange, *Towards Understanding Hindu Myths,* pp.242-252.
19. Donald Mackenzie, *Egyptian Myth and Legend,* p.190.
20. *Ibid.*, p.197.
21. R.T. Rundle Clark, *Myth and Symbol in Ancient Egypt,* Thames and Hudson, London, 1959, p.50.
22. *Ibid.*, p. 51, where the figure occurs.

23. *Ibid.,* p. 80.
24. *Ibid.,* p. 90.
25. In one depiction at Thebes (XVIII dynasty), this creature has wings. In a necklace from the tomb of Tutankhamen, the figures of Khopri are set in precious stones, the period being 1358-1349 B.C. This necklace is from Cairo Museum; and its picture is card-printed by Hermer Verlag (Hermer Publishing House), München, Germany.
26. Donald Mackenzie, *Egyptian Myth and Legend,* p.69.
27. Donald Mackenzie, *Myths of Crete and Pre-Hellenic Europe,* p.180.
28. Edith Hamilton, *Mythology,* Little Brown & Company, Boston, 1942, p.376; cf. the winged lion from Persia mentioned earlier.
29. Winged bulls, with the face of a bearded man, appear also at the entrance to the throne-room in the place of Sargaon II; cf. No.A 7369 at the Oriental Instt. Museum, University of Chicago. The date is 721-705 B.C.
30. H.A. Davis, *op. cit.,* p.64.
31. Edith Hamilton, *op. cit.,* p.34; also p.203.
32. *Ibid.,* p.193.
33. Khojeste Mistree, *op.cit.,* pp.41 and 48;32, 122;30, 58.
34. *Śat.Br.* I.2.5.5 *vāmano vā viṣṇur āsa.*
35. *Ibid.* V.3.1.5; VII.3.2. 14-16.
36. *Śiva-purāṇa* II. 42.7; R.C. Agrawal, "Agni in Early Indian Art", *Journal of Indian History,* Trivandrum, April 1965, p.53, Figs.2 and 3.
37. Dange, *Ency. P.B. & P.,* Vol.IV, New Delhi, 1989, pp. 1314-1316.
38. *Ibid.,* Vol. III, 1987, p.1053f.
39. *Ibid.,* Vol. IV, p.1221; also *Śiva P.* II.42.7 *dakṣasya yajñaśīrṣṇo hi bhavatvajāmukham śiraḥ.*
40. Dange, *Ency. P.B. & P.,* Vol.III, pp.820 and 781; Vol.II, p.693.
41. *Ibid.,* Vol. II, pp.717, 729; also *Skanda P.* VI. 25.3 and VII.1.185.2.
42. Dange, *Ency. P.B. & P.,* Vol. II, p.515ff.; *Skanda P.* VI. 149.33 *trinetras triśirā hrasvas tripādo barkarākṛtiḥ; Agni P.,* 300.31.
43. S.A. Dange, *Ency. P.B. & P.,* Vol. I, p.201 (ass-head); p.198 (horse-head) and tiger-head at the same place; for actual text, see p.207, notes6 and 8; p.208 n.12.

44. *Viṣṇudharmottara Purāṇa* (Gaikwad Or. Ser.) III. 44.11. The date of this text is A.D. 400-500 according to R. C. Hazra. According to Kane it is A.D. 600-900. See P.V. Kane, *History of Dharmaśāstra,* Vol.V, Pt. II, *BORI,* Second ed., Poona, 1977 pp.872 and 910.
45. *Viṣṇudharmottara Purāṇa, loc.cit.,* vv 44[cd]-45. See Devangana Desai, "Hayagrīva in the Vaikuṇṭha Pantheon of Khajuraho", *Colloquiem on Viṣṇu,* Birla Archaeological and Cultural Research Institute, Hyderabad, 1993, pp.47-50; Devendra Handa, "Vaikuṇṭha Images from Panjab", *Ajaya-Śrī,* Recent Studies in Indology (Prof. Ajaya Mitra Shastri Fel.Vol.), Sundeep Prakashan, Delhi, 1989, pp.502ff.; Krishna Deva, "Images of Hayagrīva as Vaikuṇṭha", *Viśvambharā* (Prof. V.S. Pathak Fel. Vol.), Harman Publications, New Delhi, 1995, pp.275-278.
46. Devendra Handa, *op.cit., loc.cit.*
47. Devangana Desai, "An Unpublished Viśvarūpa Sculpture in the Khajuraho Museum", *Journal of the Asiatic Society of Bombay,* Vol.72, 1997 (New Series), p.53.
48. Devangana Desai, "Hayagrīva in the Vaikuṇṭha..." (noted at 45 *supra*), p.49, where she refers to Krishna Deva.
49. S.A. Dange, *Ency. P.B. & P.,* Vol.II, pp.717;718, n.1; Vol.V, 1990, p. 1398; *Skanda P.* VI. 25.3;84. 4.ff. Mr. Lance Dane (from Bombay), who has collection of terracotta figurines, informed the present writer that one of these shows Viṣṇu's feet being massaged by a woman with the face of a mare. The period, according to him, may be early Śunga.
50. S.R. Rao, *The Decipherment of the Indus Script,* Asia Publishing House, Bombay (Calcutta, Delhi, Lucknow), 1982, pl.VII-A; XXI. 17, etc.
51. As in Malabar (Kerala) India; see Frits Stall, *Agni* (The Vedic Ritual of the Fire-altar), Vols.I & II, Motilal Banarsidass, Delhi, Vol.I, p.44ff.
52. As Devangana Desai proposes in *JASB,* 72, 1997, p.52, para 2.
53. *Good News Bible,* Delhi, 1988 (1970), p.347 (Kings I.14.18f.).
54. *Ibid.,* p.799 (Ezekiel I.1.4-27).
55. Hajime Nakamura, *A Comparative History of Ideas,* Motilal Banarsidass, Delhi, 1992 (foreign 1975), p.58; for

details, Dange, *Towards Understanding Hindu Myths,* p.10f; p.33, n.19.

56. C.J. Clement Webb, *A History of Philosophy,* Thornton Butterworth Ltd., London, 1937 (1915), pp.33, 37.

* Included here from the *Journal of the Asiatic Society of Bombay*, Mumbai, Vol.73 (for 1998) (New Series), 1998.

Chapter 9

The Abduction of Sītā

One of the most thrilling incidents in the *Rāmāyaṇa,* or, rather, the Rāma-story, is the abduction of Sītā by Rāvaṇa. The *Rāmāyaṇa* of Vālmīki, which is only one version of the *Rāmāyaṇa* story, has the episode as follows: On learning about the insult of his sister, Śūrpaṇakhā, Rāvaṇa decides to abduct Sītā. It appears that he got the clue of the plan to abduct Sītā from Akampana, who tells Rāvaṇa that Rāma, being very much attached to Sītā would die a natural death in the absence of Sītā; hence, it would be wise to abduct Sītā (Araṇyakāṇḍa 31.31-32). Rāvaṇa, then, goes to Mārīca and asks him to execute the plan. Mārīca does not agree, remembering how he was thrown into the ocean by Rāma at the earlier occasion. But, ultimately he agrees. Rāvaṇa unfolds the whole plan, also indicating how Rāma, Lakṣmaṇa and Sītā would behave. He says, "O Mārīca, on seeing you prancing as the golden deer, Sītā will urge Rāma to catch you and bring you (the deer) to her. Rāma would run after you. You should take him in the depth of the forest; and, as he shoots you, you should give out the call for help calling the names of Sītā and Lakṣmaṇa. On hearing that, Sītā would send Lakṣmaṇa after the call, being afraid that Rāma is in danger. When Sītā is rendered thus alone, I shall carry her away" (*ib.* 40.17-22). He also promises Mārīca that he would give him half of his kingdom (*ib.*

23). In the subsequent chapters, we are told that Mārīca is brought to the vicinity of the cottage of Rāma by Rāvaṇa. Sītā sees the gold-backed deer and says that Rāma should fetch it for her; and she would be glad to play with him in the forest-cottage, and would take him to Ayodhyā later on; that, if the deer is unable to be caught alive, he should be killed, so that his hide would be a unique gain (*ib.* 42.1-20). Rāma is convinced by the plea of Sītā, due to love for her. He instructs Lakṣmaṇa to take care of Sītā, and runs after the deer. Deep in the forest, he shoots the deer, who releases the loud cry, "O Sītā, O Lakṣmaṇa",. Being urged by Sītā, Lakṣmaṇa runs away to the forest. Rāvaṇa comes on the scene (*ib.* 44-46).

These two accounts would show that the main characters of the *Rām.* are behaving exactly as the villain has told his accomplice, Mārīca. The fact seems, however, to be that the story was already very popular in the period of Vālmīki, and the poet's depiction of Rāvaṇa explaining the plan of the plot to Mārīca was based on this already popular episode. Otherwise, we would have to believe that the main characters were puppets in the hands of the villain, which is hardly acceptable! That the Rāma-story was fluid is clear from the fact that Vālmīki's version and details are not followed exactly in the Hindu tradition itself. Thus, for example, the *Mb.* has it, that Rāvaṇa came to the forest-resort of Rāma with his head tonsured, taking a *kuṇḍa* and *tridaṇḍa* (*Mb.* Vana. 278.16 *yatir bhūtvā muṇḍaḥ kuṇḍī tridaṇḍa-dhṛk*), while the *Rām.* has it that he came wearing a fine tawny-coloured cloak, having an umbrella, with sandals in his feet, sporting a pigtail (*śikhī*), a *kamaṇḍalu* and a staff slung to his shoulder (*Rām.* Araṇya. 46.1-3). The *Rām.* does not speak of Mārīca staying nearabout the Janasthāna; it speaks of the *āśrama* of Mārīca to be somewhere beyond the sea. Mārīca stays there as a hermit subsisting on frugal rations, though he welcomes Rāvaṇa to a good meal (*Rām. loc.cit.*, 25.37-40). The *Mb.,* however, mentions the hermitage of Mārīca at Gokarṇa (*loc.cit.*, 277.56); and he treats Rāvaṇa with food prepared from flesh (*māṁsaudana*). *Rām.* has Rāvaṇa as characterized with his chariot drawn by donkeys having faces like ghosts (*loc.cit.* 34.1ff) and he enters the forest where Rāma has his cottage with this typical chariot, which is able to move in the sky and everywhere,[1] a point rather unbelievable, and discarded by *Mb.* One would expect him to take his air-car, *Puṣpaka*, as we have it in the Jain versions. Some such details are enough to show that Vālmīki's Rāma-story was not his own; it was a fluid popular narration, though he is credited with having "composed" the *Rāmāyaṇa*, which means, in metrical form. The *Rāmāyana* that goes in the name of Vālmīki clearly mentiones that he later composed it in the *'śloka'* metre, the first narrator being Nārada; then he was advised by Brahmā himself to narrate the story of Rāma in his new metre (*Rām.* Bāla. Cantos 1 and 2). In the earliest mention it was simply called *Rāmakathā* (*loc.cit.* 2.36 *kuru rāmakathām puṇyām*). As it is a *kathā*, elaborated later, many mythical elements are added to the original historical facts. As such, sticking to the episode of abduction, the facts seem to be as follows (taking a clue from the *Rām.* of Vālmīki).

Rāvana was concerned about the destruction of his power in the Janasthāna. He was also worried about the punishment meted out to his sister Śūrpaṇakhā, who according to a plan, was sent to entice Rāma and Lakṣmaṇa, but failed. Rāvaṇa, then, took advice from Akampana who suggested to him to abduct Sītā, so that Rāma would automatically get extinct. So, the main plan was to do away with Rāma and Lakṣmaṇa; and the abduction of Sītā was only secondary to this aim. As such, the proposal of Rāvaṇa to Sītā, that she should be his wife, etc., and the advances to her are to be taken as a ploy to insult Rāma, rather than the lust of Rāvaṇa. This is clear from the fact that he never actually molested Sītā even though she was in his full control, once in Laṅkā.

This thread of the account is very important, though subtle; and it can be said to be a faint suggestion for Sītā being shown as actually Rāvaṇa's own daughter, in certain non-Hindu traditions.[2] As it was impossible for Rāvaṇa to kill, or vanquish Rāma, or Lakṣmaṇa, in a face-to-face fight, he hatched a plan to deceive them. For this Rāvaṇa came in the guise of a recluse, as is mentioned above. The variation from *śikhī* to *muṇḍi* (at *Rām.* and *Mb.* respectively)[3] shows probably the influence of Buddhistic customs at the period when the text of *Mb.* was formulated. The guise of the deer on the part of Mārīca and the mention of the all-direction-moving chariot of Rāvaṇa have to be taken only as mythical elements. Now, we come to the actual abduction.

The *Rām.* states that Rāvaṇa had a good talk with Sītā, who was beguiled by his ascetic appearance,[4] prior to his proposal of taking her as wife. When she refused, and was about to enter the cottage, he is said to have assumed a huge form, after clapping one of his palms with the other (Araṇya, 49.1 *haste hastam samāhatya cakāra sumahad vapuḥ*). This is as mythical as the all-moving chariot with the ghost-faced donkeys, worked on the basis of the metaphor of a *rākṣasa* on the human Rāvaṇa, with a tinge of magic. The *Rām.* and *Mb.* are one in saying that Sītā was alone in the cottage; also that Rāvaṇa rushed towards Sītā and even followed her into the cottage. He took her by her hair and dragged her out (*Rām. loc.cit.* 16-17; 17d *abhigamya... jagrāha rāvaṇaḥ sītām... mūrdhajeṣu kareṇa saḥ; Mb.* Vana. 278.41 *iti sā tam samābhāṣya praviveśa āśramam tataḥ;* 42 *tām abhidrutya suśroṇīm rāvaṇaḥ pratyaṣedhayat*). An interesting point is to be noted. According to the *Rām.* and *Mb.* which are generally followed by the later tradition, Rāma goes after the deer leaving Sītā in the care of Lakṣmaṇa. However, Lakṣmaṇa is not seen in the picture according to a variation of the episode. Thus, Bhāsa keeps Lakṣmaṇa out of the cottage already, as he is said to have gone to receive the *kulapati.* Again, Rāvaṇa does not take the help of Mārīca to beguile Rāma. He comes himself and creates the deer with his magic. Would this indicate a slightly different version of the abduction (and the Rāma-story, for that matter?), current in folk-tradition at the period, which overlaps that of the *Mb.*, which itself shows slight variations from the *Rām.* in certain details, as we have noted above? This is the case with the Jain version of Puṣpadanta also (*Rāmāyaṇa* 72.3ff). There, having asked Mārīca to take away Rāma in the form of a deer, Rāvaṇa himself approaches Sītā, the wonderful deer going along with him prancing before him, in the guise of Rāma (cf. Indra approaching Ahalyā in the guise of her husband, Gautama,[5] or Viṣṇu approaching Tulasī in the form of her husband Śaṅkhacūḍa).[6] Lakṣmaṇa is not on the scene at all. Rāvaṇa (Rāma) tells Sītā, "O beloved, look! I have brought the deer for you (*ib.*5, *āṇiam maye hariṇa-poyayam*). Bad days have gone; see the *(puṣpaka ?)* air-car. *(savimāṇam sibiyāsamam).*" Beguiled completely, Sītā sits in the air-car; and she is taken to Laṅkā, though she was told to be heading for Ayodhyā. One should not ask the question- "How did Sītā not ask Rāma (here Rāvaṇa in essence) as to how the air-car came into his possession." In reality, the air-car *puṣpaka* was in the possession of Rāvaṇa prior to his defeat by Rāma; and, here, Rāma had gone only to fetch the deer, and not to defeat Rāvaṇa directly. It is difficult to account for the guise of Rāma on the part of Rāvaṇa, and not of a recluse, in this Jain version. Probably, a recluse might have been misinterpreted as a Jain monk himself, in spite of the difference in the colour of the cloak. It is also not improbable, that to show a Hindu recluse in the Jain work would have been objectionable.

The patterns in the account of abduction are as follows:

1. Rāma runs after a unique deer on the desire of Sītā. Lakṣmaṇa is on the scene; but taken away craftily.

2. Lakṣmaṇa is not at all on the scene (Bhāsa; Puṣpadanta).
3. Mārīca is on the scene, and is killed by Rāma.
4. Mārīca is not on the scene (Bhāsa); he is on the scene, but, it is not clear if he is killed; he appears on the scene just to take Rāma away; (and probably vanishes in the forest, having led Rāma into its depth).

On studying the details apparently contradictory to each other, (1 contradicts 2; 3 contradicts 4), what remains is as follows:

1. Rāma was beguiled not by any Mārīca who took the guise of a deer, or was a *rākṣasa.* He was softened by love towards Sītā. It was natural for a woman to desire something that charmed her. It was wrong for Rāma to hasten to fulfil his wife's such desire. To wipe this fault in the character of Rāma, the myth of Mārīca was invented. Without this mythical innovation, Rāma would have been squarely held responsible for the whole catastrophe. So, he was shown as being deceived.
2. The mythical innovation regarding Mārīca is helpful also in taking Lakṣmaṇa away (by the cry of help in the voice of Rāma) in the accounts that have Lakṣmaṇa on the scene.
3. However, Mārīca is present except for Bhāsa; and, shorn of the mythical element of his disguise, he appears to have served as a watch-dog for Rāvaṇa, keeping a constant watch on the cottage. It is more probable that Mārīca helped Rāvaṇa in ushering a beautiful deer in the vicinity of the cottage. The clue is in the Jain version, where Rāvaṇa himself brings a deer along with him, only to show to Sītā. Having ushered the deer, and having taken Rāma out of sight, he gave the call for help to take Lakṣmaṇa also away, imitating the voice of Rāma.

It may be noted, that in all these accounts, where Lakṣmaṇa is shown to be on the scene, he never controls the actions of Sītā in view of his departure to help Rāma. In another popular version, current in Maharashtra, Lakṣmaṇa is said to have drawn a line restricting Sītā to be within it. This detail does not appear till the sixteenth century. A.D. Kālidāsa does not mention it. The *Purāṇas* do not mention it. The *Campū Rāmāyaṇa* ascribed to Bhoja (tenth century A.D.) does not speak of it. Even the *Rāmacaritamānasa* of Tulasī (sixteenth century) does not mention it. Now, as the mythical guise of a deer on the part of Mārīca was to absolve Rāma of the fault of extra attachment to his wife, the "line of Lakṣmaṇa" was innovated to show Sītā (and a woman in general, at that period) to be controlled by man; and even then, she commits a fault.[7] This is to lay the whole burden of the later calamity on her head, completely absolving the two males of the tragedy of abduction.

NOTES AND REFERENCES

1. *Rām.* Araṇya. 35.6 *kāñcanam ratham ādāya kāmagam ratnabhūṣitam piśācavadanairyuktam kharaiḥ kanakabhūṣaṇaiḥ.*
2. The *Thāi Ramakein;* also the *Jain.*
3. *Rām.* *loc.cit.* 46.2, *abhicakrāma vaidehīm parivrājakarūpadhṛk 46.3 ślakṣṇa-kāṣāya-saṁvītaḥ sikhī chatrī upānahī.* He is also said to be *brāhmaṇa, atithi, dvijāti, ib.* 32; 34; 47, which may not all go together in a person.
4. Cf. Ch. 47 where she tells all details about herself and of Rāma, including how the latter had to come to the forest due to Kaikeyī.
5. This account occurs as early as the Vedic period - *Śat. Br.*III. 3.4 18-19. *Jai. Br.* II.79 — and is popular later.
6. *Brahmavaivarta P.* II.21. 1-24. In another place (*Skanda P.* II.4.21.8-24) Vṛndā is said to be the wife of the demon Jalandhara, and Viṣṇu seduces her in the demon's disguise. These episodes cannot be taken as real. A mythical

principle is involved here. It is that, to defeat a valiant person, his power in the female form should be spoilt. For discussion on this point, see Sadashiv A. Dange, *Purākathāncā Artha - Vāda āṇi Vivecana* (Marathi), Continental Prakāśana, Pune, 1993, "Reṇukā". Also Sadashiv A. Dange, *Towards Understanding Hindu Myths*, Aryan Books International, New Delhi, 1996, "Some Unique Myths regarding Viṣṇu", p.292 f.

7. In the *Ānanda Rāmāyaṇa* (a comparatively late work), we see Lakṣmaṇa drawing a circle round the hut and warning Sītā not to transgress it. See *Āananda Rām*. Sārakāṇḍa, 7.99, 100.

* Included here from the *Journal of the Asiatic Society of Bombay*, Bombay, Vols. 64-66 (for 1989-91), (New Series) 1993.

Chapter 10

Birth and Marriage of the Pāṇḍavas — A Riddle?

In the great epic we come across various tribes which seem to have loose sexual traditions and among whom the institution of marriage was not a hindrance to sexual liberty. Thus we find Karṇa speaking to Śalya about the Madra women,

How should the Madra man speak of virtue, the son of women that throw off their clothes and so dance with their garments cast off, etc.[1]

Śalya's retort to Karṇa, that the people of the land of Aṅga sell their children and wife,[2] helps bring to our notice the conditions prevailing in that country. These remarks, though made in anger and spite, must still have some basis of truth and the people at the time of the great epic can be supposed to have accepted the traditional trend of the people mentioned above at least in their lower classes!

Side by side with these we get such accounts wherein the maidenhood of girls is not supposed to get spoiled even after copulation. The tale of the princess Mādhavī can well be an example of this.[3] Satyavatī, the mother of Vyāsa could be a maiden even after her union with Parāśara,[4] and the same is the case with Kuntī, the mother of the

Pāṇḍavas, who regained her maidenhood after being united with the Sun-god.[5]

These references and instances show how gradually the society was changing and how ideas about moral conduct were being formed. Such behaviour cannot, however, be taken to represent the whole moral code of the epic society, but glimpses can be had of the tendency to explain away such behaviour on the part of young maidens and not to take it very seriously if the relations were not of the 'Pratiloma' type. From the speech of Pāṇḍu in the Ādi-*parvan* we learn that the women were free in their sexual behaviour; for says he to Kuntī,

Harken, O Fortunate one, the code of conduct, I tell unto thee. This was fixed by the ancient sages that knew the Dharma. It is said O Beautiful-faced one! that the women, formerly, were unhindered and freely did they move about,[6] O thou of lovely smile! When they, from the time of maidenhood, did trick their husbands, no wrong was therein—nay it was the right conduct in the times long past, O lovely-hipped one![7]

Then he talks how the restrictions upon the behaviour came to be put on by Śvetaketu—the son of Uddālaka. The freedom of maidens which Pāṇḍu refers to was certainly not a fixed tradition at the time of the *Mb*; and might even be extinct though certain examples here and there might be met with as we have just seen in the case of Kuntī and Satyavatī who, it must be remembered, were afraid of the family.[8] This liberty to the women was not allowed to the married ones. It is difficult to find in the whole length of the *Mb*. a single example where a married woman has union with another man, without the express desire of her husband, and is not censured. The words of Pāṇḍu "from the time of maidenhood, did trick their husbands" are guardedly said, for they only mean that the girls had such sexual liberty in their maidenhood and by such liberty they could only trick their *future husbands*. In the case of married women, even if sexual relation with a man other than the husband was allowed, it was not with a view of pleasure but only of duty—the duty enjoined by the living husband (or the elders of the family if the husband was dead!). This duty was a religious one—the procreation of a son! This necessity of a son led the people to invent means that would be within the limits of the code of conduct generally accepted and traditionally evolved. This is no place to take a note of all the passages eulogizing the son. From the Ṛgvedic times down to the present day we have varied lamentation of the sonless for the son. Hence to procreate the son or get him procreated for the freedom from the Pitṛṛṇa[9] was a necessity and we see that, out of this, the custom of Niyoga (levirate) came into being which we clearly meet with in the great epic. In the *Ṛgveda* we read—"What sacrificer doth invite you (Aśvinā) into his abode as doth a widow call a brother-in-law onto her bed or a youthful maiden her lover?"[10]—which tends to show the reference to Niyoga, as Viśvarūpa says, rather than to a second marriage.[11] It is this practice of Niyoga that sanctioned the procreation of the Pāṇḍavas, and it is easy and natural to believe so howsoever the birth of the heroes be clad into a mythical coating. Even if the Ṛgvedic quotation be taken to indicate a second marriage in the remote past(?) and not exactly Niyoga, one can clearly see the intention for both these. The Niyoga aims at the procreation of a son and marriage also has the aim of having a son; and it is possible that the Vedic Aryans in their social evolution thought this second marriage to be a long sinful bondage once the son is born to the deceased brother's wife—nay it also might have been gradually thought to be sinful to marry the wife of the deceased brother. Thus we see Manu clearly stating that:

The elder brother uniting with the wife of the younger and also the younger uniting with the wife of the elder *in the absence of a misfortune* (i.e. sonlessness), fall into sin, even when *'niyukta'*.[12]

(In the absence of a misfortune, i.e. in the absence of there being no son, according to Kullūka) and further on:

"But when the fruit of Niyoga is achieved (i.e. the widow gets impregnated), they (the widow and the elder brother of the deceased) should behave with one another as the daughter-in-law and the father-in-law (respectively).[13]

Thus we get an idea of the evolution of the marital code amongst the Vedic Aryans. From the brother marrying the widow of the deceased brother for the procreation of sons to the custom of Niyoga authorizing him and the widow to procreate for the deceased was a gradual evolution, and such a marriage for life came to be considered not only unnecessary but also immoral. Only in the case of a 'Vāgdattā', if her betrothed husband dies, her own brother-in-law is to take her as his own uniting with her *once only* in the period of each Ṛtu (but that too) only up to impregnation.[14]

In this evolution in the method for the procreation of a son for the deceased, the brother-in-law features prominently. Gautama states that certain sages would not allow one who is not a brother-in-law; but he mentions others who can act in his place.[15]

Now there is another important point to be considered in this connection. If the *Ṛgveda* be seen as indicating a (second) marriage of the widow with the brother-in-law, it also impliedly gives the sanction of producing any number of children from her; while the laws of Niyoga laid down by the various Smṛtikāras give sanction only *for one son*[16] or at the most two sons; for. in the case of only one son there is the danger of losing him and the deceased being again without a son.[17] Thus we get a situation wherein there seems to be a gradual evolution of the idea—"*From many sons to one son for the widow.*" When we arrive at this situation which we have seen as being among the Vedic people we are in a position to imagine a stage when, in the case of the sonless, more than two sons also might be allowed under certain circumstances, though not mentioned precisely, and one of these possibly is when *though the woman is not a widow,* and her husband is powerless in procreation. Thus we see that Niyoga presents two points:

(i) The widow of the sonless deceased can be allowed to have only one (or two in the opinion of some) son.
(ii) The 'powerless' husband may have his own will in this case and get procreated *more than two sons.*

The first point we have explained. We will examine the second one.

Manu clearly says:

The desired *'prajā'* may be got procreated in the absence of an issue by the *woman* (not a widow!) well-appointed, through her brother-in-law or any other person who is a 'Sapiṇḍa'.[18] Kullūka's comment on this is that the woman in question should be appointed by the "elders including the husband."[19] (This is quite in fitness seeing the word *'by a woman'* (and not a *widow!*) in the verse of Manu.) The word *'prajā'* clearly means more than two—as Kullūka rightly interprets—*'issues* may be procreated.' He further comments upon the word—*'desired'* saying "the word 'desired', of course, has the implication of uniting again in case the *son be not a fit one*".[20] Thus he clearly means that in the case when the husband is living, more *sons* than two may be procreated.

Manu clearly makes a difference between the 'woman' (whose husband is alive but is 'powerless') and the 'widow', in the very next verse saying:

But the one appointed to a *'vidhavā'* should, anointing his body with ghee, being speechless (and approaching) in the night procreate one son and never two.[21]

Thus can be clearly seen how Manu makes a difference between the two cases of women. The restriction of 'one or two' seems to be only in the case of widows. Gautama, as we have seen does speak of the widow and lays down that not more than two may be procreated. He further speaks about the 'field of the one alive' but the restriction of two should not be taken to apply here.[22] Vasiṣṭha allows Niyoga for the widow,[23] but it is not clear whether he refers to a living husband,[24] which also is found in Baudhāyana[25] who speaks against Niyoga and hence does not give any limit in the case where the husband is living. Viṣṇu while mentioning the twelve sons, also speaks of a 'Kṣetraja' son, but does not give clearly whether of a living husband or of the dead one, nor does he give any limitation on the number.[26] We have also seen how Manu differentiates between a woman with a living husband and the widow as regards Niyoga and keeps more scope for the woman with a living husband; while in the case of the birth of the Pāṇḍavas, Kuntī accepts the wish of Pāṇḍu up to three sons but at his request again at the fourth time tells him that it would be licentious and hence sinful, says she—

"Not the fourth issue even in the time of misfortune so do they say. Hence shall she be a licentious and with the fifth a whore."[27]

It is thus clearly seen that the Pāṇḍavas were born by Niyoga and were quite legitimate. The law about the procreation limit up to three is not found to be clearly expressed but can very easily be seen as implied; and it is possible that in the compilation of the law books might have slipped off somewhere as might also some other laws which do not appear before us expressly. About the case of Mādrī having two sons by Niyoga, it is seen that the Śāstras allow it. Even in the *Mb.* it can be seen. Satyavatī asks her son Vyāsa to procreate sons from the widows of Vicitravīrya and when she knows from him that the first queen's (Ambikā) son would be blind and that of the second (Ambālikā) consumptive, she desired to send her elder daughter-in-law again for one more son. This shows that two sons from one could be easily allowed in the custom of the epic period.[28] But it can be seen that this procreation of the second son from the same woman is in the case of a widow as Vicitravīrya is dead; while in the case of Kuntī Pāṇḍu is alive and desires son after son up to three when he is checked by Kuntī. But there was no such restriction of sons by Niyoga if the husband was alive and desired it—even if he was not impotent— with the idea of having illustrious sons.[29] We can see that in the case of Pāṇḍu he is not satisfied with Dharma and wants a real *Kṣatriya* full of vigour and manly power;[30] but still his 'desired one' was not even Bhīma—the second one; and desired a third, asking her to perform penance and taking the opinion of the sages. Thus there is nothing that would go against the code of conduct as regards the birth of the Pāṇḍavas. It is easy to understand that under the cloudy mythical coating, the plain custom of Niyoga is present. Now a question that is not very important can be asked. Why is it said that these sons were the sons of divine beings and not of human beings? The answer is simple.

i. All acts of Niyoga are to be secret. We read such words as 'in the night' (*niśi*) or 'in secret' (*mithaḥ*) or 'The *muhūrta* sacred to Prajāpati', etc. So this was naturally kept up a secret.

ii. To give divine halo to the heroes. The idea seems to have been taken from popular Vedic gods and their characteristics resembling those of these five sons. Yama is also called Dharma. Especially the Aśvinā and the twin sons can be easily coupled up together.

iii. Being a kingly family ordinary *brāhmaṇa-s* being appointed as the *bījin* ('seeder') would have been humiliating. In the case of Vicitravīrya, Vyāsa was a famous sage and there was nothing humiliating about union with him. But Pāṇḍu being far off in the Himālayas, the sages there being quite unknown, it was found necessary to weave a net of divine myth around their birth. The same mystery is purposely kept up; for we see the Himālayan sages escorting the Pāṇḍavas and Kuntī to Hastināpura; but without much explanation they take leave.[31]

It is not intended to take a note of all the instances of Niyoga here,[32] the main idea being to see whether Pāṇḍu's getting three sons procreated by Niyoga was according to the Aryan custom; and we have seen how during the evolution of the moral code of the Vedic Aryans a stage permitting three sons might have been in existence. Pāṇḍu's words to Kuntī about Śāradaṇḍāyanī[33] getting three sons by being appointed to a brāhmin (i.e. by Niyoga) probably refer to this rule which might have slipped off in the reshuffling of the Dharmasūtras. It is to be noted again here that Śāradaṇḍāyanī is ordered for the Niyoga by her husband Śāradaṇḍāyana who is alive! Possibly this is the reason why three sons were procreated. From the account of Niyoga given by Bhīṣma we learn that Dīrghatamas begot five sons on Sudeṣṇā—the wife of king Bali at the latter's request.[34] Here also the husband is alive. Though Bali is a Daitya King we cannot put this fact aside simply saying it to be a custom among the Daityas. We have already seen how the Aryans might gradually have changed their moral customs.

Thus we have seen that in the case of the widow, from her being taken for wife by the brother-in-law to the permission of one (or two at the most) son by Niyoga was a gradual evolution; we can also believe that even more than two sons were allowed if the husband was alive and if he desired so; and hence Pāṇḍu[35] was perfectly on the legal path in getting three sons from Kuntī by Niyoga, backed by the Aryans of India.

The question whether Niyoga was generally upheld or not is beyond the scope of the present discussion; but we can see that it was both allowed and criticized by Manu.[35]

The second debatable point is the marriage of the five Pāṇḍavas with one woman—Draupadī, which stands as an example of polyandry that is not found among the Vedic Aryans. The gradually evolved moral code of the Vedic Aryans does not give any place to such a practice. The oft quoted passage of the *Taittirīya Saṁhitā* allowing two wives for one man but not allowing a woman to have two husbands puts it in the form of a simile taking the sacrificial post as the standard of comparison.[37] We shall first see whether we get any semblance of the system of polyandry in the *Mb.*itself.

(*i*) In the Ādi *Parvan* King Pāṇḍu refers to one great sage Uddālaka whose son was Śvetaketu, stating that once a *brāhmaṇa* took Śvetaketu's mother by the hand before his eyes and bade her to go with him. To the enraged Śvetaketu his father said that it was the eternal law and that the female beings of all kinds were unhindered.[38] Since then Śvetaketu put restrictions upon women that they should not trick their husbands lest they should acquire the sin of killing an embryo; the same for the man tricking his faithful wife. But he enjoined that the woman must go to another person if ordered by her husband;[39] if not she acquired sin!

One can see that there is no reference to polyandry here; the words 'trick their husbands'[40] mark a difference between the husband and another man who is not a husband, thus showing only sexual freedom for ladies. Sexual freedom and polyandry are different from one another. The whole of this passage is for the support of Niyoga and Pāṇḍu's reference to the Uttarakurus[41] and its free women should not be taken as an example of polyandry, but only as liberty of sexual relations on the part of women.

(*ii*) Bhīṣma tells Kuntī about the birth of Dīrghatamas and the cause of his blindness as the curse of Bṛhaspati. Bṛhaspati, the younger brother of Utathya demanded sexual pleasure of the latter's wife—

Mamatā—which she denied saying that she had already in her womb the flower from Utathya. But then overwhelmed with passion Bṛhaspati—the priest of gods—tried to unite with her, when the embryo in the womb said that there was not more space in the womb and he was the first occupant of it. Bṛhaspati still went ahead and copulated with Mamatā, his seed being checked by the embryo with both of his feet and thus getting out, at which the sage Bṛhaspati cursed him to be blind.[42] Now if we examine this episode we cannot definitely call it a case of polyandry, though we see that Mamatā's objection seems only that she was already impregnated and was carrying and that there was no room there in her womb for two; thus giving rise to the doubt whether Bṛhaspati also be the husband of Mamatā. But, in the absence of an express mention to that effect this cannot be taken to be a reference to polyandry or group marriage, as Meyer does.[43] At the best it can illustrate the right of the younger brother to beget a son from the wife of his elder brother, which later on developed into the full custom of Niyoga. And even Bhīṣma makes use of this whole tale to support Niyoga.

Not only was polyandry[44] absent among the Vedic Aryans but was looked upon with contempt; and yet the Pāṇḍavas—the heroes of the Bhārata war—marry one woman giving proof of a polyandric marriage. Now the situation is like this:—

The Pāṇḍava marriage was polyandric. Polyandry was foreign to the Vedic Aryans. Hence the Pāṇḍavas were foreign to the Vedic Aryans.

In short, the Pāṇḍavas were not Aryans. This is how many scholars propound.[45] They have also other grounds to prove this. With the other grounds we are not presently concerned. The question is—can we conclude from the marriage that the Pāṇḍavas were not Aryans?

Many are the explanations given to solve this riddle; and to retain the Pāṇḍava heroes in the Aryan fold. That this marriage was considered awkward and out of the way by important members of the royal families can easily be seen from the *Mb,* itself:

(i) Kuntī herself realizes her mistake and repents over her words 'enjoy together'; and going to Dharma asks him a way to keep herself away from falsehood (i.e. not to disprove her words 'enjoy together') and at the same time to steer Draupadī away from the sin of violating the 'Dharma'.[46] This can be taken as a later interpolation purposely adjusted by the editor of the *Mb.* to give Kuntī a chance to keep her conscience clear by uttering the doubt! But this only strengthens the view that this marriage was considered to be alien to the then Aryans.

(ii) Dhṛṣṭadyumna objects to the marriage by saying—'How could the virtuous elder brother go to (and unite with) the wife of his younger brother'?[47] Does his objection relate *only* to the fact that the elder cannot approach the younger's wife, and can we conclude that he has no objection if the younger ones go to the wife of the elder? It is not correct to conclude so as J.J. Meyer does.[48] It should be clearly remembered that Dhṛṣṭadyumna's speech is in continuation to the argument of Drupada who strongly opposes this marriage calling it an '*adharma*' for a woman to have more husbands than one. The main point to be noted is that Dhṛṣṭadyumna has Arjuna, who won his sister, in his mind and he objects to Dharma's intention to himself marry Draupadī alongwith his brothers; for says Dharma, "I am as yet a bachelor and so is Bhīma"[49] and this Dhṛṣṭadyumna has in mind when he rather mildly rebukes Dharmarāja. To take it to mean the other way will be to stretch it too far.

Hence it is clear that Dhṛṣṭadyumna does not tolerate the idea of such a marriage and is one with his father who allows Draupadī to be married to any of the Pāṇḍavas but not to all the five!

(iii) Karṇa also abhors the marriage and calls Draupadī a '*bandhakī*' (a harlot).[50]

So we have to take it as it is—i.e. the marriage was a polyandric one and it was abhorred by the Aryan society at that time. But because of this to say that the Pāṇḍavas themselves were non-Aryan is quite a hasty conclusion. Various explanations were given to cut this knot. The *Mb.* tried to give a divine tinge to the whole episode and it went well with the religious-minded people in general, but we can see that these explanations are not quite logical. They were in short:

(i) That Draupadī was a *brāhmaṇa* girl in her former birth and asked for a husband when Lord Śiva presented himself before her being pleased with her penance. She said, 'Give me a husband' and said it five times.[51]

(ii) That the five Pāṇḍavas were really five Indras cursed to be mortal by Śiva and Draupadī was the divine Lakṣmī of the heavens (the personified glory—not the goddess of that name).[52]

Kumārila Bhaṭṭa in his *Tantravārtika* explains by saying that there were many Draupadīs, all similar to one another.[53] But this explanation also seems to be fantastic.

Thus we can see that all these explanations are not apt. Then should the Pāṇḍavas be really taken to be non-Aryans on the basis of this marriage? No. The Pāṇḍavas were perfect Aryans, but they probably had to resort to this sort of polyandric marriage which was not the custom of the Aryans. This can be seen from the peculiar circumstances the Pāṇḍavas were in. The scholars who think the Pāṇḍavas to be non-Aryans and those who are sure of their being Aryan but are puzzled at this marriage.

have missed certain points which are of utmost importance. It cannot be that Pāṇḍavas did not know that this was not the Aryan type, but the peculiar circumstances they were in made them accept this form of marriage, even against the wishes of their near relations and well-wishers who afterwards gave their whole-hearted consent. Let us examine these circumstances. First the home front:

(i) The problem created by the arrival of the sons of Pāṇḍu to Hastināpura was quite a grave one. Dhṛtarāṣṭra and his sons never liked these heirs to the throne and but for Bhīṣma, the good old man, would have refused them entry into their fold.
(ii) The Pāṇḍavas' superiority over the sons of Dhṛtarāṣṭra was proclaimed on the final day of the military training and Droṇa's partiality for them and especially for Arjuna was a constant thorn in the mind of the sons of Dhṛtarāṣṭra.
(iii) Naturally the Kauravas wanted to get rid of the Pāṇḍavas.
(iv) The 'Gurudakṣiṇā' episode and the defeat of the sons of Dhṛtarāṣṭra at the hands of Drupada and the subsequent victory over and subjugation of Drupada by the Pāṇḍavas (esp.Arjuna) added plumes to their helmets and thorns to the hearts of the Kauravas.[54] The result was a series of efforts on the part of the Kauravas to kill the five by poisoning, burning, etc.

Thus the Kauravas and the Pāṇḍavas were now avowed enemies. Let us now see the position on the Pāñcāla front:

(i) We are told that Droṇa and Drupada were formerly friends and played together when Drupada's father—Pṛṣat—was the king of Pāñcāla; but when in later years Droṇa returned to Pāñcāla after getting military training from Paraśurāma and went to Drupada and called him 'friend', the latter insulted him.[55] Droṇa came to Hastināpura and avenged the insult by asking his royal disciples the capture of Drupada as the 'Gurudakṣiṇā' as we have seen above.

(ii) After his subjugation by Droṇa, Drupada tried hard to get a son who would destroy Droṇa and getting 'Yāja' and 'Upayāja' as preceptors performed a sacrifice which gave him Dhṛṣṭadyumna and Draupadī.[56]

(iii) Droṇa was in the service of the Kauravas whom Drupada himself had defeated in the 'Dakṣiṇā' episode and who were the cause of his humiliation.

Thus Drupada became an avowed enemy of the Kauravas. He was naturally interested in the friendship of the mighty Pāṇḍavas, probably at any cost. Wẹ have references in *Mb.*, that show him interested in Arjuna and that he had got prepared a strong bow for that purpose.[57] We also have him worried at the victory of an unknown archer (really Arjuna in *brāhmaṇa*-disguise). He is quite zealous to have matrimonial relations with the Pāṇḍavas and though expressing his disinclination towards the polyandric marriage, shows his readiness to have any one of the Pāṇḍavas—either Dharma or Bhīma or Arjuna for that matter— and speaks out his thought to Yudhiṣṭhira.[58] The purpose of this zeal can easily be discerned. It is to win the Pāṇḍavas in case the Kauravas might make it difficult to punish Droṇa.

On the Pāṇḍava front:

The Pāṇḍavas now had to carve out their own prestige with the royal families of India. Most of the royal families were on the side of the Kauravas; and naturally to save themselves from being crushed was the upper thought. It is at this stage do they hear about the 'Svayaṁvara' of Draupadī and desiring to win over political alliance through the matrimonial one if it could be had by sheer strength of valour, they turn to the Pāñcāla. This occasion only was a proper one to win over both fame and firmness. It is a matter of great importance to note that without such chance to issue forth as supreme warriors, their approach to any royal family would have possibly been difficult and doubtful about the desired alliance. During the long absence of Pāṇḍu from Hastināpura the Dhārtarāṣṭras had full scope to increase their influence and alliances and hence even to think of a royal assistance would have been difficult at that stage of their life! What about Kṛṣṇa? He himself with Balarāma had receded far into the background losing ground to Jarāsandha. At least it was natural for the Pāṇḍavas not to expect help anywhere except the good-hearted *brāhmaṇa*[59] and potter[60] alike! This also shows the elasticity of their nature to adjust to any circumstances.

They then decided to take up this chance of showing their mettle and thus probably winning a royal alliance.

Thus, both the sides had the desire to join hand, Drupada—the king of Pāñcāla—and the five Pāṇḍavas. And it came about successfully and Arjuna, the Pāṇḍava won Draupadī—the Pāñcālī! But could he marry her? Not before his two elder brothers who were yet unmarried; for that would be quite against the Dharmaśāstras. It would mean the sin of 'Parivedana'.[61]

Now the situation stands thus:

(i) To avoid the sin of Parivedana, Dharmarāja and Bhīma must get married before Arjuna,
(ii) Arjuna should give up the prize and walk off with his brothers.

The first was not possible: because:

(i) As we have seen the Pāṇḍavas' peculiar circumstances would not have seen them easily married in royal homes;
(ii) secondly, at this particular time the whole galaxy of the kings was against them (Kṛṣṇa had not yet met them) not recognizing them because of their *brāhmaṇa*-attire; and
(iii) for Dharma and Bhīma to marry before Arjuna, the time even was not sufficient. We do not read the Pāñcāla king having daughters ready for marriages

as Janaka, the Videha had in the case of Rāma and his brothers.

The Second was also not possible, for:

(i) As we have already seen, the Pāṇḍavas seized this opportunity and hastened to the Pāncālas;[62]
(ii) Drupada would not allow Arjuna to do so both for fear of being thus insulted and also losing the mighty alliance; and
(iii) it would mean humiliation of Draupadī.

Being thus on the horns of the dilemma, the only course open to Arjuna was to offer the prize to his eldest brother—Dharmarāja; for though Arjuna had won her, he was not obliged to marry her himself; and in not marrying her himself but offering her to his eldest brother, he has acted quite like his great-grandfather, Bhīṣma.[63] Thus he offers Draupadī to Yudhiṣṭhira, rather than incur the sin of 'Parivedana.' But Yudhiṣṭhira himself would not like to take Draupadī as his own wife and so too Bhīma when Arjuna won her with his own might and skill; and out of this fix the only way open was to call her the wife of all the three; and when she could be the wife of three she could as well be the wife of all the five! It was with the precise consent of Kuntī and the order of the eldest Pāṇḍavas; and the peculiar circumstances forced the Pāṇḍavas to take up this form of marriage which was not common amongst the then-Aryans, but which the Pāṇḍavas could imitate from the aboriginal tribes. It was a step besides the track, but political pressure and the contracted social status forced the Pāṇḍavas to take it, and they took it boldly!

Drupada ultimately saw the situation and had to submit for fear of losing the alliance of the Pāṇḍavas who were thus driven by sheer necessity. Moreover we have grounds to suppose that Draupadī was not his own daughter; and she, with her brother Dhṛṣṭadyumna, might have been adopted for political ends. That these two came out of the sacrificial altar is clearly a myth.[64] We can suppose that they were adopted before fire with a sort of a sacrifice. At the time of adoption they might be quite grown up. The description of these two when they came from Agni can bear testimony to it.[65] That these two were adopted can also be seen from the words of the queen of the Pāñcālas who requests the preceptor to grant her the desire that these two should not call any other woman except herself, mother.[66] We learn from *Mb.* that Drupada got these two after a long search for the preceptor with the particular aim of getting a son who would kill Droṇa. If we look at the whole affair we can even see a motive in the Draupadī-affair. Thus we are inclined to think—

(i) Drupada knew that the Pāṇḍavas escaped the tortures at the hands of Kauravas, who were a common enemy.
(ii) He wanted to strike an alliance with the Pāṇḍavas, as he had already seen their valour.
(iii) For this, it was necessary to find them out.
(iv) So the Svayaṁvara was to be arranged; and if a daughter was not already there, one could be adopted!
(v) Hence Draupadī was adopted.

The plan to be successful must be arranged well; and we have seen how Drupada purposely set up a bow-test that would help him detect Arjuna. We also see how Karṇa was denied by Draupadī even when he was successful in the test. Draupadī's objection to him was that he was a 'Sūtaputra'.[67] Thus was Karṇa avoided, and it was definitely for getting Arjuna, if he was present! It was all a politically planned affair. It was this political consideration that led Drupada to accept the Pāṇḍavas with their peculiar decision. It was again this consideration of political alliance mixed with the sense of duty to his brothers that Yudhiṣṭhira was forced to accept Draupadī in a polyandric marriage.

Even if we look to the 'Svayaṁvara', we do not find its parallel anywhere. The well known 'Svayaṁvaras' are

(i) Sitā-Svayaṁvara
(ii) Sāvitrī-Svayaṁvara
(iii) Damayantī-Svayaṁvara
(iv) Rukmiṇī-Svayaṁvara, etc.

But in none of these do we find a batch of brothers going to choose; and there is no question of the sin of Parivedana or any fix about the affair. In the Sītā-Svayaṁvara only the two brothers go; but as it is the elder one that wins there is no conflict; and even if there was, Janaka's daughters were there to solve it. Here, the case is quite different. It is not the eldest that is the winner and Drupada has no daughters to solve the problem easily. It would not have been proper to marry them to girls who were of less than a royal birth or who could not at least show a royal parentage.

Thus, we can see that the whole case of the Pāṇḍavas is peculiar; and this peculiarity of the social and political contraction is at the back of their polyandric marriage — a custom they were forced to take resort to. Even in this marriage there is a point peculiar to the Pāṇḍavas. Though Draupadī is the wife of five husbands, she gets only one son from each of her husbands, as if by a moral code decided by the brothers amongst themselves. Without taking these things into consideration to try to explain away the marriage is sure to lead us astray. The references of Jaṭilā who was the wife of seven sages and the daughter of Vṛkṣa who married ten Pracetasa brothers[68] also seem obviously to be later interpolations which only confused the matters. It is this confusion that has caused many scholars to doubt the Aryan origin of the Pāṇḍavas; but on seeing clearly through the whole mist, we can understand how hasty it is to call them non-Aryans; and then the riddle about them ceases to be a riddle.

* While dealing with this topic, the Chitrashala edition of the *Mb.* is used.

NOTES AND REFERENCES

1. *Mb.* Karṇa *parvan* 40.35 ff.
2. *Ibid.,* 45.40.
3. See Sadashiv A. Dange, *Myths from the Mahābhārata*, Vol.2, Aryan Books International, New Delhi, 2001, Chapter on "Tests".

   For the account of Mādhavī, see *Mb.* Udyoga *parvan* chapters 114-119; later her marriage by self-choosing was proposed, but she preferred forest-life. See *Ibid.,* 120.1-5.
4. *Ibid.,* Ādi 63.70-83.
5. *Ibid.,* Ādi III.17.
6. Cf. Yule's *Marco Polo* ii.40, "In Tibet every girl got a ring from each man that had enjoyed her; and unless she could show at least twenty she did not find a husband."
7. *Mb.* Ādi 122.3-5 (not given in the Gita Press ed. of the *Mb.*).
8. *Ibid.* Ādi III.16 - *bandhupakṣabhayādbhītā lajjayā tu yaśasvinī;*
   also *ibid.,* 105.10 - *tamaham śāpabhītā pitṛbhītā ca bhārata.*
9. Cf. *Ait.Br.* VII. 13 = 33.1.
10. *ṚV* X.40.2.
11. *Yāj. Sm.* I.69; see also Medhātithi on *Manu Sm.* IX.66. About remarriage the picture is not very clear in that period. However, an earlier text, *Vasiṣṭha Dh. S.* allows remarriage for child-widows (XVII.74) and also *niyoga* (XVII.56ff); see P.V. Kane, *Hist. of Dh. S.*, Vol.I, pt.I, Poona, 1968, p.105; Kauṭilya allows it even for grown up women (*ibid.*, p.205).
12. *Manu Sm.* IX. 50.
13. *Ibid.,* IX.62.
14. *Ibid.,* IX.69,70.
15. *Gaut. Dh. S.* XVIII. 6.8 - *piṇḍagotrarṣisambandhebhyo yonimātrād vā / nādevarādityeke*
16. Cf. *Manu Sm.* IX.60^{cd}
    ekamutpādayet putram na dvitīyam kadācana/
17. *Ibid.* IX.61 ab —
    dvitīyameke prajanam manyante strīṣu tadvidaḥ /
    and Kullūka's comment - *aputra ekaputra iti śiṣṭapravādāt;* also *Gaut.Dh.S.* XVIII.8. *nātidvitīyam*
18. *Manu Sm.* IX. 59 —

devarād vā sapiṇḍād vā striyā samyanniyuktayā / prajepsitādhigantavyā santānasya parikṣaye

19. *patyādiguruniyuktayā*
20. Kullūka on *Manu Sm.* IX.59 - *iṣṭāḥ prajā utpādayitavyāḥ* / (Mark the *plural no.*) *'īpsitā' ityabhidhānam arthāt kāryākṣamaputrotpattau punargamanārtham* /
21. *Manu Sm.* IX.60a — *vidhavāyām niyuktastu*...etc. (Mark *'tu'* to show difference).
    While commenting on *Manu Sm.* IX.60, Kullūka clearly contradicts his own comment on *Manu Sm.* IX.59 see - notes 19 and 20 *supra*; and *'vidhavāyām' ityapatyotpādanayogyapatyabhāvaparamidam / jīvatyapi patyau ayogyapatyādiguruniyukto ... ekam putram janayet na katham-cana dvitīyam* /
    The *pati* in IX.59 is also to be necessarily *apatyotpādana-ayogya* and also living. His interpretation of *'vidhavā'* seems to be laboured and unnecessary.
22. *jīvataśca kṣetre parasmāt* / (*Gaut. Dh.Ś.* XVIII.18) goes with *'tasya dvayorvā'* and not with *'nātidvitīyam'* which lays down a restriction of number for one who is *apatiḥ*. See *apatirapatyalipsurdevarāt,* etc. (*ibid.,* XVIII.2).
23. *Vas.Dh.S.* XVII.55.
24. *Ibid.,* XVII.9.
25. *Baudh.Dh.S.* II. 2.41.
26. *Viṣṇu Dh.S.* XV.3.
27. *Mb.* Ādi 123.76 - *nātaścaturtham prasavamāpatsvapi vadantyuta / ataḥ param svairiṇī syād bandhakī pañcame bhavet //*
28. Cf. *Mb.* Ādi 106.11-21. It is a different thing that the elder queen refused remembering the repulsive appearance of Vyāsa.
29. See how Dīrghatamas begets eleven and five sons on the Dāsī and the wife of Bali resp. *Mb.* Ādi 104.41-55 (This is not given in the Gita Press ed. of the *Mb.*).
30. *Ibid.,* 123.10.
31. *Ibid.,* 126.35.
32. To mention some instances of Niyoga in the epic—
    Ibid., Ādi 104.41-50 — Dīrghatamas procreating for Bali.
    Ibid., 182.1-26 — Vasiṣṭha procreating for Kalmāṣapāda.
33. *Ibid.,* Ādi 120.38-40 — A *brāhmaṇa* procreating for

Śāradaṇḍāyanī.

34. See note 32 *supra*.
35. Pāṇḍu's being forced to Niyoga by a curse has a parallel in Kalmāṣapāda. The two episodes are almost similar in the purport; see *Mb.* Ādi 182, where we read Kalmāṣapāda getting a curse from a *brāhmaṇī* engaged in love-sport with her husband.
36. For discussion about Niyoga being allowed and criticized — vide P.V. Kane, *Hist. of Dh.S.*, Vol. II, pt.I, pp.599-607.
37. *Tait.Sam.* VI.6.4.3.
38. *Mb.* Ādi 122.9-19.
39. We read just after that, he himself appointed his wife to Vasiṣṭha and got a son by Niyoga *Ibid.,* 122.20-22.
40. *Ibid.,* Ādi 122.17 —
    vyuccarantyāḥ patim nāryā adyaprabhṛti pātakam/
41. Cf. The boast of the husband in having a 'wife' attracting many persons and giving a proof likewise by her many sexual unions - see J.J. Meyer, *Sexual Life in Ancient India,* Calcutta, 1952, p.121 notes.
42. Mb. Ādi 104.8-22.
43. J.J. Meyer, *op.cit.*, p.113f.
44. P.V. Kane, finds traces of the knowledge of polyandry in the Dharmaśāstra works - for a short discussion on polyandry, see *Hist. of Dh.S;* Vol.II, pt.II, p.555.
45. J.J. Meyer, *op.cit.*, p.108 and E.W. Hopkins, *The Great Epic,* pp.376, 400.
46. *Mb.* Ādi 191.2 —
    paścācca kuntī prasamīkṣya kṛṣṇām kaṣṭam mayā bhāṣitamityuvāca / and reading further see — *yathocitam putra mayāpi coktam sametya bhuṅkteti nṛpa pramādāt.*
47. *Ibid.,* Ādi 196.10.
48. *Sexual Life in Ancient India*, p.113. Here Meyer (quite unnecessarily and inaptly) finds a parallel in the Mamatā-Bṛhaspati episode calling it a case of 'Fellowship-marriage' and is surprised (p.114) to see this in ancient Indian literature. We have already seen that it should not be taken as a reference to such polyandric marriage.
49. *Mb.* Ādi 195.24 —
    aham cāpyaniviṣṭo vai bhīmasenaśca pāṇḍavaḥ /
50. *Ibid.,* Sabhā 68.35 —
    iyam tvanekavaśagā bandhakīti viniścitā /

51. *Ibid.,* Ādi 168.5-15 and 197.44-51.
52. Cf. *Ibid.,* Ādi 197 which contains an artistically woven account of the birth not only of the Pāṇḍavas and Draupadī, but also of Kṛṣṇa.
53. For this see P.V. Kane, *op.cit.,* Vol.II, pt.II, p.555.

    Such explanations are apologistic, as Andrew Lang would say. He branded the scholars and commentators who resorted to such explanation as 'Apologists'. See Andrew Lang, *Myth, Ritual and Religion,* Vol.I, London, 1913 (1887), p.15f.
54. *Mb.* Ādi Chap.138.
55. *Ibid.,* 130.41; 131.1-7; also 166.4-16.
56. See Ādi 167.1-40.
57. *Ibid.,* 185.7-8. *so'nveṣamāṇaḥ kaunteyam pāñcālyo janamejaya / dṛḍham dhanuranānamyam kārayāmāsa bhārata / /*
58. *Ibid.,* 195.22 —

    bhavān vā vidhivat pāṇim gṛhṇātu duhiturmama / yasya vā manyase vīra tasya kṛṣṇāmupādiśa / /
59. The Pāṇḍavas were given escort by the *brāhmaṇa* to the Pāñcāla country. See *ibid* chap.184
60. See *Ibid.,* 185.6
61. For a fuller idea of a Parivedana, see P.V. Kane, *op.cit.,* Vol.II, pt.II, p.547.
62. *Mb.* Ādi 167.1-2
63. *Ibid.,* 102.2-65. Bhīṣma carried off the three daughters of Kāśīrāja and offered two to Vicitravīrya — one of them left to go away to her lover.
64. See Dange, *Myths from the Mahābhārata,* Vol.2, Aryan Books International, New Delhi, 2001, Chap. on "Supranormal Birth", (iv) Sacrificial Altar, p.162f.
65. *Mb.* Ādi 167.40 and 45.
66. *Ibid.,* 165.50.
67. *Ibid.,* 187.22.
68. *Ibid.,* 196.12-15.

* Included here from the *Journal of the University of Bombay,* Bombay, Vol.XXVI, pt.2, September 1957.

Chapter 11

The "Bodies" of Pāṇḍu and Mādrī and the Funeral Rites

The discussion to follow refers to an *apparent* contradiction in two passages from the *Mb*. The passages come immediately after one another; and, it would appear that they indicate two different versions of the death and the subsequent cremation of Pāṇḍu and Mādrī, the latter's following her husband in the same pyre liable to be questioned. On the one hand, we read that Mādrī followed her husband in the same pyre (*satī*) (Ādi, 116.31: *madra-rāja-sutā tūrṇam anvārohad yaśasvinī;* also 117.28: *praviṣṭā pāvakaṁ mādrī hitvā jīvitam ātmanaḥ).*[1] On the other hand, immediately afterwards it is said that the sages brought their "bodies" to Hastināpura for further funeral rites (*ibid.*, 29-31: *ime tayoḥ śarīre dve).* The point is whether these two places are to be taken as contradictory to one another, indicating that Mādrī did not really get herself burnt in the same pyre as that of her husband, according to one version, and that the bodies of these two were *actually* brought to Hastināpura, by some process of embalming which is not mentioned in the text or, for that matter, in the whole of the tradition.

The problem was touched recently by M.A. Mehendale,[2] who stated that these are two different versions, and that, the version mentioning the bodies could also be equally authentic, thus suggesting, on the one hand, that Mādrī did not go as *satī*, and that, on the other hand, the cremation of Pāṇḍu (along with Mādrī) did not take place where they died (at the remote Śataśṛṅga), but that the dead bodies were brought to Hastināpura for cremation. Mehendale writes that some details in the accounts were lost, viz. (i) how the dead bodies remained fresh (at least without decay) for seventeen days, which was the time for bringing the bodies from the mountain Śataśṛṅga to Hastināpura; and (ii) Mādrī died of intense grief (and was cremated later, like her husband, at Hastināpura). He criticises the famous commentator of the *Mahābhārata,* Nilakaṇṭha, saying that he sought to avert the contradiction in these two accounts by rendering the word *śarīre* (dual) as *asthi*, and doubts how only two bones (one each of Pāṇḍu and Mādrī) could be called *śarīra,* and how elaborate funeral rites, mentioned by the *Mb*., could be done on *one bone* each. He is aware of the tradition of second cremation in case an *agnihotrin* (a person who keeps fire for life) dies in travel away from his residence, and rightly says that, in such cases, he is cremated at the place of death and his bones are brought to his usual place and re-cremated. But, says he, in such references there is mention of many bones, the word used being *śarīrāṇi*. According to him the account from the *Mb*. has the dual (*śarīre*); hence, the word must indicate two actual bodies. He states that the description of the funeral rites from the *Mb*. (Ādi, 118) does not suit the "one bone"; for here we have Mādrī's body covered all over lest it should be seen by the sun or the wind-god; also that when the body of Pāṇḍu was covered with cloth he appeared to be as if alive. This does not suit the "one bone". Citing the authority of Sukthankar, who believes that not much of corpse would remain after the first burning for wrapping it with clothes and the application of sandal paste, he asserts, though guardedly, the second account has to be taken as more plausible. At the same time, he accepts Sukthankar's plea that there is no help from the text itself, and that there is no room for taking the first account as an interpolation! Both appear in all the manuscripts from the North as well as the South. As there is absolutely no help from the manuscripts, Mehendale resorts to interpretative arguments, with which we are not concerned here,[3] as they are based on imagination, which might be considered in the absence of direct evidence. Here, we are face to face with an equally authentic account of the bodies being burnt together before the sages arrived at Hastināpura. The conflict appears due to there being no word *śarīra* (singular), according to Mehendale, indicating the whole body in the ritual context. But, then, if we hunt it out the conflict gets automatically resolved! A point to be remembered is that, in such cases where both accounts are equally authentic, the contradiction has to be taken as only apparent; and it is better to probe further rather than resorting to arguments based on imagination. Let us examine the ritual references. These pertain to the death of the person away from his residence.

The *Ait. Br.* says that in such an event, somebody should go on pouring milk-offering in his regular fire at his place, up to the time the bones of the person cremated elsewhere in travel are brought (*Ait. Br.* VII.3 = 32.2: *āśarīrāṇām āhartoḥ*). Sāyaṇa renders the word *śarīrāṇām* as "bones" (*asthyādīnām*). While mentioning what is to be done to reconstruct the body symbolically, in the event of even the bones not being available, we have the expression *yadi śarīrāṇi na vidyeran (ib.)*. The *Kātyāyana Śrauta-sūtra* has *śarīrāṇi grāmasamīpam āhṛtya* (21.3.7). From these bones the figure of the dead was reconstructed (*ib.*, 25.8.14: *śarīrāṇī āhṛtya kṛṣṇājine puruṣavidhim vidhāya)*. Though this is all said for the *agnihotrin,* there is ground to hold that this practice was followed in the case of important persons (including women).[4] Well, here we have the word '*śarīra*' in the plural; and the *śarīra* at the *Mb.* would not get help from these expressions. But not also we do have the word *śarīra* (singular) indicating a jar wherein the bones (*śarīrāṇi*) were collected. Thus, at the *Baudhāyana-pitṛmedha-sūtra*, we have the following ritual. After the bones of the person, after the first cremation, are placed in a jar (starting from the feet-bones and going up to the head-bone), they are sprinkled over with milk to purify them. After that, liquid ghee is to be poured in the jar, on the arranged bones; this liquid symbolized the soul. The jar was the symbolic "body" (a symbol common throughout the Hindu tradition).[5] After the ghee was poured, or as it was being poured, the following was the address to be recited:

> This is the body of your own; this (ghee) is your soul; from your body does Brahmā distinguish your soul. (*idaṁ ta ātmanaḥ śarīram, ayaṁ ta ātmā; ātmanas ta ātmānaṁ śarīrād brahmā nirbhinatti; Bau. P.S.,* 3.10).

This would indicate that the jar containing bones (*śarīrāṇi*) was believed to be the very *śarīra*.

When this *śarīra* was re-made (in the form of a jar), it was coated with food-paste; it was then buried into the ground to be taken out for re-cremation whenever it was convenient. We have a similar concept and practice from the *K.Ś.S.* (21.3.7). Here it is prescribed that the *śarīrāṇi* (i.e., burnt bones) be brought from the place (where they were buried in a jar) to the village of the person; they were to be placed in a new jar on a pre-arranged cot; it was to be covered with new cloth; near-relatives would go round it from left to right (i.e., opposite the usual *pradakṣiṇā*, as it is the funeral), sounding small drums[6], etc., and fanning it. This would go on for the whole of the night. It was then taken to the place where it was to be finally buried and a mound (*śmaśāna*) was to be structured upon it. It could also be re-cremated.[7] The instruction at its being led away finally to the southern quarter is: "They go to the south along with the body" (in the form of the jar; *ib.* 13: *sa-śarīā dakṣiṇā gacchanti*). The word *sa-*

śarīrāḥ does not have the bones in view, but the unit of bones—the jar; and the commentator rightly explains it as *"saha śarīreṇa"*, which refers to the jar of bones. That the *śarīra* here is the jar of bones (as one unit) is clear from the fact, that it was offered food (*ib., annam asmā upa-haranty 'eke;* and comm. *asma asthikumbhāya...*). The jar in such cases had signs to indicate the gender of the person.[8] In an alternate practice, when the bones could not be had, a "body" was to be structured with the help of the twigs of *palāśa (Butea Frondosa),* numbering 360; they were arranged so as to make the human figure; and it was coated with barley-flour paste. When dried, cloth was wrapped over it (*Śāṅkhāyana Ś.S.,* IV. 15.20:... *yavacūrṇaiḥ pralipya).* This was the "body".[9]

What has been said above, would show that the "body" (*śarīra,* in the singular) was conceived to be in the form of the jar. The "two bodies" (*śarīre*) mentioned in the *Mb.* were of the sort described above; and there can be no question (or, even doubt) of "one bone" being taken as one "body". Nīlakaṇṭha, the commentator of the *Mb.*, has the right understanding of this tradition when he renders *śarīra* as *asthi*. As such, there is no contradiction between the two accounts from the *Mb.* that follow one another. There is, hence, no question of the second falsifying the first. Hence, also, there is no need to censure Nīlakaṇṭha as trying to gloss over the contradiction. The plea that certain portion has been lost is untenable, nor is it necessary to ask how the bodies could be without any decay for seventeen days and to believe that the passages mentioning the remedy to preserve them were also lost! Thus, the "bodies" could be either the jars containing bones, or the "body" made from the twigs of *palāśa*. The fact that the sages and Kuntī were witness to the death, and also the *sahagamana* (burning with the husband) of Mādrī, the other alternative (*palāśa*-twigs) has no place. One need not ask the question as to how the bones of the two could have been differentiated. After the jar-bodies were brought, they appear to have been re-made into big jars (though it is not specifically mentioned being unnecessary), which were later covered with fresh cloth and ornaments to give the semblance of actual bodies. The act for semblance, however, was not done for the jar-body of Mādrī; hence the mention that the sun and the wind-god could not see her. With ornaments on, Pāṇḍu's "body" taken in procession could well give the semblance of reality, with the royal umbrella and other things, poetic fancy allowed due scope! There is subtle similarity between the description at the *K.Ś.S.* and that at the *Mb.* Both have this rite as the *pitṛmedha.*

Mb.	*K.Ś.S.*
(1) *pitṛmedhaṁ labhatām* (117.33)	(1) *pitṛmedhaḥ saṁvatsarāt* (21.3.1)
(2) *amātya-jñātayaścaiva* (118.8)	(2) *amātyāḥ* (*ib.*, 8)
(At both places the meaning of this word is near-relations, *amā+tya*).	
(3) *ātapatra, cāmara, vyajana, vāditra* (*ib.*,10-11)	(3) *āyasa-vādya, vīṇā, chatrāṇi* (*ib.*,6); also *nṛttagītavāditra* (*ib.*, 11)
(4) *śātakumbha-ghaṭaiḥ* (sprinkling water from golden jars, 19)	(4) *kumbhān ādāya* (*ib.*, 6)

The things mentioned at the *K.Ś.S.* are necessary for the rite. The mention of these at the funeral procession at the *Mb.* also must be taken as necessary for the rite of re-cremation,[10] though royalty may have added to the things. When the procession reached the bank of the Gaṅgā, the "body" of Pāṇḍu is said to have been smeared with fragrant ointments; it was decorated with sandal paste and was covered with white cloth (118.20ff). But, this need not be the actual body; and, it was not! This could be equally true in the case of a big (life-size) jar. Such jars do obtain in rituals; and the ritual-performer has to sit in such jars.[11] When covered with cloth and decorated, it could very much give an *idea* of the very person.

Now, the point about Mādrī's *sahagamana*. The first account clearly mentions it. But, even in the second account, which would misguide a less careful reader in believing that actual dead bodies were brought (*tayoḥ śarīre*), we have a clear hint of *sahagamana*. After the "bodies" were brought to the bank of the Gaṅgā, and were treated with the unguents and cloth, the following is said:

> *ghṛtāvasiktaṁ rājānaṁ saha mādryā su-alaṅkṛtam /*
> *vidhinā samadāhayan / /*
> (*ib.*, 22-23)

"The people cremated the king together with Mādrī, after sprinkling him with ghee". The expression *saha samadāhayan* shows that both "bodies" were put on the same pyre.[12] If this was not the case of *sahagamana* where was the necessity of cremating the actual bodies (if at all they were actual) in the same pyre? Actually, the re-cremation of the jar-bodies was a re-enactment of the earlier cremation, wherein the two were cremated together. It has to be noted that there was only one carrier (*śibikā*) for both (*ib.*, 7: *śibikāṁ tām alaṅkṛtya)*, in which the king was tied up and carried with Mādrī (9: *avahan yānamukhyena saha mādryā su-saṁyatam;* this is more suitable for two jars placed side by side), thus showing the *sahatva*. When all this is taken into consideration, one more detail may be noted, which is that both the "bodies", when they were placed in the same '*śibikā*', were driven to the Gaṅgā in a vehicle drawn by men (*ib.,* 8-9: *nara-yuktena....yānamukhyena*). Whether this would be possible with the bodies that remained lifeless for (now) more than about three weeks, and had become heavy, is anybody's guess![13]

In this connection it will be proper to take note of the views expressed in an article, written subsequently, by Prof. Mehendale in which he has referred to my views on the topic. This is his paper read at a Seminar at the University of Poona, included later in the *Proceedings*.[14] This paper in English is a version of his article in Marathi, mentioned earlier. In both these his aim has been to take a wider survey of the custom of satī in ancient India, the episode of Mādrī being a part of it, though very striking. His observation that, the custom of satī (*saha-gamana*), "which was prevalent in the very distant past among the people who came to India had become obsolete at a time very much prior to the Vedic period" is totally acceptable. There can be no difference of opinion about the view that the custom was never an obligatory rule. A step further and one should say that *it should never be encouraged.* But, the reality in the *sahagamana* in the case of Mādrī has not been set aside successfully. It is not necessary to defend Nīlakaṇṭha, the commentator of the *Mb.,* but Mehendale's criticism of him has to be scrutinized. He criticizes Nīlakaṇṭha: (i) for interpreting the word *śarīra*, in the second narrative, as 'bone' (p.165) and questions the propriety of the sages bringing not two bodies but two bones, one each of Mādrī and Pāṇḍu; and (ii) for interpreting the word *deha* (Ādi I.26.4) as 'bones' (*asthi*), with the gloss that *deha* be taken as *dehayoḥ* (as indicating two bodies) finally meaning 'bones' (*asthīni*). Prof. Mehendale argues, "Now although, as noted above, the word *śarīra* in a definite context is found used in the meaning 'bone', the word *deha* is never so found. Secondly, in the description of the funeral rites that follow there is no reference to the *saṁskāra* having been done with the *agnihotra* fire" (p.167), while the commentary of Nīlakaṇṭha says that it should be so done (actually, the words of Nīlakaṇṭha are — *dehaṁ dehayor asthīni agnihotrāgnibhiḥ saṁskāra-lambhanārtham.* Prof. Mehendale also quotes them). It should be noted that there is no other place where the word *deha* occurs in this account. It is clear, that though the word *deha* (sing.) here is in respect of Pāṇḍu, Nīlakaṇṭha takes it in the sense of the dual, with the inclusion of Mādrī; then he gives the explanation *asthīni* to suggest that actual bodies were not meant, obviously in view of the first account, the one of *sahagamana*. Prof. Mehendale remarks that "Nīlakaṇṭha has interpreted the word *deha* as 'bone' under the influence of his knowledge of the *agnisaṁskāra* of an *agnihotrī* Brahmin" (*ib.*) The fact is that Nīlakaṇṭha has interpreted *deha* as "bones" (*asthīni*) indicating even one *deha* as a unit of bones; such two units, not one or two bones!

Now, there can be no doubt that the account of Pāṇḍu and Mādrī, like the ancient accounts, came through the oral tradition, prior to being set to writing. It is not, hence, probable that the bard who sang (may be after considerable lapse of time) would know the exact difference between the technical word *śarīra* (used at all other places in the account —which may even be a pretty earlier version) and the popular word *deha*, though he uses both these words (but *deha* only once).[15] It is not enough to say that Nīlakaṇṭha is influenced by his knowledge of the *agnisaṁskāra* of an *agnihotrī* Brahmin, in the sense of the word in his time, or even in the very modern times. In the ancient context, not excluding the *Mahābhārata,* one has to make a difference between the modern word Brahmin and a *dvija.* A *kṣatriya*—and a king to wit—was a *dvija*; and the preceptor of a king could certainly keep the fires.[16] This apart, the account of the *saṁskāra* in the case of Pāṇḍu, together with that of Mādrī (as noted earlier), has close similarity to the *saṁskāra* or re-cremation of an *agnihotrin* in the Śrauta-sūtras (as noted by me earlier). Prof. Mehendale does not take into account this point in my paper. Moreover, re-cremation was not restricted to an *agnihotrin.*[17] Not mentioning the jar on the part of Nīlakaṇṭha, as I have done, as pointed out by Prof. Mehendale (p.168) should not matter in the least. Nīlakaṇṭha's intention, obviously, was to help understanding the account rather than entering into a critical *śāstric* discussion (say, like a commentator of a Smṛti text). As to the statement of Prof. Mehendale, "(Prof. Dange) maintains that *śarīra* is after all used in the sense of 'bone' *even when used in the singular*" (his paper, p.167, where he mentions p.3 of my paper, now included here; italics mine), it has to be made clear that this statement is incorrect (as can be verified, as the said paper is included here without any change, whatsoever; see p.143f *supra*). It is to be stressed, that I have nowhere said, far less 'maintained' that the word *śarīra* (singular) is used in the sense of 'bone' (one may compare Prof. Mehendale's criticism of Nīlakaṇṭha - one 'bone'). I repeat what I said (for convenience of ready reference): "(*ib.*25.8.14 *śarīrāṇi āhṛtya kṛṣṇājine ...vidhāya*)... Well, here we have the word *śarīra* in the plural; and the *śarīra* at the *Mb.* would not get help from these expressions. But, we do have the word *śarīra* (singular) indicating a jar wherein the bones (*śarīrāṇi*) were collected." Further, Prof. Mehendale changes "we do have" in my paper to "we also have", attributing them to me, to suggest that I 'maintain': (i) that the word *śarīra* (singular) is used in the sense of 'bone'; and (ii) "also" that I take the word *śarīra* to indicate a jar (see his paper, p.167). To quote: "He (Dr.Dange) says that "...we also have the word *śarīra* (singular) indicating, etc." Prof. Mehendale leaves away the word "But" in my statement; further he inserts dots (...); and changes "we do have" to "... we also have". Why should these changes be made is unthinkable for me. Prof. Mehendale further remarks, "Dr. Dange also refers to the *Kātyāyana–Śrauta Sūtra* 21.3.7-13, and the *Śāṅkhāyana-Śrauta-Sūtra* (4.15.20), but in both these passages we do not have the use of the word *śarīram* (sing) in the sense of 'bone'." This, again, is not exactly correct. It is apt to misrepresent my stand like that of Nilakaṇṭha. One can see from my article that after referring to the Baudhāyana-Pitṛmedha-sūtra (3.10), where the word *śarīra* (singular) indicates a jar wherein the bones (*śarīrāṇi*) were collected, I mentioned the *Kātyāyana-śrauta-sūtra* (21.3.7) for a "similar concept and practice" for "re-making" the *śarīra (*body) *in the form of a jar* (see my article). Here also I never said that these two Sūtra-texts "use the word *śarīra (*sing) in the sense 'bone'." I have, all along, 'maintained' that the jar containing the bones (plural) was conceived as the body. I am happy to note that Prof. Mehendale accepts the reference to the *Bau.P.S.* where the word *śarīra* (singular) occurs in the sense of a *jar filled with bones*, after the first cremation. On the basis of this concept I explained the word *sa-śarīrāḥ* in *Kātyāyana-Ś.S.* (*loc.cit.*,13) as "They go... with the body (in the form of the jar)".[18] In this I have not to "rely on the commentator" (as Mehendale writes, see note 8, p.171 of his paper); it is to show how even the commentator thought likewise. I have also mentioned the other alternative of the 'body' being formed from the twigs of *palāśa*, not accepting it, as the sages and Kuntī are said to be witness to the cremation which took place earlier, and the alternative of the twig-body is when even the bones are not found indicating some mishap in a distant place. In the present case, at the most, there could be room for this second alternative in the absence of the clear words 'jar of bones', and the word *deha* (in the verse not accepted by the Crit.ed.) and the *śarīre* (two) could be taken as those formed from the twigs and coated with flour-paste, and the cloths, to give a semblance of an actual body. But, the bringing of actual bodies, which took seventeen days, does not appear feasible in spite of the second narration. It is not necessary to believe, with Prof. Mehendale, if we take note of other passages in the *Mb.*, that: (i) Mādrī died of a serious shock and that "since in the first narration it has been stated that Mādrī committed *satī*, the redactor responsible for the combination of the two versions could not retain the stanza in the second narration informing us that Mādrī died a natural death";[19] and (ii) that the dead bodies could be preserved by some method known to "the *tāpasas* living on the Himalayas or that here some element of the supernatural is involved since the sages who brought the bodies appear to be siddhas since they are said to have disappeared." These explanations, together with the so-called second version indicating that actual bodies were brought can only be termed 'apologetic', to refer to Andrew Lang, the famous mytho-anthropologist.[20] The second version appears to be an effort to negate the truth of the *sahagamana* of Mādrī, as it was a unique case (to take a clue from Prof. Mehendale's own argument of its being out of the common); it reflects only an 'effort to show' resentment towards the act, at the best. Looked from this angle, the probability is not of the redactor feeling shy of the express mention of the *sahagamana* of Mādrī and dropping the stanza (if it, at all existed) informing us of Mādrī's death by shock; on the contrary, the probability is of *sahagamana* and a subsequent cremation of the 'bodies' formed in the manner mentioned above. As the conventionalised words for body were pretty well known, there was hardly any need to use an expression such as 'jars containing the bones' (or *palāśa-śarīra*) and the like.

It is to be noted that, even earlier, the *Mb.* mentions the words of Mādrī which would leave no doubt about the reality that it was a case of *sahagamana* or *satī*, which is also *anugamana*. Thus, the sage who curses Pāṇḍu as he was disturbed and killed in the act of mating with a female-deer, himself in the form of a deer, says to him, "She (Mādrī, certainly will follow you in the pyre (*tvām anugamiṣyati*), when you go to the region of the god of the dead." Later we have Mādrī speaking to Kuntī, just after the sudden death of Pāṇḍu, "I shall alone follow (*anuyāsyāmi*) my dead husband;" and further, "With the king's body my body also should be burnt, well concealed with his; O lady, do this, which is to my liking";[21] and, just after this we have, "Saying this, that righteous wife, that daughter of the king of the Madras, swiftly ascended to the mighty king posited on the funeral fire".[22] This would set aside the shock -death suggestion, along with the plea that a stanza to that effect might have been dropped by the redactor. Why should this conversation of Mādrī with Kuntī, whom she is said to have called upon to approach her leaving the children, immediately after the death of her husband, be set aside? It shows Mādrī fully determined, after her initial shock, to ascend the pyre. Hence, the puzzling question of preserving the bodies does not arise. For the sudden death of Pāṇḍu and Mādrī's (desire and) getting burnt along with him the myth of the sage, Kindam, in the form of a deer, is introduced. The word *anugamiṣyati* cannot be taken to mean, simply, 'will die'. It has the sense of *anugamana*. Thus, the fact of the death of Pāṇḍu and the burning of Mādrī is couched in the myth. This was to explain the, rather, uncommon event of the *satī* of a woman in the royal family of the Kurus.[23] Needless to say that a supernatural element in a narration has to be taken as mythical in a scientific study. To take it as real is not acceptable. So is the case of the *siddhas*, who are said to have disappeared suddenly, along with the *tāpasa*-s, and that it was a miracle like *gandharvanagara*.

NOTES AND REFERENCES

1. The references are to the Crit. Ed. BORI, Poona.
2. His article in Marathi, "Satī—Kāhīn Prācīna Sandarbha", *Navabhārata,* Wai (Maharashtra), Jan.1988. This stand he maintains even in his later article. See note 14 *infra.*
3. *Ibid.*, pp.6ff. of his article. To mention one example: that, as no other woman from the Kuru family performed *satī*, it is more probable that Mādrī must not have done so.
4. See *Garuḍa P.,* II. 16.45:

   kṛṣṇājinaṁ samāstīrya kuśaiśca puruṣākṛtim / śata-traya - ṣaṣṭi-yutair vṛntaiḥ prokto' sthisañcayaḥ / /

   See. P.V. Kane, *Hist. of Dh.S.*, Vol.IV, Poona, 1973 (1946), p.225
5. We may compare such expressions as *ghaṭasphoṭa,* meaning severance of marital relationship, indicating a symbolic rite; also such as *ghaṭa ghaṭa hai antaryāmī* ('God is in every *ghaṭa'*, i.e., in every human body). The belief

is reflected in the *Garuḍa P.* II.27.7:

mānuṣasya śarīre tu asthnām eve ca sañcayaḥ /
udakumbhena puṣṭāni tāny' asthīni bhavanti hi / /

6. The words are: *āyaseṣu vādyamāneṣu;* and the commentator explains as, *vāditreṣu paṭahādiṣu* for *āyaseṣu;* Weber explains *āyaseṣu* as *lohamayeṣu*, indicating that the drums were made of iron; see *K.Ś.S*, ed. by Albert Weber with extracts from the commentaries of Karka and Yājñikadeva, Chawkhamba, Varanasi (New print), 1972.
7. *K.Ś.S.* 25.8.7: *kumbhe sañcayanam;* and 14; *pūrvavad dāhaḥ*
8. *Āśv. G.S.* IV.5.2.
9. Also compare *K.Ś.S,. loc.cit.* (quoted earlier above); *Śat.Br.* has about the same passage (XII.5.1.13) except that it has the word *asthīni* for the usual *śarīrāṇi.*
10. It may be of interest to note in this connection, that these details are not mentioned at the funeral of Daśaratha (*Rām.* Ayodhyā, 76.13ff) and also of Prabhākaravardhana at the *Harṣacaritam* (5); there it is not re-cremation.
11. *Matya P.*, 274.4-13; see Dange, *Ency. P.B. & P.,* Vol.III, New Delhi, 1986, p.934 f.
12. Even Mehendale renders this passage to mean that both the bodies were placed on the same pyre and consigned to flames; see p.4 of his article.
13. There is no mention of any remedy to keep the corpses free from decay. To imagine that the verses to that effect might have been lost is too spacious a suggestion.
14. "The custom of Sahagamana, some early references", *Proceedings* of The National Seminar on Living Customs and Their Ancient Indian Sources, Centre of Advanced Study in Sanskrit, University of Poona, 1991, pp.159-171.
15. The verse with the word *deha*, hence, seems doubtful. It does not occur in the Critical ed.
16. The *Mb.*, Āśramavāsika, 37.11 says that Dhṛtarāṣṭra stayed in the forest, with Gāndhārī, Kuntī and Sañjaya with his *agnihotra* fire and with the sacrificing priests; cf. *sāgnihotraḥ sayājakaḥ;* he was burnt in the wild fire caused by his 'own fire', cf. 39.5 *agninā...svena;* also 39.7 *svenāgninā*; even in the present context, the fires that were taken out of the city for the re-cremation were his own and carried by his priests, Ādi 126.6. (Here I am referring to the Gorakhpur Ed., which is ready at hand.)

17. Cf. P.V. Kane, *Hist. of Dh.S.* Vol.IV, 2nd Ed., 1973, Poona, p.225, where he refers to the *Vaikhānasa-smārta-sūtra* (V.12) to say that the burning of an effigy was a meritorious act for every one and, further (referring to the Śuddhiprakāśa, p.187) that it was to be followed even in the case of one who has not consecrated Śrauta fires.
18. The text is *saśarīrā gacchanti;* see my main article.
19. Mehendale, *op.cit.,* p.168.
20. *Myth, Ritual* and *Religion,* London, 1913 (1887), p.11f.
21. Ādi., 124.29 (Crit. ed. 116.29).
22. *Ibid.*, v31 (Crit. ed. 116.31). This seems to be the version accepted by the *Mahābhārata;* cf. also Ādi (Gorakhpur ed.) 95.65, the speech of Mādrī, *tatraiva citāgnistham mādrī samanvāruroha;*66, where the *tāpasa*-s are mentioned as going to Hāstinapura, telling about the incident and disappearing; but there is no mention of the dead bodies being taken to Hāstinapura.
23. Kane refers to the *Bhāgavata* P. I.13.57 to state in the context of *satī,* that Gāndhārī burnt herself on the death of her husband; for this he mentions Raghunandana (Śuddhitattva), stating that he quotes the passage from the *Bhāgavata P.* However, it is doubtful if that passage could be taken as an example of *satī.* It says that Dhṛtarāṣṭra got burnt in his cottage in the forest; Gāndhārī was standing outside; when she saw her husband being enveloped in fire in the cottage, she also entered it. The *Mb.* Āśramavāsika, 37.29-36, however, says that Dhṛtarāṣṭra and Gāndhārī, along with Kuntī, were burnt by the forest-fire.

* Included here from *Bhāratī* (*Bulletin of the College of Indology,* Banaras Hindu University), Vol.17, Varanasi, 1987.

Chapter 12

Stūpa — Vedic and Buddhistic

As the evidence stands, the word *stūpa* has been associated mostly with the Buddhistic structure of a peculiar type, in the post-Buddhistic period. It is also well known, that the word *stūpa* was not restricted to the funeral mounds even in the Buddhistic context. Some *stūpa*-s came to be built even on the belongings of the dead *arhat*, or even with nothing inside. It is proposed by some scholars that the Buddhistic *stūpa*-s were the result of imitation of the Vedic funeral mounds.[1] The same is the opinion about the *caitya,* the difference being only structural rather than conceptual. Though, as mentioned above, it was pointed out that the *stūpa* was an imitation of the Vedic funeral mounds, it is necessary to go into the details, which have not been worked out by scholars. It is also said that the *stūpa* was the direct descendant of the sepulchral mounds of the Turanians, because the Hindus never buried, but burned their dead, and hence, there was not tumuli in the latter practice.[2] The similarity between the Buddhistic *stūpa* was, further, said to be that the Turanian mound was based on the practice of the tent-burial and the hut-burial.[3] However, even if one tolerates this suggestion, the question is, why was the Buddhistic *stūpa* called *stūpa?* It is also suggested, that the *stūpa* has Persian affinities. It is proposed that the Persians migrated to the Panjab (India), and further still to

Magadha, which was inhabited by the Vrātyas.[4] The indication is, that the Licchavis were (influenced by?) the Vrātyas and imitated the Turanian custom; or, that the Licchavis borrowed the custom of the Turanians through the Vrātyas, and the Buddhistic custom of the *stūpa* was influenced by the Licchavis. This is a rather spacious argument; and, in the absence of a solid proof of the Turanian remains of that period, it is difficult to accept it. About the suggestion of the Persian influence the same is true; and that the Hindus never buried their dead is an example of incomplete observation of a time (1876) when Hindu practices do not seem to have been fully known by the author.[5]

The Buddhistic *stūpa* is of two types: one with the square base and the other with the round base. Both these types show a rounded or elongated top, surmounted by the *harmikā* or the *chatra*. The *chatra* or the *harmikā*, however, cannot be taken as the original integral part of the *stūpa*. The essential *stūpa*-structure has to be taken as either a rounded top or as an elongated one, over a square or a rounded base. If we try to get some clue from the elongated top *stūpa* of Svayambhūnātha in Nepal, we might say that the top formed the head superimposed by a conic helmet; the square frame just below it serves for the face of the Buddha. The antiquity of the belief cannot be determined with certainty; but, it must be said that it is very old.[6] It appears that *stūpa* is mentioned, for the first time, in the Vinaya texts. The Chabbaggiya nuns are said to have made a *stūpa* over the remains of their leader.[7]

The Buddha himself mentions the *thūpa* and recommends it for the Tathāgata, the Arhat, and the Paccekabuddha, the structure being over the remains of the dead (*śarīra-stūpa*). In this context he says, that these persons deserve the *stūpa* as does a king, indicating thereby that the construction of the *stūpa* was not for an ordinary person, but for one of high rank including a respectable mendicant.[8]

A very ticklish problem presents itself if one traces the source of the practice and the name *thūpa*. There is no doubt that the word *thūpa* has its origin in the Vedic word *stūpa*. However, the Vedic evidence hardly supports the equation of *stūpa* with any funeral mound. The point deserves close study. It is said that Varuṇa, the king, established the *stūpa* in the form of a 'tree' in the bottomless void (*Ṛgveda* = *ṚV*. 1.24.7: *vanasya stūpam*). This is the earliest concept of the world tree, a veritable *axis mundi*; but the 'tree' is not an ordinary one. Its shoots spread downwards, while its root is up. This is also not a naturally grown tree; because, Varuṇa is said to have *placed* it (*dadate;* and Sāyaṇa *dhārayati*). It should be noted, that the *Kaṭha-upaniṣad* (II.3.1) and the *Bhagavadgītā* (XV.1) which borrow the same imagery, replace the word *stūpa* with *aśvattha*, which, unlike the former (i.e. *stūpa*) is the name of a tree. The *stūpa* is not indicative of 'tree' as such, though in the expression *vanasya stūpam* the former would indicate 'wood'. The primary meaning of *stūpa* is 'collection' (fr. √*styai*); and, in this case, 'an arrangement in the form of a tree'. However, this 'tree' has its supporting bottom (*budhna*) up in the sky. The later texts, mentioned above, change the word *budhna* to *mūla* (root-source). If one fixes one's attention on the Vedic image alone, the *stūpa* of Varuṇa would have a rounded bottom up. From it the streaks of light (*ketavaḥ*) would shoot down (*nīcīnāḥ syuḥ*). These streaks of light were changed to 'branches' in the later texts, as they changed the *stūpa* to the *aśvattha* tree. In the original (Vedic) image, *the budhna* is the sun-disk, or the curved canopy of the sky; and the *stūpa* is the mass (collection) of light-rays that shoot from it and reach the earth. There is another place in *ṚV* where Agni is described as *aruṣa-stūpa* (III.29.3), where the *stūpa* is sought to be differentiated from the deity, the fire-god, and appears to indicate the tuft of hair, or helmet, in the form of flames. This gets support from the name Hiraṇyastūpa, where also the *stūpa* occurs as the second member of the compound. The word *hiraṇyastūpa* would mean 'one having the *stūpa* of gold'. Hiraṇyastūpa was the seer of *ṚV* X.149 (see esp. verse 5) and was from the family of Aṅgiras. The word *stūpa* here would indicate a helmet, or a cap, or even the bunch of hair tied in a knot on the head. This would give a twofold image of *stūpa:* (i) elongated mass (cf. *stūpa* of Varuṇa) with a separate *budhna;* and (ii) a canopy-like, or hair-knot like rounded top (as we see in the case of the hair of the Buddha). The latter gets support where *stūpa* is the word used for the upper back portion of the head, along with the knot of hair tied up (*Taitt. Br.* III.3.6.5; *Pañcaviṁśa-brāhmaṇa* XIII.4.4). At the *Pañcaviṁśa-brāhmaṇa* noted above, there is a graphic suggestion for *stūpa* being the rounded upper portion of the head. In the context of a ritual, it is said, as an explanation, that the horns are more pointed than the *stūpa* and the commentator, Sāyaṇa, explains: "*stūpa* is the central portion between the horns" (*stūpaḥ śṛṅgayor madhyaḥ saṁhito deśaḥ*). This is in the case of the actual head. By extension to a cover on the head, it would mean that a rounded helmet is the *stūpa;* or, any rounded cover, or a canopy would be *stūpa*. This is one aspect. But, when the fire is said to be *aruṣa-stūpa*, as noted above, or at another place Agni is invoked to touch the top of heaven with his *stūpa*-s (*ṚV* VII.2.1:*upa spṛśa divyam sānu stūpaiḥ*), the *stūpa*-s are the formation of the tapering flames that rise upwards. In the first case (the *stūpa* of Varuṇa) the Buddhist *stūpa* with the rounded dome is answered; in the second the one that is conic.

How are we to explain the fact, that, though the word *stūpa* is known to the *Ṛgveda*, and even the later texts mention it, it does not occur in the funeral context in the Vedic tradition, while in the Buddhist tradition it is so used? Taking the clue from what the Buddha has said, and noted above, in the case of the *stūpa* for special persons, we could say that the Vedic custom was to build some sort of a mound over the ashes of the dead; but, in some special cases such a mound might have been more spectacular, with a tapering or dome-like canopy-like structure. But, it was not given the name *stūpa*, as the word was used in auspicious contexts, like the flames of the sacrificial fire, or a divine pole, as noted above. The rounded or canopy-like structure might have been made for kings or special priests. An interesting indication to that effect is in the request of the sage Vasiṣṭha, who implores on Varuṇa to see that he (Vasiṣṭha) does not go to the house made of clay (*ṚV*. VII.89.1: *mo ṣu varuṇa mṛṇmayaṁ gṛhaṁ rājann ahaṁ gamam*). The clay-house is the monument on the ashes of the dead. That this prayer is in view of the impending death is clear from the words in a later verse from the same hymn, "As I am getting swelled like a leather-bag bloated with air" (*ibid*.2), indicating dropsy or some such terminal disease. This hymn was for a person suffering from dropsy.[9] Though the custom was to collect the bones, after cremation, in an urn, it is not probable that the word *gṛha* 'house' refers to the small urn. It is more probable, that it refers to a bigger structure on the urn after it was buried in the earth. Though it is not called *stūpa*, for the probable reason given above, it brings to our mind the *maṭṭikā-thūpa* of the Buddhistic tradition. This structure, called *gṛha*, must have been in appearance like a small house with a thatched dome and held inside in the urn. This must have been for special persons, while for the commoners there was the less elaborate mound called *śmaśāna*, which was the 'resting place for the body' (cf. Yāska, *Nirukta* III.1: *śma= śarīra+śāna = śayanam),* or the mound whereunder the body (in the form of the bones collected after cremation) 'slept'. As the Vedic ritual texts deal with the sacrificial aspect of life, and the practices that are commonly followed, there is hardly any room for royal and stately funeral monuments. But, indications in the *mṛṇmayam-gṛham* can not be bypassed. The *śmaśāna*, and likewise the 'clay-house' was not built immediately after the cremation and the collection of the bones. It was built after some period had passed, and away from the locality. The *śmaśāna* was of two types: the square one and the round one. The square one was for the followers of the Vedic gods (*daivyāḥ prajāḥ*) and the round one was for those belonging to the *asura*-s (*asuryāḥ prajāḥ*). It is further said, that the one for the 'godly people' (i.e., Vedic) was not separated from the ground, while the other one was separated (*Sat. Br.* XIII.8.1.1ff). The Vedic *śmaśāna*-s were of different sizes, depending upon the *varṇa* of a person. For a *brāhmaṇa* it was high up to the mouth of a person; that for a *kṣatriya* it was up to the chest; for a *vaiśya* it was up to the thighs and for a *śudra* it had to be up to the knees. For a woman (of all *varṇa*-s) it was to be up to the hips.

From what has been noted above, the Buddhistic *stūpa* appears to have been evolved from the *śmaśāna* structure mentioned in the Vedic texts. It is not improbable that the *asurya* type mentioned therein, the round one, was borrowed by the Buddhists from a non-Vedic practice. It is not necessary to believe that the *asurya* practice was of a non-Indian origin; and, though it was non-Vedic, there was a continuous effort for the assimilation of the Vedic and the non-Vedic. The post-Ṛgvedic texts on ritual, as a rule, stress that the gods and the *asura*-s were both sons of Prajāpati, though they always contested. As has been said earlier, there seems a probability of the *stūpa*-like structure being prevalent even among the more affluent and honoured persons who followed the Vedic religion. This structure called *gṛha* must have been over and above the *śmaśāna;* but the word *stūpa* was not popularly used for it. However, there is no doubt that the Buddhistic word *stūpa* presupposes its use even among the Vedic people, though it is not recorded. How else could the word be suddenly seen used for such a structure in the Buddhistic literature? It is clear that, like the word *vihāra*, they adopted it from the usage of the Vedic people. The word *vihāra* is also from the Vedic sacrificial context;[10] it is for the enclosure where the fires were kept. The Buddhists adopted such word for status.

Another word to be considered in this context is *caitya*. This word does not occur in the Vedic texts as such. It is seen used in the Sūtra period, which concurs with the rise of the Buddha and the Buddhistic faith, and also with the rise of the Jain faith. However, *caitya* was more prevalent in the Jain faith, and among all these faiths it was not restricted to the mound or structure over the ashes of the dead. As in the later period the *stūpa* was erected even on a hair or a nail of a living Buddha, the *caitya* came to be any thing including a hall, a tree and a shrine. The later Buddhistic faith applied the term *caitya* also for a funeral mound. This is clear from the account that a Bodhisattva called Sarvasattva Priyadarśana wrapped his body with the cloth steeped in aromatic oils and set fire to it, and caused to be erected as many as 84,000 (obviously a mythical number!) *caitya*-s.[11] A regular practice of preparing *caitya-s* from the clay mixed with oil and honey and cutting them lengthwise obtains in the later Buddhistic period among the Buddhists of Nepal, along with the gift of such miniature *caitya*-s.[12] Among the Jains initiation took place in a *caityālaya*,[13] and one Hindu *Gṛhyasūtra* speaks of *Caitya-yajña*. It is the *Āśvalāyana G.S.* (I.12.1-4) which recommends even sending an offering to a *caitya*, if it is in a far off place. In any case, the origin of the *caitya* is in *citi* or *cita*, which is 'pile'; and the earliest concept of the *citi*, and hence of the *caitya*, is in the Vedic rite of *Agnicayana*. The *Śat. Br.* (VI.2.3.1) uses the word *citi*. There is mention of various such *citi*-s or *cita*-s in the context of the *Agnicayana*, including the *śmaśāna-cita*;[14] and the *Agnicayana* rite goes back far prior to the pre-Buddhistic period, as it is mentioned in the post-Ṛgvedic Saṁhitās. The *Agnicayana* is, virtually, *Agniciti*; or, in other words, we may call it *Agnicaitya*, though no structure remained at the place after the rite was over. The worship of the *caitya* continued in the Hindu tradition. The *Rām* (Ayodhyā 56.33)[15] and the *Mb*. (Vana

190.67) mention it. In fine we could say, that the *stūpa*[16] and the *caitya* have their origin in the Vedic practice and concept.

NOTES AND REFERENCES

1. T.N. Ramachandran, "A Brief Survey of Buddhistic Art", in: *2500 Years of Buddhism,* Govt. of India Pbn., New Delhi, 1976 (1959), p.247.
2. J. Fergusson, *History of Indian and Eastern Architecture,* Vol.I, Delhi, 1967, p.65.
3. *Ibid.*
4. S. Vidyabhusana, "Persian Affinities of the Licchavis", in: *Indian Antiquary,* Vol.37, 1908, p.79.
5. The author was, obviously, speaking about the general practice in ancient India. There are some castes among the Hindus who practise burial; and, with children burial is the general practice.
6. J. Fergusson, *op.cit.* p.276.
7. Meena V. Talim, "Origin of the Chabbaggiyas", *Proceedings of the Prakrit Seminar,* University of Bombay, Bombay, 1971, p.214.
8. *Mahāparinirvāṇasūtra,* ed. Bhiksu Kittima, published by U.Kyo-Zan, Akyab, Burma, printed at the Indian Press Ltd., Benares, Vikrama Saṁvat 1998 (= A.D. 1941), pp. 110-112 (sūtra-s 191-195).
9. H.D. Velankar, *Ṛgveda - Maṇḍala VII*, Bharatiya Vidya Bhavan, Bombay, 1963, p.195.
10. P.V. Kane, *History of Dharmaśāstra*, Vol.II, pt.II, B.O.R.I., Second edn., Poona, 1974, p.984.
11. Rajendralal Mitra, *Sanskrit Buddhist Literature of Nepal*, Cosmo Pbn., Delhi, 1981 (1882), p.206. The number is mythical; cf. 84,000 years of separation between the Buddha and Śreṇiya Bimbisāra; also the Hindu concept of a cycle of 84000 births (*yoni*-s). Fergusson, *op.cit.,* p.67, appears to take the number as real.
12. Rajendralal Mitra, *op.cit.,* p.256; gifts of clay-*caityas*, p.229; *caitya-vrata,* p.279, etc.
13. Sindhu S. Dange, *Jaina Dharma āṇi Tattvajñāna,* Continental Prakashan, Pune, 1980, p.138.
14. Cf. *Taitt. Sam,* V.4.10 where the word is *cita;* some of the

cita-s mentioned are *śyenacita, kaṅkacita, droṇacita;* and *śmaśānacita.*

15. The *Rām.* mentions here the establishing of Vedic altars along with the *caityasthāna*-s.
16. It may be noted that a *stūpa* found in the precincts of Vat Vishun in Luang Prabang (Laos) has a flame-like projection at the top. Otherwise it is similar to the *stūpa* at Sanchi, which has a rounded top; see T.N Ramachandran, *op.cit.,* p.265.

* Included here from the *Oriental Journal,* Sri Venkateswara University, Vol. XXXVII, Jan.-Dec.1994, pts. 1 & 2.

Chapter 13

Purāṇa and Śāstra*

Like many words that have come down to us, and have lost their original connotation, the word Purāṇa has had some shifts in its meaning. The general meaning of this word is 'old'. It is also used in common language to indicate a much prolonged (or, we may coin a new word, prolengthened) discourse, or narration. However, in the context of this paper the word has the connotation of a particular type of literature or, better, a mass of traditional knowledge. In this sense, Purāṇa is first mentioned in the *Atharvaveda* (XI.7.24), where it says that, along with other things, the *ṛc*-s, *sāman*-s, *chandas*-es (i.e. the metres), the Purāṇa and the *yajus* formulas were created from the principle called *ucchiṣṭa* ('that which remains'). At another place this Veda includes the Purāṇa in the list where other types of lore are mentioned, such as *gāthā*-s, *nārāśaṁsī*-s, and also *itihāsa* (XV.6.11,12). At this time, the nature of Purāṇa was not strictly defined yet it was known as an important branch of knowledge. This is clear from the fact that, like other types mentioned above, Purāṇa is also included in the list of such types that are said to follow the Vrātya, wherever

* Keynote Address at the Seminar on "Purāṇaśāstra", Sanskrit Sahitya Academy, Gandhinagar and North Gujarath University, Patan, Jan., 4-5, 1998.

he went (*AV* XV.6.11,12). The *Śat.Br.* mentions Purāṇa (XI.5.6.8); and, in the context of the Pāriplava, the cycle of narrations to be recited daily at the Horse-sacrifice till the released horse came back after one year, various lores are prescribed to be recited for various tribes of men (XIII.4.3.2ff.). These are all common people, and it is prescribed that the king and the other people who gathered there should be entertained "with some *purāṇa*" (*ib.* XIII.4.3.13 *kañ* cit *purāṇam ācakṣīta*). The reason for reciting a Purāṇa is as interesting as it is illuminating. It is said, that at this daily congregation, many persons would be coming together; and many of them might not know the Veda and the Vedic language. Among them, for one tribe, on a particular day, some Purāṇa was to be recited, as its special *'veda'*. Here, the word used for knowers of the Veda is *śrotriya*. Many in this assemblage would be *aśrotriya*. Hence the prescription of Purāṇa.[1] This marks a clear difference, that the type of lore called Purāṇa was meant for the common masses. This difference between the elite and the common has been prevalent in all societies, and at all ages. Thus, we speak of King's English and the common English, the former being for the elite and those associated with the royal court. The case of the Sanskrit language is the same. Prākṛta is for the commoners, while Saṁskṛta is for the elite, as the very names show. Hence, even the language of the extant Purāṇa texts shows a trend which, at many places, diverges from the Sanskṛta written, or spoken, according to the normative Pāṇinian rules formulated two thousand and more years ago. Though the language of the Purāṇas is not Prākṛta, as such, there is no doubt that this type of lore was meant for the commoners.[2]

The point to be noted in this connection, i.e., of the relationship between the language of the *śrotriya*-s and that of the other lores, including that of the Purāṇa, even in the ancient Vedic period, is that the *śrotriya*-s could understand the language in which the other lores, including the Purāṇa, was recited. It could also be a language akin to the Vedic Sanskrit, though not strictly the Sanskrit of the Vedas. There is indication, that these lores were recited by the Hotṛ priest on the command of the Adhvaryu. This means that this language had become also of the commoners. Actually the *śrotriya* was the one who had the knowledge of Vedic language and could recite the *chandas* in addition to his ability to speak and also understand the language of the common people. Like the Purāṇa, which had the connotation of 'the lore of the common people', *śrotra* denoted a class of lore (and Vedic lore, for that matter), which included Vedic lauds, other verses and ritual-*mantras*. The Ṛgveda is clear about this concept of the *śrotra*, as is clear in the description of the car of Sūryā at her marriage, where its wheels are said to comprise the *śrotra* (*ṚV* X.85.11[c] *śrotram te cakre āstām*).[3] It should be noted that, the *śrotra* is differentiated from the *ṚC* and the *Sāman,* which are said to be tethers of the bullocks at the car (*ib. ṛksāmābhyām abhihitau),* the bullocks being the sun and the moon (as Sāyaṇa thinks). Thus, *śrotra*, as distinct from the *Ṛgveda* and other Saṁhitās, spoken of individually, is the whole class of Vedic lore, including the ritual. The one who knows the *śrotra* is the *śrotriya.* This word occurs first in the *AV* (IX. 6.37; X.2.20.21), and got currency in the later literature. The *Śat.Br.*, as we have noted above, makes a difference between the *śrotriya* and the commoner, and prescribes Purāṇa for the latter, which could also be understood by the *śrotriya.* This prescription is in view of the fact, that, on that day, the commoners came to attend the Pāriplava.

A finer analysis of the concept behind the word *purāṇa,* and of the nature of the lore called Purāṇa, is suggested by Yāska. He mentions (as seen from the com.) other alternative words for *purāṇa*, such as *pratna, pradivas, pravayas* and so on; but, for the lore, known in his time as Purāṇa, he has an explanation which hints at the nature of Purāṇa. He asks, *"purāṇam kasmāt?"* and explains, *"purā navam bhavati*", i.e., the lore which is called Purāṇa is both *purā* and also *nava* (*Nir*. III.19 *purā navam bhavati*). He further explains the word *nava,* by saying that it is 'brought forward' (*ib. navam kasmāt? ānītam bhavati)*. That serves as the exact nature of the Purāṇa. It is brought forward in the tradition; and, it is never new, in the sense that it is accepted by the later generations. In other words, it is considered as traditional belonging. The implication is that Purāṇa is as old as the Veda and also that it developed side by side with the Veda. This is why, the *Śat. Br.* (XIII.4.3. 3ff) calls these lores, including Purāṇa, Veda. This shows the sanctity that they had acquired. Though it has been difficult to give a crisp and clear definition of the term Purāṇa, one has to accept, that Yāska's was the very first attempt to define it; and he did it splendidly. To put in the style we have been accustomed to, it would be: 'Purāṇa is ancient traditional knowledge that assumes ever new gloss, being on par with the Veda, for the common people.' Having a broad base, and common appeal, this type of lore gets getting fattened with new additions, together with new interpretations of the old events. Its one foot is in the Vedic lore, while the other touches new fields. The latter foot treads on contemporary ground, while the earlier one brings with it the vestiges of the past. It, thus, assumes the nature of a compendium of the old and the new, or Vedic and Popular new factors — customs, manners, rites and so on. Here, the Purāṇa gets the status of Itihāsa. This is the reason, why at many places, Itihāsa and Purāṇa are spoken of together. The nature of the Purāṇa as a social compendium, in course of time, gave it the status of not only a *vidyāsthāna* but also of a *dharmasthāna.*[4] Kauṭilya, the date of whose *Arthaśāstra* more or less concurs with that of *Manusmṛti*, ordains that a king should regularly, and daily in the afternoon, hear the Purāṇa and the Itihāsa (*Artha*. 1.5.14). He also mentions the *paurāṇika*, who, he says, is the *sūta* or the *māgadha (ib*., III. 7.29). The indication is, that he was specially employed by the king to acquaint him with popular code of conduct and tales about the same, from the past. Here the *paurāṇika* is said to be the son of a mixed union (*paurāṇikastv-anyaḥ, sūto māgadhaś ca; brahmakṣatrād viśeṣaḥ),* and a *sūta* or a *māgadha.* However, at another place (*ib.,* V.3.13), he is differentiated from the *sūta* and the *māgadha* (cf. *kārtāntika-naimittika-mauhūrtika-paurāṇika-sūtamāgadhāḥ*).[5] The first context is of the type of sons, i.e., *pratiloma;* the second is of appointments of officers and servants (*bhṛtya-bharaṇīyam).* Even when the duty of the *paurāṇika* is stipulated, it is not clear, from these references, whether there were more than one Purāṇas. All that is clear is, that there could have been (and this is very probable) a number of floating accounts which went by the general name '*purāṇa*'. This gets support from the mention of *purāṇāni* even prior to the Christian era (cf. *Manu Sm.* III.232; *Mb.* Strī 13.2), not to speak about the *Yājñavalkyasmṛti* (III.189) of the third-fourth century A.D. The *Mb.* (Svargārohaṇa, 5.46-47) mentions the number of the Purāṇas as eighteen (*aṣṭādaśa-purāṇāni*). But their names are not yet mentioned. Even in the absence of any specific names in the texts mentioned above, it is not difficult to accept the statement, that "At least some of the extant purāṇas were composed in the first centuries of the Christian era".[6] This implies that, prior to the Christian era, the extant Purāṇas were not known; also, they were not specified as such. Before we take up the point about the Purāṇa being a *śāstra,* we shall do well to see how the spread of Puranic texts was worked out. When Purāṇas came to be classed on the names of various deities, the stage of oral transmission was already over; and these texts came to be written. It seems, rather, improbable that, at the stage of oral communication or recitation of the Purāṇas, the expanse of these texts was very large. But, when they came to be written down, their spread was brought about with a unique method. This was also the stage when the deity of the Purāṇa was believed to be present in the Purāṇa.

At this stage, it came to be faithfully believed that, by copying a Purāṇa manuscript, the deity of the Purāṇa was pleased and virtue was gained. The common method was to copy the whole, or part of a Purāṇa and gift it to a *brāhmaṇa*. It could also be kept in a temple. Various Purāṇa manuscripts, this way, came to be copied, and for various purposes. The gift of the Purāṇa, or keeping a manuscript thereof, came to be believed to ward off untimely death, atone for sins committed, and what not! Regular assemblages for the reading, and hearing, of the Purāṇas were arranged. The most popular such reading was of the *Bhāgavata Purāṇa*. The cycle of such reading, generally, comprised seven days (called *saptāha,* which term is current even today). For such *saptāha*-s arrangements were elaborately made; and the persons attending them were housed in temporarily structured sheds or tents. They had to follow strict rules during this period. They had to observe celibacy; they had to sleep on the ground, and take food in plates made of leaves *(Padma P.,* Uttarakhaṇḍa 194.47 *brahmacaryam adhaḥ-suptiḥ patrāvalyām ca bhojanam)*. Even the *Purāṇika* had to observe strict rules, being ready before sunrise. The reading had to start exactly at sunrise. His seat was on a higher level than the audience. He faced the north, while the audience faced the east. The session went on till the third part of the day, with short break at midday for taking food. The *puraṇika* was called Vyāsa, and was not to bow down to anybody once he assumed the seat. He was also to be a *brāhmaṇa* by birth and by his side there was to be a helper. He was also to be learned, able to satisfy the audience in case somebody had any doubt about any detail in the narration (*ib.*25 *paṇḍitaḥ saṁśaya-chettā lokabodhana-tatparaḥ*). The change of the caste of the *paurāṇika* from the earlier times to that of the *purāṇika*[7] of the period, when the Purāṇa texts were written down, and were classified according to the deities and on other principles, has to be noted. Interesting details of the retribution for breaking the restrictions on the part of the audience appear. It is said, that a person chewing betel leaves while hearing the Purāṇa would go to hell, after death, and would be made to eat the excreta of a dog (*Skanda P.* II. 1.27.47).[8] It was also ordained that, while the Purāṇa session went on, none should wear his turban on the head, for fear of getting born with the brain of just a child for the whole of the next birth.

THE ŚĀSTRA

The first, and the foremost, point to be sorted out is: In what way is the Purāṇa (a class-name for all the Purāṇas) a *śāstra*? According to the ancient tradition, Purāṇa is the Veda, as we have seen (cf. the context of the Pāriplava, noted above); and even the Puranic tradition calls it Veda, i.e., the fifth Veda.[9] This is because this lore comprises traditional knowledge. In common usage, Veda is differentiated from *śāstra* in which an expression as *veda-śāstra-sampanna*, which hints at a person who is well-versed in both Veda and the *śāstra*. However, Veda, in one of its aspects, is a *śāstra*. The Saṁhitā portion is, in essence, Veda, while the Brāhmaṇa portion, which forms part of the general mass known as Veda (cf. *mantra-brāhmaṇayor veda-nāmadheyam*), is the *śāstra*, though it is not so said. The reason is, that the Brāhmaṇa texts contain injunctions, to a large extent, regarding sacrifice. The Śrautasūtras take a further step in this direction and this completes the concept of *śāstra*, which, in this case, concerns sacrifice. The Purāṇa lore assumes the status of a *śāstra* because it teaches many things. We have no idea of what the nature of the lore called Purāṇa was prior to the extant texts were available (i.e. from about the fourth century A.D.); but, there is reason to believe that it gave important advice on many items of social and personal needs. The necessity of a king to listen to the Purāṇa, as enjoined by the *Arthaśāstra*, is an indication to this effect. In the later times, when the Purāṇas were specifically grouped, they, not only contained many topics from the older tradition of the Veda but, also recorded many beliefs, customs, practices and myths. This gave them a full status of a *śāstra;* because, they got the status of Dharmaśāstra.[10] Advice, guidance and hints about religious and social matters, with suitable examples from older and new myths and legends, formed their main nature. In fact, as these various items taught and guided (*śās*), in the form of a bulk compendium, the Purāṇas could rightly be called *śāstra*. The process had already started from the *Mb.* which contains such items. In that sense, it could very well be termed *śāstra*, though it is termed Itihāsa.[11] In the real sense of the term, Itihāsa is not only 'history' in the personal restricted connotation attached to it. It is a record of things as they were (*iti ha āsa*), i.e. 'this way it was', including not only lineage of kings and descriptions of war and coronations but also information of past rites, code of conduct and sacrifices. That is why, in the ancient texts, Purāṇa was often mentioned with Itihāsa, as if both formed a single whole. In the stage of further codification and this is the stage of a perfect scientific approach with the connotation of *śāstra* as a scientific treatise, Purāṇas came to be characterised with the famous *pañca-lakṣaṇa* motif. The scientific codification is marked also in the classification of the extant Purāṇas as Sāttvika, Rājasa and Tāmasa. In the Purāṇas termed Sāttvika, Hari (Viṣṇu), the greatness of whom is extolled, is the chief deity. In those termed Rājasa, Brahmā is extolled more; and in those termed Tāmasa, the greatness of Agni and of Śiva is prominent (*Matsya P.* 53.67ff.). There are some Purāṇas that are of a general (or mixed, *saṁkīrṇa*) nature, in which Sarasvatī and the manes are said to be extolled (*ib.*68). Howsoever arbitrary this classification may appear, it has a germ of scientific method of identifying the contents of the various Purāṇa texts. As such, this and such other efforts at grouping and classifying indicate that these texts got getting scientific in the modern sense of the term. Thus, in Purāṇas, in their present form, hold the double status of *śāstra:* (i) Books that preach, teach, advise, instruct and provide injunctions on a number of topics; and (ii) Books that studied and classified the collected information in various ways. This will be clear from the topics covered by them. It is difficult to give here a whole, and concise, list of the topics; it is also not necessary. But, a general idea could be had from the following. There are topics that go under Dharmaśāstra, such as adoption, adultery, Āśrama, Dharma, initiation (*dīkṣā*), king and kingship, ordeals, taboos, vows and the like. These cover the three main phases of Dharmaśāstra, viz. *Ācāra, Vyavahāra* and *Prāyaścitta.* There are instructions on building of temples and other buildings, of tanks and the rituals connected with them; on stars and planets; on horticulture and agriculture; on diseases and medicines; on the use of metals; on poetics; on the interpretation of dreams and other such topics of social importance and relevance.

An important phase of the Purāṇas is what is called mythology in modern times. In the Purāṇa texts this is covered by *sarga* and *pratisarga* from the *pañcalakṣaṇa* motif, i.e. creation and counter, or subsidiary, creation, wherein the modern concept of 'myth' holds good, though, however, the term 'myth' has a wider scope. In *manvantara* (various eras) and *vaṁśa* (genealogy), the Purāṇa leans more to history in its modern sense; and in *vaṁśā(śyā)nucarita*, the Purāṇa often mixes myth with history, the result being the formation of legends. We have seen how Yāska has explained the term *purāṇa* as *purā nava*, where he rightly takes *purā* as the base on which Purāṇa assumes the garb of traditionality. Various tales recorded by the Purāṇa texts, which are called 'myth', have to be termed *purā-kathā* (and not *purāṇa-kathā*, as is sometimes done) to keep to the original sense. Because, *purāṇa-kathā* would mean, simply, 'a tale from the Purāṇa'; and such a tale may be even a real tale, dry and factual, without the element of fancy and rearrangement, which are characteristic of a myth (*purā-kathā*). Purāṇaśāstra, in this phase of the meaning of the term, is expected to contain interpretation of old tales (*kathā*-s), together with the collection of tales. In the former, i.e. interpretation, old tales will be presented in a new light requiring the context in which they are set and also the purpose for which they are employed. This would require additions and modifications. In modern times, this process is called 'charter'. By this method old myths (or *purākathā*-s) are presented with a rearrangement. There are a number of such instances of old myths being used in a new situation. Their bulk is so great, and conspicuous, in the Puranic texts, that Purāṇas are identified with them. It is here that the Purāṇas are termed in the modern times by the general term 'Mythology', which has been taken to contain only stories of gods and demons, or such fanciful tales which were never true. This is doing injustice to the nature of the Purāṇas; it also exposes the ignorance of those who do so! The study of the Purāṇas, as a *śāstra*, cannot be profitable and worth its name without the study on a comparative basis. Single Purāṇa texts have been studied; but, study of a particular topic from all the Purāṇa texts is apt to reward the scholar and others, wherein a track of evolution of ideas and practices will show itself. A few examples would show what I propose. For example, *upanayana* is not allowed for a *śūdra*, as a general rule; and most Purāṇa texts follow the tradition handed down from the Vedic period. However, the *Varāha Purāṇa* allows it (ch.127; also 128). After prescribing the attire for the initiates of other *varṇa*-s, this text says that for the *śūdra* the covering skin should be of a black-goat; a staff of a bamboo measuring eight cubits; blue (or black, *nīla*) cloak and an umbrella also having black cloth. Interesting information about marriage obtains from the *Brahmāṇḍa Purāṇa*. According to it, a girl might be allowed to have sexual intercourse with a person with the permission of her parents, even prior to the marriage. However, at marriage with the same person, the man has to be purified by a three-day fast (*Brahmāṇḍa P.*

II.4.8.17). Like the marriage of the Tulasī plant (as a bride) with Viṣṇu, which is referred to by the Purāṇas generally, the *Skanda P.* (IV.259.62) recommends the regular marriage of a black bull. Devoid of the motif of marriage, Tulasī appears as the symbol of the vegetation spirit; and the bull symbolizes all males here. Such other symbols are strewn in the Puranic literature, another being the *bilva* or the *śrī-phala*. An interesting myth (*purā-kathā*) occurs about Kandalī, which is a plant and is also anthropomorphised as the daughter of the sage Aurva born from his knee, and was married to no less a sage than the haughty Durvāsas. Durvāsas showed his real nature and cursed her to be a heap of ashes,[12] when she used her tongue, sharp as a razor, as was her nature, to injure the feelings of people. On the compassion of the seer she was, later, born as a plant of that time. To understand the implication of such mythical accounts, a transpuranic and transcultural study is necessary. For that, it is not enough to study material from only the Hindu context. One has to take help from works on the methods of the study of myths. Works like *Vedic Mythology* (A.A. Macdonell) or *Epic Mythology* (E.W. Hopkins) and so on are preliminary and mostly of a documentative nature, in the face of modern trends of the study of myths, with the rise of such approaches as functionalism, structuralism and so on. It was pointed out by J. Gonda in his presidential address at the All India Oriental Conference, 1978, Poona (*Proceedings,* 1980, p.3) that in the study of myths (and, we may add, of mythology) new insights into the structure and functions of myths in the archaic societies gained by scholars outside the field of Sanskrit did not seem to have attracted the attention they deserved. He, probably, hinted at taking note on the study of such scholars as Malinowski and Claude Lévi Strauss. This statement, even at that time, was not exactly true, in view of efforts on similar lines by the present speaker (writer) right from 1969, which, unfortunately, did not come to the notice of Gonda, though the books were published by the Universities of Poona and Bombay, not to mention other publishers of repute. In any case, to study the Purāṇas as a *śāstra,* one has to take help from works on Dharmaśāstra, if the study concerns ancient Hindu law; and, to study them from the point of mythology, the study has to proceed on the socio-anthropological lines,[13] with comparative material from such ancient stock as the Chinese, the Middle Eastern sources like the Assyro-Babylonian and even the pre-Columbus American, such as the Aztecs and the Mayans, and also the Incan. It is unrewarding just to stop at the sources from the Avestan and the Greek mythologies. One has not only to get acquainted with the works of Dumezil, Miercia Elied, Joseph Campbell and Wendy Doniger O 'Flaherty who have studied myths from various angles but also of the structuralists. Myths have been taken as a form of language, as they have the value of communication prior to the development of language. As such, the study has to be supported by such observations. Then only will the study be *purā* and yet *nava*, to keep to the spirit of the PURĀṆA.

NOTES AND REFERENCES

1. Purāṇa is prescribed for the people called here *vayāmsi* and others, i.e. birds and bird-catchers.

   However, looking to the later tradition, Purāṇa cannot be taken as restricted to them. The groups of people mentioned in this context have to be taken as governed by the term *'aśrotriya',* mentioned above. Hence, all are common people.
2. For examples, see Sindhu S. Dange, *Puranic Etymologies and Flexible Forms,* Viveka Publications, Aligarh, 1989; cf. p.122 *vide*; p.123 *aparādham kṣamā*; *tyajase;* p. 125 *uccaritvā;* 131 *bumbārava;* p. 132 *khānapānaiś ca;* and a number of others.
3. Sāyaṇa takes the singular, *śrotram,* as *śrotre* (dual) to correspond to *abhihitau* (tied; cf. *abhidhānī*, which is a tying rope). This is not only unnecessary, but also spoils the concept, which is clear.

4. *Yājñavalkya-smṛti* I.3 *sthānāni vidyānām dharmasya ca.*
5. Whether we have to understand *paurāṇika* here as an epithet of *sūtamāgadhau* is unclear. There is another paper in this Seminar by Mrs. S.S. Dange, on this topic. The same paper - "Sūta - The Paurānika", was later on pub. in *Purāṇa,* All India Kashiraj Trust, Varanasi, Vol.XL, No.2, July 1998, pp.83-91.
6. P.V. Kane, *History of Dharma*śāstra, Vol.III, Poona (Second ed.), 1973, p.872.
7. It appears that when Kauṭilya speaks of a *paurāṇika*, it indicates the post. It was his duty to study the current lore and also to gather it and commit it to memory. The *purāṇika*, of the later period, was to read the manuscripts collected and copied.
8. For this information, see Sadashiv A. Dange, *Ency. P. B. & P.,* Navrang, New Delhi, Vol. IV, 1989, pp.1134-1140.
9. *Skanda P.* (VII.1.2.90) says that the Purāṇa is not only not inferior to the Veda, but that it is the fifth Veda *(ib.,* V.3.1.18).
10. See note 4 *supra.*
11. *Mb.* Ādi 1.9 *bhāratasyetihāsasya.*
12. Dange, *Ency. P. B. & P.* Vol.V, p.1474 for Bilva anthropomorphised as a young man.
13. For the study of Hindu myths, taking a note of various approaches, see Sadashiv A. Dange, *Towards Understanding Hindu Myths.* Aryan Books International, New Delhi, 1996.

* Included here from the Journal *Purāṇa*, All India Kashiraj Trust, Varanasi, Vol.XL, No.2, July 1998.

Chapter 14

The King with Two Faces

One of the most intriguing tales from the *Uttarādhyayana-Sūtra* is that of the king of Kāmpilya, called Domuha, which is not his real name. It is an appellative name which came to be famous. His real name was Jaya. The incident which was said to be the cause of the popular name —Domuha — is also interesting. It is said, that once this king was receiving dignitaries in the assembly-hall and asked a certain *dūta* (whether he was an ambassador from another country, or was his ambassador returned from another country, is not quite clear), "What is lacking with me which other kings possess?" The *dūta* replied, "My Lord, you do not possess a *cittasabhā" (cittasabhā tumha natthi)*. The *cittasabhā* might have been a hall of painting or a gallery with fascinating objects (a detail to be discussed later). Hearing this, the king ordered a *cittasabhā* to be built. Accordingly, when the ground was being dug up for building the *sabhā*, the workers found, on the fifth day, a crown. It was studded with all sorts of precious stones and was shining like blazing fire *(savvarayaṇāmao jaraṇovva teyasā jalanto)*. The text describes the crown as 'Great' (*mahāmauḍo*). Joyous, the workmen reported it to the king, Jaya. The king also got the 'Great Crown' brought up from the pit of the earth with shouts of joy. He rewarded the *sthapati*-s with due respect. In course of time, when the high-towering *cittasabhā* was completed, he festivated the day of first entry. After entering the *sabhā,* with all pomp, he placed the 'Great Crown' on his head, as auspicious notes of the drums were declaring the event. And, due to the prowess that was inherent (in the 'Great Crown' *tapapabhāveṇa*) the king became endowed with two faces (mouths, *dovayaṇo*). People gave him the name 'Domuha'.

The account goes on to tell us that Jaya had seven sons, but no daughter, and that, later, a daughter was born to him through the favour of a Yakṣa. As time went on, this daughter, named Mayaṇamañjarī (Madanamañjarī), blossomed into a very beautiful woman; and she was ready for marriage. This detail is not very important for our purpose here. The point is that, king Pajjoya (in fact, Caṇḍapajjoya=Caṇḍa-Pradyota) of Ujjenī (Ujjayinī) had heard about the 'Great Crown' that 'Domuha' had obtained and that, thereby, the latter developed two faces. This bit of information was given to him by his own ambassador. So, Caṇḍapajjoya coveted the wonder crown. Being super-confident of his own might, he sent his messenger (ambassador) to Jaya and insolently demanded the 'Great Crown', along with the message that, otherwise, Jaya should be ready for war. On hearing this threat, king Jaya 'Domuha' sent the messenger back with the message, that he would do so on condition that Caṇḍapajjoya should part with his elephant, named Nalagiri,[1] the excellent chariot Aggibhīru (Agnibhīru), also his wife Sivādevī (Śivādevī) and the courtwriter named Lohajaṅgha. On hearing these conditions, Caṇḍapajjoya got furious and advanced against 'Domuha' with a large army.[2] King Domuha also advanced and the armies clashed. However, through the power of a jewel in the 'Great Crown' (*mauḍa-rayaṇa-pahāveṇa*) king Domuha became invisible (*ajeho*). The army of Caṇḍapajjoya ran away (*bhaggam pajjoyassa balam).* Caṇḍapajjoya was soon fettered; was entered and marched into the city (Kāmpilya); a ring was set round his foot (as an indication of his being a captive, though not a slave, in this case).

In captivity, Pajjoya passed his time comfortably. Once he happened to see Mayaṇamañjarī and fell deeply in love and longing for her. The effect showed on his body which got emaciated. When Domuha came to know of it he enquired from the royal prisoner himself; but, the latter would not speak a word in explanation. At long last, he confessed his deep love-pangs for the victor's daughter. The latter had already formed a favourable opinion about his royal captive and fulfilled the desire of Pajjoya. Mayaṇamañjarī was given in marriage to the latter; and the couple departed to Ujjenī (Ujjayinī) with all pomp and glory.

Up-till now, the account has dwelt on the empirical status and royalty of king Jaya 'Domuha'. Suddenly, there is a turn. We read of the usual Indamausaho (Indramahotsava), the festival of the Banner of Indra.[3] So, as usual, Domuha ordered the Banner of Indra (*indakeu= indra-ketu*) to be hoisted. This was done. The banner was adorned with various types of garlands and fixed at the stipulated place with noisy welcome with the beating of drums. The streets of the capital were astir with song and merry dancing. Alms were given, presents were awarded and the fun and frolic lingered through the night till glances of the dawn came longingly to participate in the deliberations. This went on every day for seven days, until the Full-moon-day arrived. The king Domuha worshipped the banner, offering it flowers and decorating it with new robes. On the next day, however, the 'Banner of Indra' fell on the ground with a loud noise. It lay in filth and was being plundered for the gems and cloth-strips on it, by the common thieves. This king Domuha saw. A revelation dawned on his inner-conscience— "So fleeting is this world and its glory!" He decided. His enlightenment changed him into a 'Paccekabuddha' (*pratyekabuddha*).[4] He performed the *pañcamuṭṭhiyam loyam* (plucking the hair on his head in five handfuls) and renounced the world.

The account comes to a close with a dramatic

contrast, between empirical glory and the inner revelation. The banner stands as the symbol for empirical glory with all the pomp associated with it. It also symbolizes the king. The revelation appears as a reaction; but, in fact, it is suggested to be the final desired aim of fruitful human life. The account and the end here mark a well-set pattern in Jain tales; the pattern works close to the life of Mahāvīra and also of Gautama, the Buddha. The pattern is seen also in the account of Karakaṇḍu in the detail of the bull adored by him. The bull was hefty, of white colour and youthful. He was looked after by every one, by the order of Karakaṇḍu. Later, when Karakaṇḍu saw the same bull getting old and weak, he suddenly woke up to the revelation of the futility of life. The result: He at once renounced the world.[5]

In our account Caṇḍapajjoya is a historical figure. In the case of Domuha, it could be said that he has been rooted in the tradition as he is mentioned even in the Jātaka (cf. *Kumbhakāra-jātaka*),[6] though in history he appears to be unrecorded. He is said to be the king of the Pāñcālas. In the Buddhistic period the Pāñcālas were divided into the Uttara Pāñcāla, with its capital at Ahicchatra, and the Dakṣiṇa-Pāñcāla, with its capital at Kāmpilya.[7] Our account associates Jaya Domuha with this Kāmpilya. Also known as Caṇḍamahāsena due to his vast army, Caṇḍapajjoya was a senior contemporary of king Ajaya Udayana,[8] of the Vatsa country. His beloved wife was the daughter of Caṇḍamahāsena, and was the famous Vāsavadattā. The period of Caṇḍapajjoya and Udayana (sixth century B.C.) was earlier than that of the formation of the Jātakas (not before the fourth century B.C.; and about the first century B.C. the Jātakas were fully settled), though they mention earlier kings. When the *Uttarādhyayanasūtra* was known in its completed form (second to the fifth century A.D.), the Udayana-kathā was very popular. In the present tale there is a clear inversion of the Udayana-kathā. In the earlier tale (chronologically) Caṇḍapajjoya is aware of the proud nature of Udayana and contrives the capture of Udayana, whom he desires to marry his daughter Vāsavadattā but knows the pride of the former. The capture of Udayana, his being treated with all respect, and his assignment to teach lute-playing to Vāsavadattā give rise to the love between the royal captive and the captor's daughter, leading to the end that all parties ultimately desire. In the tale of Domuha the point of inversion steps in, and the elderly captor (Caṇḍapajjoya) is placed in the situation of the young captive Udayana. As is usual with such Jain tales, there are changes in certain details. In the Udayana tale, the desire of Caṇḍapajjoya (in reality, Caṇḍapradyota) to make Udayana his son-in-law, and the subsequent events were historical facts. In the present case, in spite of Caṇḍapajjoya being a historical person, the tale associated with Domuha has the status only of a myth. If, now, we fix our attention on the motive of the tale, it is clear that it is a myth of the 'charter' type, to speak in the technical terminology. To graft this myth on a historical reality of a popular narration, the episode of the 'Great Crown' was employed. The wonderful (magical?) Crown made Jaya famous. It also lured Caṇḍapajjoya, and the result was war. It is the 'Great Crown' that made Jaya Domuha invisible—another mythical employment. It is this Crown itself that, obviously, led Domuha to victory and to the capture of Caṇḍapajjoya. It is this Crown, again, that established peace — and lasting peace—with the agreeable flavour of love in the minds of the young couple and affection in the mind of the wise king Jaya Domuha. The 'Great Crown' and the status of being Domuha in the case of Jaya end here. It has nothing to do, whatsoever, with the renunciation of king Jaya. Renunciation, in his case, is associated with the hoisting and fall of the Indradhvaja; and, what happens to the 'Great Crown', so important for the first part of the tale, is not mentioned. It simply goes into the background, like an actor that has served the stage for the day and has gone back into the green-room. The tale has used the festival of Indradhvaja that has been current in the tradition. It is to be remembered that the *Uttarādhyayanasūtra* is assigned to about the second century A.D., while the Indramaha, figuring the Banner of Indra is already known to the Mahābhārata. But, what about the 'Great Crown'? The crown that is associated with the concept of two anthropomorphic faces is not known from the Indian context, though a seal from Harappa shows two non-human faces with a single neck, but without a body.[9] But, before we probe this point, let us dwell on the occasioned reason for finding for the 'Great Crown'.

According to the account, Jaya asks the *duta* (*dūya*), as he was sitting in the assembly-hall (*atthāṇamaṇḍava*), if he did not possess anything others have; and the *dūta* says that the king did not possess a *cittasabhā* (*citrasabhā*). This reminds one of a similar question Yudhiṣṭhira posed to the divine all-round messenger Nārada about his own *sabhā*. He asks, "O Brahman, you travel to many regions created by Brahmā. Have you ever seen a *sabhā* like this (of mine) or even better than this? (*Mb.* Sabhā, 6.7-8).[10] The *dū*ta (here Nārada) then tells him that among the mortals he did not see such a *sabhā*, but he asks permission to describe the *sabhā*-s of the gods: of Indra, Yama, Varuṇa and Brahmā. The *Matsya-P.* follows the description of the Indrasabhā from the *Mb.* to some extent using the same words (161.38ff). The period of the *Matsya-P.* is about A.D. 200–A.D 400 and it, more or less, corresponds to that of the *Uttarādhyayanasūtra*, while that of the *Mahābhārata* (in its final form) is from second century B.C. to the second century A.D. This would indicate, that at this period the building of the *sabhā*-s was thought to be a matter of prestige and affluence for the kings. In the mythical account of king Jaya Domuha, the narrator, or the composer, appears to have followed the motif from the *Mahābhārata,* as did the *Matsya P.* What was the nature of the *citta-sabhā*? It does not appear to be a gallery of paintings,[11] as it may be mistaken to appear. The word *citra* does not get exhausted with the meaning 'picture'. In fact, the very question indicates that it must have been a spacious apartment filled with curious objects. The description from the *Mahābhārata* and the *Matsya-P.* lends support to this. It is said, that at the request of Kṛṣṇa the *asura* Maya built the said *sabhā*, where divine splendrous objects could be witnessed (*loc.cit.*, 1. 13 *yatra divyān abhiprāyān paśyema*). The same *sabhā* is described as *bahucitrā bahudhanā* and *ratnaprākāra-toraṇā* (*ib.*, 3.26), also *citra-sphaṭika-sopānā* and *paṅkajaiś citrā* (*ib.*, 31). In all these places the word *citra* indicates variety of attractiveness; not mere 'picture' or 'paintings'. The very fact that the whole book is called 'Sabhā-parvan' would show how, during that period, the building of a *sabhā*—and a *citra-sabhā*, for that matter—was viewed as a mark of great distinction. The corroboration for this comes from the temples of that period, where a separate *sabhā-maṇḍapa* was a prominent feature. That the composer of the Jain tale in question is definitely influenced by, and that he is copying, the description from the *Mahābhārata* is clear from another detail: *uttuṅgasiharā cittasabhā* here is the expression reflecting *divam āvṛtya viṣṭhitā* (*Mb. loc.cit.*, 3.25) or *mahāratnavatī citrā... sitābhra-śikharākārā* (having many attractive things, attractive and high like the tips of the white clouds) (*ib.*, 10.4). The *Matsya P.*, noted above, describing the *sabhā* of Hiraṇyakaśipu, uses: *nānārūpair upakṛtām* (endowed with various forms and objects) and *nākapṛṣṭhasthā* (standing on the plane of heaven; *ib.*, 45-46). It was for constructing such a lofty wonder-*sabhā*, which would be the envy of any monarch, that Jaya gave orders to dig the earth. And, while the clods of earth were being cleared from the excavated portion, the crown was found—itself a unique object and a great wonder!

In any case, the find of the Crown was an event of great wonder; and the narrator reflects the feelings of the then society. It is also clear that the object found was of an unseen nature theretofore. The appellation Domuha warrants actual two faces; and there seems to be the least possibility of its being due to the actual face or head of the king plus its reflection in the crown. As such, our search must go in the direction of examining the actual two faces in one unit. In narrative literature another such example is that of the bird known as *bhāraṇda*, which is ficticious though the idea is charming. This bird is said to have had two heads with a common neck; and, in a didactic tale from the *Pañcatantra* (Aparīkṣita-kāritva, Tale No.13) the quarrel between these two heads leads to the death of both, and, of course, of the bird, here *bhāraṇḍa*. A similar bird is mentioned in the legend of Udāyana. Though the bird is mentioned as *bhāruṇḍa* here, it is said that a pair of *bhāruṇḍa*-s had three legs between them. The question is, "How many faces?" This shows that the bird is mythical; and, even in this latter case, there has to be a pair of heads with one neck. The bird-pair in the Udāyana legend is said to be able to carry a man who gets tied to the three legs.[12] We have already noted the double-headed figure from a seal at Harappa. However, the heads there appear to be of beasts. In such cases, it is much more probable that in narration such descriptions appear due to actual observation in figures rather than pure imagination, though, in the very earliest stage imagination cannot be ruled out. Considering the age of the *Pañcatantra*[13] it appears that the double-headed bird *bhāraṇḍa* was suggested from the double-headed bird on a *stūpa* at Takṣaśilā (Taxila), under the influence of the Śakas, in the first century A.D.[14] But, the motif goes far back; and we have the ancient Egyptian double-headed Horus,[15] though with hawk-heads, as Horus was conceived as a man-form with hawk-head. Similarly, the Assyrian god Marduk is pictured as having two heads, though of birds. However, the body is anthropomorphic.[16] A further stage, in such representations, is of two human heads. In a more polished, or sophisticated, form of religious belief the centre of power and prowess changes from the theriomorphic head of a god to the human. Thus, in the

Sumerian mythology itself, we have the god Ismud having two human heads.[17] A more sophisticated example is of the ancient Italian god Janus, who gave the name January[18] to the month that is the start of the year. This god is important from our point of view. The position of the month of January is such that it starts the new year, as also it is nearest to the year that has ended. This way, this month is a door which ushers in the new year and also acts as the exit for the last. This is exactly the reason why the god Janus was called 'God of doors', or 'God of beginnings'. His temple in Rome was open east-west; and his idol was placed in the centre of these doors. Another important trait of this god is that his temple was closed only in times of peace. This means that it was never closed in times of war.[19] The belief was that, in war, it was thought beneficial to keep the god in a position to see the events of war so that he would give victory, and peace. It is said, that during seven hundred years of the establishment of Rome, the temple was closed only thrice: in the reign of king Numa; after the defeat of Carthage in 241 B.C.; and in the reign of Augustus (31 B.C.-A.D.14).[20] The period of king Numa is, obviously, anterior to the Republic of Rome. Though king Numa is not so much remembered in the din of the republic, mythologically he has a sound base; for, he was closely believed to be divine. His name is close to the concept of *numina*, which word means 'god' in the Latin language (cf. Latin *numen, numinis*= divinity), and with *numisma* (in Latin, meaning 'current coin'; cf. numismatic), which indicates riches. No doubt, in the sphere of mythology, Janus and Numa got closely associated, and the association lingered on with a complexity of Victory and Wealth. Roman contact with India goes back, at least as far back as, to the first century A.D., when Roman gold began to be poured into India in return for Indian silk, spices, etc., in the reign of emperor Tiberius (A.D. 14-38); and the 'dīnār' (Roman, Denarius) was quite popular in A.D. 100.[21] Roman influence on Indian culture and coinage continued till the end of the fourth century A.D.[22] And, it is not improbable that Roman myths and folk-tales, together with their beliefs, percolated and settled in India by that period.

If we review the detail of the two faces of king Jaya, it appears that the idea of the two faces was suggested from something like a crown having two faces. Looking to the contacts of the Romans, it is not improbable that the myth regarding the Roman god Janus was familiar here; and it was imagined that the god with two faces must have a crown that suited his two heads. It should be particularly noted that, though the 'double-face' of Jaya was the reason for the strife, the end was in peace. This is exactly the trait of Janus. Even in our account, the jewel in the so-called 'Great Crown' leads to the invisibility of Jaya resulting in the welcome capture of his would-be son-in-law. It is of further interest to note, that the victory-trait of the Roman god Janus appears to be reflected in the name of Domuha, which is Jaya-(=victory). This mythical account about king Jaya Domuha was softly transplanted on the earlier legend of king Caṇḍapajjoya, with the inversion of the Udayana account as far as the relationship is considered. In this graft, the 'Great Crown', suggested from the double-faced Janus, played a twofold symbolic role: (i) to further enhance the glorious character of Jaya to show that *even he* renounced the world; and (ii) to explain the name 'Domuha', which was current and popular long before the compilation of the *Uttarādhyayanasūtra,* and which was the substitute for the original — Dummuha — as it had a tinge of censure (cf. *durmukha).*

To recapitulate and examine the structures involved in the tale:

A. The main function of the tale, as it appears here, is to highlight the point of renunciation. Towards this aim, the popular festival of Indramaha was used.
B. For the aim noted above, according to a set pattern, here Jaya Domuha was cast in the central place. To

elevate him yet further, he was depicted as building a *sabhā;* and for this, the pattern of the period and information drawn from the known source was used.

C. The name Domuha was sought to be explained by taking resort to a mythical narration, built on the myths about the double-faced birds[23] and, in all probability, on the beliefs about the Roman god Janus that might have travelled through Roman contacts in India at that period. The myth of the 'Great Crown' was floated on the basis of the same beliefs.

D. The mythical crown was sought to serve the purpose and the basis for the inversion of the earlier popular legend of Caṇḍapajjoya, Udayana and Vāsavadattā. However, here the tale shows a defect. According to the tale, much time was gone after the finding of the crown (*aikkanto koi kālo*) and before the birth of seven sons and a daughter to Jaya Domuha. This would mean that Caṇḍapajjoya never knew about the 'Great Crown' all these years, or that he reserved his jealousy till the daughter of Jaya developed into a young girl!

This would show that the whole account is artificial and not properly smoothened. The result is that it has used older motifs, but the narration is smothered by function.

NOTES AND REFERENCES

1. The wording here is *nalagirihatthi,* i.e. originally, Nalagiri as the name of the elephant. Actually, this is a shadow of the elephant named Nālagiri that was sent to destroy the Buddha by Devadatta, but which was subdued by the Buddha with his loving glance; cf. *Cullavagga* VII.2.5. At the *Pratijñāyaugandharāyaṇa* (Act III) the name appears as Nalāgiri. At the *Meghadūta* (Pūrvamegha, 34) the name is Nalagiri.
2. The largeness of the army can be seen from the (fanciful)

description: two lakh elephants, two thousand chariots, fifty thousand horsemen and so on.

3. The first mention of the Banner of Indra occurs in the *Mb.* where Indra is said to have given the staff of bamboo (*yaṣṭim vaiṇavīm*) to king Vasu Uparicara; see *Mb.*Ādi 63.17-28. However, the earliest suggestion of the Indra-staff occurs at *ṚV* I.10.1 *brahmāṇas tvā śatakrato ud vaṁśam iva yemire.*
4. The *pratyekabuddha* is an individual who is enlightened. He is lower than the Bodhisattva but higher than the *arhat* or *śrāvaka.* See P.V. Bapat in *2500 Years of Buddhism*, Gen. Ed. P.V. Bapat, Publications Division, Ministry of Information and Broadcasting, Govt. of India, New Delhi, 1976 (1959), p.145; also (Mrs.) Sindhu S. Dange, *Bauddha Dharma āṇi Tattvajñāna*, Continental Prakashan, Pune, 1980, p.221, where she mentions the *Milindapañha* (105) where he is said to be called '*sayambhu anācariyaka*'. Here the Buddhistic influence on Jain thought can be noted.
5. Cf. the story as it occurs in Devendra's Commentary on *Uttarādhyayanasūtra; pecchai mahākāyam juṇṇvasabham .... tam tārisam pecchiya gayo visāyam,* etc. In the Karaṇḍu-kathā in the Kumbhakāra-jātaka, a mango tree with full fruits and then without fruits figures.
6. Cf. Kumbhakāra-jātaka, which mentions four famous kings:

   karaṇḍunāma kaliṅgānam gandhārāṇam ca niggai
   nimirājā vedēhānam pañcālānam ca dummukho

   In *A Treasury of Jain Tales* (Ed. V.M.Kulkarni), Sharadaben Chimanbhai Educational Research Centre, Ahmedabad, 1994, p.12, *dummuho* is rendered in Sanskrit as Dvimukha; see also in the title on p.127. Hiralal Jain renders it as Durmukha; see his ed. of *Karakaṇḍacariu*, Bhāratīya Jñānapīṭha Prakashan, Varanasi (Calcutta), Second ed. 1964, p.229. One feels the rendering Durmukha belies the original name. The story, as it occurs in the *Uttarādhyayanasūtra*, starts with the words, *sampai dummuhacariyam;* and goes on, immediately, to relate the story: *do-vayaṇo* so *rāyā jāo.... loyeṇa tassa domoho tti nāma. kayam.* It is probable that in speech, here, *du* changed to *do* and *mu* to *mo*. But the reduplication in *mm* (*dummuho*) remains un-answered. Is it probable that the original *dummuha* (= *dur-mukha*) caused unease in the later period; hence *domuha* got currency; and to explain it the myth was created on purpose? The case is like 'Suyodhana' in Bhāsa's *Dūtāvākyam,* v.18.

7. A.D. Pusalkar, *Bhāsa — A Study,* Munshiram Manoharlal, Delhi, Second ed., 1968 (1940), p.341; also S. Muzafer Ali, *The Geography of the Purāṇas*, People's Publishing House, New Delhi, Ahmedabad, Bombay, Second ed., 1973 (1966), p.135.
8. The name Ajaya Vatsarāja appears in the *Dīghanikāya,* for which see R.G. Kolangade, *Tyāgarāja Bhagavān Gotama Buddha* (in Marathi), who is also the publisher, Mumbai, 1946, p.20.
9. Madho Sarup Vats, *Excavations at Harappa* (Vols. I-II), Vol. I, Calcutta, 1940, plate LXXIX, Fig. 88. He calls it an animal figurine.
10. *bhavān sañcarate lokān sadā nānāvidhān bahūn* /
    īdṛśī bhavatā kācid dṛṣṭapūrvā sabhā kvacit /
    ito vā śreyasī brahmans tanmamācakṣva pṛcchataḥ /
    Cf. our present story:
    kim natthi mama jam anna-rāiṇam atthi
11. As rendered by G.S. Bedagkar in *A Treasury of Jain Tales,* p.127.
12. V.M. Kulkarni, *op.cit.,* p.15.
13. It existed long before its Pehlevi version in A.D. 570. According to Hertel, however, *Tantrākhyāyikā*, which existed as early as 200 B.C., is the earliest available recension of the *Pañcatantra;* see *A History of Sanskrit Literature — Classical Period,* Vol. I, Ed. S.N. Dasgupta, University of Calcutta, 1947, pp.87, 705.
14. J. Petrocinio De Souza, "The Symbol of the Double-headed Eagle: Its Origin, Diffusion and Significance", *Journal of the University of Bombay*, Bombay, Oct. 1969 (No.74, Vol.XXXVIII), p.125.
15. *Ibid.,* p.131, where the figure occurs.
16. *Ibid.*, p.130, where the figure occurs.
17. S.N. Kramer, *Sumerian Mythology*, American Philosophical Society, Philadelphia, 1944, p.32.
18. Edith Hamilton, *Mythology*, Little Brown and Company, Boston, 1942, p.51.
19. *Ibid.*

20. *Ibid.*
21. S.N. Dasgupta, *op.cit.,* p.82.
22. R.D. Banerji, *Prehistoric Ancient and Hindu India,* Blackie and Son (India) Limited, Bombay, Calcutta and Madras, 1950 (1914), p.147.
23. The influence of the concept of the double-head can also be marked in the description of the buffalo-demon, Mahiṣa, in the *Matsya P.* (260.61) which, as we have noted earlier, was compiled during A.D. 200-400. In the context of preparing the image of the goddess it is prescribed here that Mahiṣa should be shown as having two heads: *adhastān mahiṣam tadvad dviśiraskam pradarśayet.* The motif appears even earlier in the *Suparṇādhyāya,* which is a work after the period of the Brāhmaṇa texts; cf. *madhye dvivaktrā bhujagendrarājiḥ* (XIV.28.1). These are, however, examples of the theriomorphism. See Sadashiv A. Dange, *Legends in the Mahābhārata,* Motilal Banarsidass, Delhi, 1969, p.36, n.91, or his *Myths from the Mahābhārata,* Vol.1, Aryan, New Delhi, 1997, p.129, n.91.

* *Uttarajjhayaṇasutta* Ed. Nirnayasagara, Poona, 1937, pp.125-135.

Chapter 15

Woman's Share and the Mīmāṁsā Rule at "Dvayoḥ Praṇayanti" (An Examination)

While discussing the rite of a widow to her husband's wealth, in the event of her being issueless (actually, without a son), Yājñavalkya states that such a widow gets it (*Yajñ. Sm.*, II.135). This is understood by some authorities, like Dhāreśvara as that she gets the share due to her husband in the family-property, or her husband's wealth, under some conditions, such as submitting to *niyoga*. This has been refuted by Vijñāneśvara, the commentator of the *Yājñ.Sm.* He points out that Yājñavalkya himself has said, that the wife (wives) gets a share equal to that of her sons, if the husband, when living, divides his property (II.115 *patnyaḥ kāryāḥ samāṁśikāḥ*), and if the property is divided after the death of a man, his sons and his wife get equal share (*ib.*, 123 *pitur ūrdhvam vibhajatām mātā'py'aṁśam samam haret*). Vijñāneśvara argues that, if the woman is eligible for the wealth of her husband in his lifetime or when he is dead, and even when the sons are there to share, why could she not get the husband's share (or wealth) in the event of her husband being dead without living male children. In this context, he docs not state whether this gain on the part of the woman is conditioned by the *strīdhana*. Actually, at the passages he refers to, there is the condition of the *strīdhana,* as he himself has pointed out. If she has *strīdhana* she would get a share equal to the half of that of a son (115cd *na dattam strīdhanam yāsām bhartrā vā śvaśureṇa vā;* here he comments that in that case she gets only a half, quoting from v.148 *datte tv'ardham prakalpayet*). The point has not been clarified by him in the context of a widow's case. What if the widow, having no male child, has *strīdhana?* Vijñāneśvara is silent about the matter, which means that, according to him *strīdhana* is no bar for the issueless woman getting the share (from the family-property) due to her dead husband. The silence of Vijñāneśvara in the context of the right of a son-less widow about the *strīdhana* is to be explained by saying, that he cites the other example (share of a woman with sons living, and the husband being alive or dead, as noted above, v. 115 and 123, along with v. 148) only to indicate that she is eligible to a share; and, on that analogy, he stresses a share for the widow, with the help of an argument which is like the *kaimutika-nyāya:* 'When the husband himself has to give her a share (equal to that of a son, in spite of the presence of the son), who could deny this share to her when he is no more?, Hence, he does not touch the condition of *strīdhana* in the context of the widow's share—as also because Yājñavalkya himself does not mention it in this context! It is to be noted, that *strīdhana* in the context mentioned above is only from the husband's side, or from the father-in-law only. Hence is the question of adjustment with a share from the husband.

Having referred to the other two verses mentioned above, Vijñāneśvara tries to refute the wrong interpretation that may, probably, be given (with the words *syān matam...*). According to this (hypothetical) interpretation of these verses, the woman gets a share equal to that of the son, if the wealth of the husband is meagre. This would mean, the husband, or the sons after him, might give her a definite share. But, if the wealth is much, she would get only so much as is sufficient for her maintenance (comm. on v.137, *bahudhane jīvanopayuktam dhanam gṛhṇāti, alpe tu putrāñśa-samamamamśam gṛhṇāti iti*). This position is refuted by Vijñāneśvara, as it involves anomaly in law (*vidhivaiṣamya*). How? Because, the words *samam* and *añśa* are to be understood in two different senses—(i) equal share; and (ii) just maintenance. To explain the anomaly he gives an example from the ritual context on which a rule is based. The ritual is from the Cāturmāsya sacrifices. The Cāturmāsya has four parts (*parvan*): Vaiśvadeva, Varuṇapraghāsa, Sākamedha and the Śunāsīrīya. Actually, the name *cāturmāsya* indicates that every *parvan* was to be performed once in four months (*catur-māsāḥ*); hence, originally there were only three *parvan*-s—the first three; and the last one (Śunāsīrīya) was added later. Out of the four, only in two the *uttaravedi* was to be filled in (i.e., constructed and filled with sand, etc. to make it elevated). There is also a rite called *praṇayana,* wherein the fire from the Gārhapatya fireplace is to be carried onto the Āhavanīya fireplace, which is in the centre of this *uttaravedi.*[1] To this effect there is the injunction, "they carry the fire only in the two (*parvan-s).*" The whole passage is:

They carry forward the fire in the two; hence, they march on two (legs, thighs); these two are the thighs of the sacrifice — the Varuṇa-praghāsa and the Sākamedha; hence do they march with the two; here do they fill (the *uttaravedi*); they do not fill the *uttaravedi* in the Vaiśvadeva, nor in the Śunāsīrīya.[2]

In the passage above, there is an injunction (*vidhi*) in the words, "here do they fill" indicating that the *uttaravedi* is to be filled in at the two middle *parvan*-s (Varuṇapraghāsa and Sākamedha). About the other two, the first and the last (i.e. Vaiśvadeva and Śunāsīrīya) there is a prohibition (*pratiṣedha*). Along with the filling of the *uttaravedi* there is the *praṇayana;* and it would be also at the middle two, naturally. Now, the point is this: The norm for the Cāturmāsya is the Darśapūrṇamāsa (New-and-Full-moon sacrifices). According to a general Mimāṁsā rule, the norm (*prakṛti*) is followed by other rituals that are its modifications (*prakṛtivad vikṛtiḥ kartavyā*). In the present case, as the Darśapūrṇamāsa has no *uttaravedi*, there is the difficulty. The *uttaravedi* is a mark of the Soma sacrifice, of which the Agniṣṭoma is the *prakṛti*. According to the general rule about the *prakṛti-vikṛti*, whatever is not enjoined in the *vikṛti* is to be taken from the *prakṛti*. But, here *praṇayana* and the *uttara-vedi* are actually enjoined in the two *parvan*-s; and they are not enjoined in the *prakṛti,* the Darśapūrṇamāsa! The position is reversed! Hence, there is nothing to be taken from the Darśapūrṇamāsa. Therefore one view (*Pūrvapakṣa*) is that, here there is mention of the *praṇayana*. Now, there is *praṇayana* also in the Darśapūrṇamāsa, but that is of a simple nature. When the *prakṛti* already has *praṇayana*, it is not necessary to mention it again in the two which is the *vikṛti*; for it would automatically come on the basis of the rule *prakṛtivad vikṛtiḥ kartavyā*. Hence, this *praṇayana* must be from some other context. And that is the context of the Soma sacrifice. The view further says, that the suggestion of the Soma-context is valid even in the case of the prohibition of the *uttaravedi* (that obtains only at the Soma sacrifice); for, without the prohibition, *uttaravedi* would have been filled in at all the four *parvan*-s, as enjoined from the (new) *prakṛti*-context of the Soma sacrifice (also, there is the rule that prohibition is only true when there is the possibility of prescription, *na a-prasaktasya pratiṣedhaḥ*).

This argument is purely academic, and does not much concern the matter in hand, i.e. the woman's share. What concerns it is another view, which is *supposed* to support the final and true view (termed *rāddhāntaikadeśin*). According to this view, there is no extension (*atideśa*) from the Soma sacrifice. What, then?

According to this view, the word "they fill in here" (*upātra vapanti*) in relation to the *uttaravedi* are from the same context (i.e. of the Caturmāsya),[3] as they are uttered in this connection (*prākaraṇikena vacanena;* i.e. they are *prakaraṇa-prāpta*). As such, they are to be taken for all the four *parvan*-s of the Cāturmāsya; and they would be so taken; hence the prohibition in the case of the two — first and the last. In other words, they are *prasakta*—indicative; hence there is the *pratiṣedha* (for the *parvan*-s covered by the *pratiṣedha*).

But, this view, rightly rejected by the Siddhānta itself, is open to the fault of *vidhi-vaiṣamya*, as is rightly pointed out by the *Pūrvapakṣin*. How? The words *upātra vapanti* would be applicable to the two middle *parvan*-s without the expectation of the prohibition; and, to the other two, with the expectation of the prohibition. Thus, in the case of the first and the last *parvan*-s, there will be an option for the filling of the *uttaravedi,* because there is the injunction by the general instruction (*upātra vapanti*) and also prohibition. This is exactly the case with the interpretation of the words *sama aṁśa* (which is understood as "equal share" and also "unequal share" = only maintenance) by some authorities. The final *siddhānta* view in the context of the *uttaravedi* at the Cāturmāsya is that the negation in the case of first and the last is not a prohibition; it is only an explanation of the injunction of filling the *uttaravedi* at the middle two. In other words, it is an *anuvāda*. Hence, there is no ground for *vidhi-vaiṣamya,* as in the case of the interpretation of the woman's share. The passage is brought in by Vijñāneśvara to stress that even a semblance of *vidhivaiṣamya* even in the *rāddhāntika* – supporter is discarded. So, an actual *vidhivaiṣamya* as in the case of the meaning of *sama-aṁśa* has to be totally discarded.

Here the point of the woman's share ends; and we now enter the details of the actual ritual, that is associated with the Mimāṁsā-rule quoted by

Vijñāneśvara in parts and quoted by us in full. Kane, who gives the discussion in detail, says that the passage is from the Veda, and is quoted by Śabara and others.[4] The point has to be examined. Kane does not mention the exact Vedic text where one could find this passage. The fact is that the passage is only a paraphrase from Vedic texts; and if this point is understood, it would be clear that there is hardly any *pratiṣedha* in the real sense of the term, and that the Pūrvapakṣa and the *rāddhāntaikadeśa* presented by the authorities on Dharmaśāstra, including Vijñāneśvara are quite unnecessary, even misleading and cannot be strictly accepted. In the Brāhmaṇa texts, the sentence indicating the negation of the filling of the *uttaravedi* hardly comes after the sentence indicative of injunction — *upātra vapanti,* or *upakirati.* Thus, the *Śat. Br.* (II.5.2.5) which mentions that there are two *vedi*-s in the Varuṇapraghāsa says: *uttarasyām eva vedau uttaravedim upakirati na dakṣiṇasyām.* Here the *pratiṣedha* does not concern the two other *parvan*-s but to the *dakṣiṇa-vedi,* that is to be constructed to the south of the *uttaravedi* in this *parvan.*[5] The *Mait-Sam.* (I.10.13) has: *na vaiśvadeva uttaravedim upavapanti, upā'tra vapanti.* The *Taitt. Br.* (I.6.4.3) has: *uttarasyām vedyām uttaravedim upavapanti,* which is very much the same as the *Śat. Br.* However, in the context of the earlier Vaiśvadeva *parvan,* it says: *na uttaravedim upavapanti* (*Taitt. Br.* I.6.3.7). Thus, the sentences of negation of the *uttaravedi* at the Vaiśvadeva and the prescription of it at the Varuṇapraghāsa are far removed, even here the negation coming prior to the prescription. The *Śat. Br.* has the negation coming prior to the prescription. The *Śat. Br.* has the negation in the context of the last *parvan, Śunāsīrīya,* thus: *tasyā āvṛt* (i.e. *kriyā* according to Sāyaṇa), *na upakiranty 'uttaravedim.* Here the negation comes after the prescription; but, after various passages, and in the fourth *parvan.* All these have been used to form a whole sentence: *dvayoḥ praṇayanti,* etc. as noted earlier. This sentence is a later formation, and is not a

Vedic passage! The Brāhmaṇa texts and the Samhitā deal with the *parvan*-s separately; and there is no ground for a statement concerning all these *parvan*-s in one, as we find in the long sentence, under discussion (= n.2). Actually there is hardly any text to enjoin the *uttaravedi* even in the Sākamedha *parvan*. But, then, how is the passage which speaks of the two being the thighs of the Sacrifice (here the Cāturmāsya) to be reconciled with the actual Vedic texts? The explanation may be given as follows.

We have noted that the texts clearly mention that the *uttaravedi* is to be filled in at the Varuṇapraghāsa. The three texts, taken as examples, state that this *vedi* is not to be filled in at the first *parvan,* which is the Vaiśvadeva. This is followed by the instruction *upātra vapanti,* which concerns the second *parvan*, the Varuṇapraghāsa; then there is no mention of the *uttaravedi* in the third *parvan*; this has to be taken as the *atideśa* (extension) of the *uttaravedi* in the third *parvan*, the Sākamedha. Finally, there is the negation of the *uttaravedi* in the Śunāsīrīya. Thus, the 'filling' is only in the middle *parvan*-s. If we follow the order of the Vedic texts, there is no room for *pratiṣedha*, as we have already noted. But, also, there is no need to understand the *rāddhāntaikadeśa* (the partisan of the real position, the *siddhānta*). It becomes clear that the 'partisan' is not sound. How? Here is the explanation. The position of the partisan is that the injunction of the *uttaravedi* is obtained from the context which is clear in *upātra vapanti* (*upātra vapantīti prākaraṇikena vacanena prāptāyā uttaravedyāḥ*); and this he takes as an injunction for all the four *parvan*-s. This position is accepted by Vijñāneśvara and others, which is also followed by Kane. But, this position is unreal; for, in that case, the question is, which context (*prakaraṇa*)? The context cannot be the Darśapūrṇamāsa, as there is no *uttaravedi*, and, naturally, the 'filling in' there. The context (*prakaraṇa)* must be the Cāturmāsya itself.[6] But, as we have seen, the words *upātra vapanti* ("here do they fill") actually come at the second (Varuṇapraghāsa) *parvan,* leaving the first (Vaiśvadeva). Hence, the injunction to fill cannot be taken for all the four *parvan*-s, as is maintained by the commentator, Vijñāneśvara, and accepted by the whole tradition of authorities! As such, the whole argument, and fear of the *Siddhānta* (*Rāddhānta*) that the 'filling' is enjoined for the four, and narrowed to two, collapses, so goes also the fear that there could be *vidhivaiṣamya.* The example contained in *dvayoḥ praṇayanti,* is, thus, unsound, if we follow strictly the Vedic data.

The long passage *dvayoḥ praṇayanti,* etc. has been formulated by Jaimini on the basis of the Vedic injunctions, with his own innovation of order, to explain some ritual details; and there, in such innovations—and not strictly in the Vedic texts—is the basis of the Mimāmsā rules.

NOTES AND REFERENCES

1. The Varuṇapraghāsa (and the Sākamedha) has two new *vedi*-s established, to the east of the usual → Āhavanīya, their position being one to the north of the other; the one to the north is called the (new) Uttaravedi; the one to the south is termed Dakṣiṇavedi. Referring to my article, "Religious Suicide in the Vedic Period (?)", *Indologia Tauriensia,* 8-9 (1980-81), Torino, Italy, H.W. Bodewitz, "What did Indra do with the Yatis", *Amṛtadhārā,* Delhi, 1984, p.66, n.9, says that the Uttaravedi and Dakṣiṇavedi do not occur in the context (Indra-sālāvṛka and Varuṇapraghāsa). His statement is unsound, as is clear. I have taken a full note of this in another article contributed to the *Haryana Research J.* I-i.
2. *dvayoḥ praṇayanti / tasmād dvābhyām yanti ūrū vā etau yajñasya yad varuṇapraghāsaśca sākamedhaśca / tasmād dvābhyām yanti / upātra vapanti / na vaiśvadeve uttaravedimupa kiranti na śunāsīrīye /*
   The first occurrence of the concept of '*ūrū*' comes at *Śat.Br* .XI.5.2.2-4.

3. See P.V. Kane, *Hist. of Dh.S.*, Vol.III, p.705, n.also; but, he refers to the Darśapūrṇamāsa also for *praṇayana.*
4. Kane, *op.cit.,* p.704.
5. *Uttaravedi* is a technical term in the Soma sacrifice; and it is to the east; here, it is a descriptive term; hence to the north. This point is not grasped by Bodewitz (note 1 *supra*), who simply says that the *uttaravedi* is to the east.
6. Actually, the *praṇayana* and the *uttaravedi* are a new feature here, and expect no *atideśa* or *prakṛti*. This is clear also from the Dakṣiṇavedi, which is found nowhere else. This is why Kumārila says that here we have an *apūrva* (special) kind of a *vedi*; see Kane, *op.cit.*, p.705, n.

* Included here from *Bhāratīya Vidyā,* Vols. XLV-XLVII, 1 to 4 (*J.H. Dave Fel.Vol.)*, Bombay, 1987.

Chapter 16

Moral Value and the Pūrva-Mīmāṁsā

The concept of morality, or value, cannot be thought of in isolation; it presupposes a definite context. That context may be a social one, or a ritual one. Though it may look like duplicity to talk of a social context as different from the ritual one, in terms of morality, or value, it has to be remembered that, in practically all societies, a difference is maintained between these two strata. That is the reason, why the values reflected in rituals are not on the same level as those of a particular society in its modern phase.[1] The same is the case with myths. Restricting ourselves to the Vedic, and there too the Mīmāṁsaka tradition, it is necessary to examine the concept of Dharma and Ṛta. It is a known fact that the Mīmāṁsaka school is embedded in ritualism; and it does not accept any other authority than the Veda and the Vedic tradition. Its concept of Dharma is plain. Jaimini established a system, after a thorough churning of ritualistic material; and it clearly says, "Sacrifice is itself Dharma".[2] This shows that the tradition accepts the wide connotation of the term Dharma, and yet restricts it to sacrifice and the various rituals in the sacrificial system. For that matter, the term *dharma* is very difficult to be explained in a fixed unit of words, or a short measured expression, that would contain all it implies. But, the *Ṛgveda,* at most places, shows that Dharma was, for the seers, a commonly accepted rule of conduct. This rule of conduct was twofold: (i) the ritual-conduct; and (ii) social conduct. The latter was, more or less, seen as in the society of gods. Thus, when a particular god is said to have "his" *dharma*, it shows his distinguishing characteristic as seen in his action, or conduct. There are also instances where a *dharman* is common with various gods. That the concept of value is fully realized by the Vedic seers is clear in such expression as "*those were the first dharman*-s" (*ṚV* I.164.43 and 50, where the reference is to ritual-value), and "If we transgress your *dharman*-s unmindfully" (*ṚV* VII. 89.5; cf. *AV* VI.51.3). The *AV* shows a difference between Dharma and *karma* (XI.7.17), indicating that *dharma* was an established code of conduct, while *karma* was an act of an individual; here, *dharma* has the implication of value; and, this value is in the social context. The *Bṛhad. Up.* (1.4.14) shows that the word *dharma* was seen in the context of social value, when it says, that there is nothing beyond Dharma; that it is on the basis of Dharma that even a weak person can subdue a strong one.[3] It identifies Satya and Dharma (Truth, the ever-lasting principle, and the fixed code of conduct). And when the *Ait. Br.* (VIII.12 = 38.1) says for consecrated king, "Born is the protector of Dharma", the Dharma refers to the code of conduct of the society. Value and social conduct are clearly reflected in the expression of the *ṚV*, where it is said that a person (normally) does not commit sin by himself; nay, it is not in his power (VII.86.6 *na sa svo dakṣaḥ*); he does it when he is beside himself in the power of wine, wrath, or dice; or, when his mind goes astray; moreover, in the sin of a younger one the elder one is associated; again, stupor (sleep) mixes sin (*an-ṛta*) (with the normal conduct of a person).

The passage is as interesting as it is important. It suggests, that for the Vedic people, normal social behaviour was a fact of life.[4] It was *Ṛta*. A behaviour against it was *an-ṛta*. But, *an-ṛta* (or sin) was an outside contamination; it was like a virus. Normal behaviour was moral; behaviour against it was immoral. It has to be particularly noticed, that here the conviction is that man is by nature not immoral. Another very important point is, that for the contamination of sin, or immorality, the elders in the society are as responsible as the person who gets contaminated through being off-guard, himself. The thought holds good at all times; and it holds good even today. Poverty may lead to sin; but, it is the responsibility of the "Elders" (the kings, or politicians) who rule to see to it that equal amenities are made available, so that the deprived person should not get any chance to get contaminated by desire to transgress the established moral code. As one of the most striking examples, in our own days, having the same motif, may be taken of a conscientious leader undertaking fast for the atonement for the bad behaviour of his followers. This concept of Dharma lies at the base of the multitudes of expiations (*prāyaścitta*-s). The *prāyaścitta*-s cannot be taken to be restricted to the religious context alone; they have an equally sound social context. As a flaw in ritual required a *prāyaścitta* for the wholesomeness and holiness of the ritual, a *prāyaścitta* in the social context absolved the person of calumny in the eyes of the society. Even the *prāyaścitta*-s undergone secretly, for lesser flaws which others might not have even known, had an immense moral value; for they gave the performer the tranqullity of mind, which is a coveted desire of an individual. In the case of *prāyaścitta*-s prescribed and performed openly, the readiness of the defaulter to undergo them indicated repentance, which was a welcome step towards the gain of social sympathy, and even status. The texts on rituals, right from the Saṁhitā and the Brāhmaṇa texts, are replete with *prāyaścitta*-s of various types.[5] These relate to ritual behaviour and have association with a code of conduct, though it is restricted to sacrifice. *Prāyaścitta*-s that have association with social conduct are mentioned in the Smṛti texts. However, the principle underlying both the sets is the same, which is, behavioural value.

The point of *an-ṛta*, as something astray from the moral, or the established order, brings us to the concept of Ṛta. This is no place to examine the various stages of the concept of Ṛta.[6] It is, however, necessary to know, that, primarily, Ṛta was the Order—both cosmic and socio-ritual, against which it was not advisable to go. The gods abide by Ṛta; hence, some of them are specially called *ṛtavān*; so is the case with the ancient seers.[7] The term, in this case, included the moral values of the society, together with the cosmic order. The sun, moon and the rivers went on their course regularly, because they followed Ṛta. Every behaviour was controlled by Ṛta, which, on the ethical plane, indicated certain fixed code of conduct. To transgress it was following *an-ṛta*. Though the word Ṛta went out of vogue in later times, it is constantly indicated in the word *an-ṛta*, which is current even this day. The highest god of the Vedic people, Agni, is described as "The First-born of Ṛta" (*ṚV* X.5.7), and the seer calls himself by the same epithet (X.61.19), as he is confident that he knows the working of the cosmos. On the practical side, Brahman, which is nothing but sacrifice for the earliest Vedic thinkers, is closely associated with Ṛta; because, Brahman is said to come from the abode of Ṛta (VII.36.1). On the other hand, Ṛta and Satya (Truth) are said to be cognates being born from cosmic brilliance (X.190.1). In the later Vedic stage of the ritual-texts, and further, Ṛta completely gave place to Satya as a social value. And, now, *an-ṛta* came to be juxtaposed with Satya, rather than Ṛta. But, the process had already started in the times of the *Ṛgveda* itself; it has the expression *satyānṛte* (VII.49.3). But, surprisingly, it does not have the most naturally expected expression *ṛtānṛte*. This will show that Truth as the principle of everlasting value was fully understood by the Vedic Hindus; and the fact was also expressed proverbially, when it is said, that the "Earth is propelled by Truth"

(X.85.1). The expression is important, if we consider the whole verse. It says, "The earth is propelled by Truth; sky is propelled by the sun; the sons of Aditi (the gods) stand firm due to Ṛta; Soma is stationed in heaven." It will be seen that the world of the mortals is said to rest on Truth, which is its utmost moral value. Thus, in the Vedic tradition Dharma, Ṛta, Satya and Brahman were more important than the gods; for, the gods had to abide by the value indicated by these concepts. Brahman was something to be performed, and the word had a different connotation from what was attached to it in the pure philosophical context. Brahman, as something to be performed, came to be the sacrifice which was the holiest act on the earth; and it is not to be wondered that the sacrificer was ordained to speak truth during (at least!) the period of the sacrificial session.[8] The Mīmāṁsakas, having heavy leaning onto the sacrificial tradition, understood Dharma as sacrifice itself. Hence it is stressed, "*yāgādir eva dharmaḥ*"; and that Dharma is the one that is propounded by (in) the Veda alone!

The march from the Vedic texts, through the ritual texts, to the period of Jaimini, who was the founder of the Mīmāṁsā doctrine (between 400 B.C and 200 B.C) was a very long one. Ritual texts showed variations at various rituals; and many are the authorities mentioned by these texts. Ritual also got gradually evolved. It was, hence, necessary to give a general code for the performance of sacrifices. Jaimini did it and others expounded the subject. But, the suggestions and instructions given while doing it have been of immense use in getting at the moral values the Mīmāṁsā system stood for. That the Mīmāṁsā school started from ritual and entered social behaviour and law is attested by Colebrooke who says that the logic of the Mīmāṁsā is the logic of the law, and that a keen study of the application of the maxims of the Mīmāṁsā would constitute the philosophy of law.[9] However, the law reflected in the Vedic texts and the later Smṛti texts is not the same in all cases.[10] As we shall see later on in our discussion, the Smṛtis discard some of the practices found in Veda; and, yet, the general gloss is that the Smṛtis are based on the Vedas! At the moment, we may just point out that the change of moral values reflected in certain cases in the Veda and the later Smṛti texts is obvious; and here is the real problem. One of the most glaring examples of this change is what is called "Kali-varjya" (practices to be discarded in the Kali age), such as Niyoga. But, before coming to that, it is better to note some unique *dicta* which indicate the concept of value and morality according to the Mīmāṁsakas.

The most important principle is that of *a-pūrva*. Apūrva is said to be the capacity that accrues to a person who performs a sacrifice. The Mīmāṁsakas believe that the Veda, which is the supreme authority, brings sacrifice and heaven, which is the fruit of sacrifice, together. Now, a sacrifice is a collection of many rites, and one rite does not remain when the new rite is performed. Also, the fruit of heaven does not accrue to the performer immediately after the sacrifice is over. Yet, in the injunction, "a person desirous of heaven should sacrifice" heaven is aimed at; and as it is so aimed at by the Veda, it is sure to accrue to the performer. To this end we have to presume the rise of a power that brings about the gain of heaven; the power, once created, gets stored in the performer (some say in the sacrifice itself, though ended); and this power results in the reward of heaven after the death of the sacrificer. There are two points in this assumption: (i) the power that is created was not there prior to the performance of the sacrifice, i.e. it is *a-pūrva*; and (ii) when it is said that it abides in the performer, even after his death, it is clear that it gets attached to the soul, which would enjoy it in heaven. Jaimini says that even the very injunction, which causes the intense desire to perform a sacrifice (*codanā*) is the source of Apūrva; and Śabara (about A.D. 200) says that *codanā* itself should be termed Apūrva.[11] This is so, because the *codanā* presupposes a link between the fruit and the act of sacrifice. It is here, that the statement, or a definition we may say, of Dharma—*codanālakṣaṇo 'rtho dharmaḥ* — has its base. Having taken the base on the Veda and its injunctions (such as stated just above), the Mīmāṁasakas do not see any necessity of God. It is the Apūrva itself that is the dispenser of fruits. In the body of a whole sacrifice, Apūrva accrues at various levels right from the sprinkling of the grain for preparing the offering to the last offering. It has to be remembered, however, that Jaimini never mentions soul in any of his *sūtras*. But, non-mention of soul by Jaimini should not be taken as his belief in there being no soul, and that he was an atheist, an allegation levelled against him in the tradition.[12] Actually Śabara propounds the existence of the soul;[13] and for that the best testimony is of Śaṅkara himself (*Vedāntasūtra* III.3.53). Later Mīmāṁsakas believed not only in the individual soul, but also in the plurality of souls. On the lines of the Apūrva, they also believed that the individual soul is the performer as well as the enjoyer (*kartṛ* and *bhoktṛ*). Beyond the individual soul, and those in all beings separately, they have no need to believe in the Supreme Soul, where the individual soul should merge.[14] From this point of view, the Mīmāṁsā is the most practical and earthly system. In the social context, the principle of Apūrva does not separate the soul from what a person does, though it separates it (i.e. soul) from the body. The difference in the conditions of human beings (*vaiṣamya*) gets explained this way, as there is no *kartṛ* beyond the mortal performer; and moral values are only to be expected; because, the Veda never *enjoins* something that would be immoral. Even if somebody may point out to the various accounts about the gods in the Veda, referred to in the ritual-texts, the answer is that they are *arthavādas* which extol the rites prescribed, or deprecate rites that are to be avoided. At any rate, God not being believed in as the Creator, there is no plight in explaining the diversity and disparity in the world, as is seen in Śaṅkara, who, though on the authority of the *Kauṣītakibrāhmaṇa Up.* (III.8), had to admit the covert will of God to this result, even averring that He is like rain showering equally![15]

It may be of interest to know, in this connection, that Jaimini's concept of human values (*puruṣārtha*-s) included only the Dharma, Artha and Kāma; the first was the supreme, and the next two were subservient to it. Dharma comprised the following of the injunctions of the *śāstra*-s, which, in the case of the Mīmāṁsakas, was the conduct according to the injunctions of the Veda; these were mainly the daily rites. Artha included the conduct according to legal authorities; and Kāma comprised enjoyments of life.[16] But these latter two were to be not in contravention to Dharma. It is only later, the Mokṣa (release) was added, on the analogy of the Vedānta; and this was done by Kumārila and Prabhākara (seventh century A.D. and the twelfth century A.D. respectively, leaving the divergence of opinion about the date of the latter). Kumārila stresses that what relates to Dharma and Mokṣa is known from the Veda, and that what relates to Artha and Kāma is known from worldly discourse (*Tantravārtika* I.111.2). This would *apparently* indicate that Dharma has nothing to do with the norms of worldly life, which embraces only Artha and Kāma. But this is not the case. Purity, in acts in the wordly life is closely associated with the Veda; for it is specifically said that the Vedas do not purify the unrighteous. Thus, purity, which presupposes behaviour according to the fixed norms of the society, is held to be absolutely necessary for the study of the Veda and the following of the Dharma. However, the question may arise when the sacrificial rituals expect acts that are not attested by the current practices. In such a situation, the traditional ritual has to be followed; for the ritual stratum has always to be separate from the normal social one. From Jaimini to the period of Kumārila, there is a shift in the aim of life, from *svarga* to *apavarga* (release, which is only another term for *mokṣa*). We have already noted, that *svarga* was not the immediate gain; and, hence the principle of Apūrva was a necessity. Conceptually, though *svarga* was a thing to be desired, it was only an inducement for the performance of sacrifice which is supreme.[17] In *mokṣa*, for the Mīmāṁsakas, there is no sublation of the world unlike the Vedāntins. For them *jñāna* is only an indirect means to *mokṣa*. According to them, this *jñāna* is the means to know the difference of the soul from the body. *Mokṣa*, for the Mīmāṁsakas, is the state where the soul is free from pain, yet being conscious of the world.[18] This is done by the adherence to the acts that are obligatory (*nitya-karman*) which are the injunctions of the Veda, and such acts as Agnihotra where there is no desire for any fruit. This is not to be confused with the principle of *niṣkāma karma,* where a person is advised to do his duty without expecting the fruit. The concept of *niṣkāma karman* is a further step from the Mīmāṁsā principle of adherence to the *nitya-karman*. It is the extension of *nitya-karman* from the context of the Vedic injunctions to the social stratum of the world. As such, it has to be accepted that the Mīmāṁsā concept of adherence to *nitya-karman* gave rise to that of *niṣkāma karma*. The discussion on the concept of value according to the Mīmāṁsakas, for whom the authority of the Veda is supreme, would show that those who did not have the access to the Veda, or its injunctions, would not get freedom from pain, which is *mokṣa* for them. Under this category would come the Śūdras and women. Jaimini has plainly said so, and has quoted the authority of Ātreya.[19] But, the basis for this explanation is psychological, rather than caste itself; and this has also been made clear by Jaimini. The four *varṇa*-s are classified on the basis of: intelligence (Brāhmaṇa), *ahaṁkāra* and mind (Kṣatriya), senses (Vaiśya) and the objects of senses (Śūdra). The last *varṇa* being mere object of senses, has no capacity for intelligence or sense or thinking, which fact is arrived at by the keen observation of the Vedic texts. Hence the Śūdras have no access to the Veda; and as they are the objects, they can be acquired; they cannot acquire anything. This, however, has to be seen in the context of the then society and its structure. But, if somehow the Śūdra can be proved to have intelligence, it will mean that he could have access to the Veda, as is the case in these days. The circular argument of no Veda, no intelligence, and no intelligence no Veda was true in the ancient times. Already there has been a change in the position of the Mīmāṁsakas as to various values, as history shows; and with the example of *mokṣa* being already given above, there is no room to doubt why this could not be expected from the Mīmāṁsaka of modern times.

Another important contribution of the Mīmāṁsakas is the principles of *kratvartha* and *puruṣārtha*. As in the case of Apūrva, the twin-concept of *kratvartha* and *puruṣārtha* was primarily set in the context of ritual; but, it got extended to the social context. Jaimini defines *puruṣārtha* as "that in which there is the desired happiness of man, etc."[20] Thus, all main sacrifices are included in *puruṣārtha*. In *kratvartha* ("conducive to the sacrifice") are included all details and auxiliary acts that have the purpose of accomplishing the main sacrifice. They include such rites as fore-offerings, etc. What is *kratvartha* renders the whole sacrifice defective if it is, itself, defective. If what is *puruṣārtha* is not followed, the performer gets the blemish, while there is no defect in the sacrifice. Śabara applies these principles, on the social stratum, to the acquisition of wealth. Now, if one acquires wealth by means not sanctioned by the *śāstras* and performs a holy act, such as sacrifice, the placement of defect will depend on whether the rules for the gain of wealth are *kratvartha* or *puruṣārtha*. If the acquisition of wealth is *kratvartha*, wealth obtained by means not prescribed by the *śāstras* will be defective, with the result that the sacrifice will be defective. But, if the acquisition of wealth is *puruṣārtha,* such wealth could be used for any holy act, and the act will be meritorious. The performer may undergo an expiation. This twin principle has been used in the Dharmaśāstra; and it is decided, that the gain of wealth is *puruṣārtha* and not *kratvartha*, as the tendency to acquire wealth is natural to man, and no *śāstra* is required for it. An extension of this concept further has been helpful. As the gain of money is *puruṣārtha* one may gain money by any means and do a pious act. The act has existing value. Thus, if a dacoit builds a temple, the temple remains intact as a place of respect; the dacoit may be punished for his act of dacoity. The same will be (and is) true in the case of many businessmen (who are termed *prakāśa vañcaka* by Manu)[21] who build temples or construct places of public utility. It will be noticed that this plea of the Mīmāṁsakas has a great social value. Likewise, marriage is said to be *puruṣārtha*, which is a way to explain the change in the laws of marriage, based on a variety of customs. Hence, though the consideration of *gotra* is *kratvartha* marrying a diseased girl, against the caution of the *śāstra* is *puruṣārtha*. Though it is not stated clearly, marriage with a maternal uncle's daughter prevalent in some parts of the country could be explained on this plea, though some texts censure it as void. Actually, though writers on Dharmaśāstra did not specifically state it, the scope of *kratvartha-puruṣārtha* is very wide. As mentioned above, it explains almost all changes, what is *kratvartha* and what is *puruṣārtha* being decided by the thinkers of a specific period.[22] This brings us to a very ticklish problem, which is, of the practices reflected as prescribed in the Veda but not accepted by later law-givers. It is not necessary to go into details, which are termed *kalivarjya* (abandoned in the Kali age).[23] We may refer to just one detail, the *niyoga*. Long discussions are found in this regard, Manu enjoining it and forbidding it; and, in that case, whether it is optional! The proper answer would be to say, that the purpose of *niyoga* (which is the appointment of a person. preferably younger brother of a deceased person, or of an impotent person, to beget a son on the latter's wife) is to procreate a son for another person; the gain of a son is a necessity for the gain of heaven; hence, this depends on the natural desire of a man. Hence, the gain of a son, by whatever means, is *puruṣārtha*. Therefore, there is no defect in such a son and in such a method. In the event of change in values and concepts, say in the Kaliyuga and modern times, the same is not *puruṣārtha*. Then it is viewed as *kratvartha;* and the resulting birth of such a son and the son himself becomes defective. What is the *kratu* in this case of a sexual act? Well, a sexual act is not itself censurable, if it is within the accepted norms of a society. According to the Hindu tradition, all *saṁskāra*-s, including the *garbhādhāna* are ritual acts. Even in *niyoga* the act was supposed to be holy; and the person 'appointed' had to do it in a particular discipline, and the period for the act was called Brāhma. Hence, it was a veritable *kratu*. Actually, in changed times, this act will even cease to be viewed as a *kratu*.

What has been said above as regards *kratvartha* and *puruṣārtha* would explain the Mīmāṁsā position as regards Vedic rituals (and not mere mythical accounts referred to as *arthavāda*-s), which are unpalatable to-day. The *kratvartha-puruṣārtha* concept is fluid and suits the change in value.

NOTES AND REFERENCES

1. For such rituals and their study, see, S.A. Dange, *Sexual Symbolism from the Vedic Ritual,* Delhi, 1979, esp. pp.1-82.
2. Cf. Laugākṣibhāskara, *Arthasaṅgraha*, ed. S.M. Paranjape, Bombay, 1927, p.10.
3. Cf. *atho abalīyān balīyānsaṁ āśaṁsate dharmeṇa.*
4. The *Ṛgveda* says that a person who eats without caring for others eats food that is of no use to him, *ṚV* X.117.6.
5. For a treatment of this topic, see P.V. Kane, *History of Dharmaśāstra,* Vol. IV, Poona, 1973, pp.1-152.
6. See Dange, *op.cit.*, pp.8-14, where other views are noted.

7. *ṚV* II.28.6; V.65.2; II.24.7, etc.
8. *Ait.Br* I.6; *Taitt Sam.* II.5.5.6.
9. *Miscellaneous Essays*, Vol.I, Madras, 1837, pp.316-17
10. P.V. Kane, *op.cit.,* Vol. V, pt.II, p.1260ff.
11. *Jaim.*, *Pūrvamīmāṁsāsūtra,* Anandashram, Poona. II.1.5, *codanā punar ārambhaḥ*; and Śabara, *codanety, apūrvaṁ brūmaḥ.*
12. *Padma Purāṇa,* VI.263.74-76.
13. On *Jaimini* I.1.5; Anandashram, ed., pp.60-72.
14. See P.V. Kane, *op.cit.*, Vol. V, pt.II, p.1206; see also S.Cromwell Crawford, *The Evolution of Hindu Ethical Ideas,* Hawaii, 1982 (1974), p.102
15. Cf. *eṣa hy 'evainaṁ sādhu karma kārayati* ... and *eṣa hy' evainam asādhu karma kārayati.*
16. P.V. Kane, *op.cit.*, p.1216; C. Crawford, *op.cit.*, pp.102-104.
17. The injunction *svarga-kāmo yajeta* is explained by the Mīmāṁsakas as: *yāgena svargaṁ bhāvayet,* where *yāga* has higher status.
18. *Pūrva M.S.* (Jaimini) IV. 3.15 and Śabara.
19. *Ibid.*, VI.1.26.
20. *Ibid.*, IV.1.2 *yasmin prītiḥ puruṣasya.....*
21. *Manu Sm.* IX.257 *prakāśavañcakās teṣām nānāpaṇyopajīvinaḥ.*
22. Thus at various places in the Brāhmaṇa texts we have mention of a practice, which is advised to be discarded with the words *tan na ādṛtyam*, or *tad u tathā na kuryāt.* The present writer has taken up a project on such variations, now published. See S.A. Dange, *Vedic Sacrifices — Early Nature*, Vols. I & II, Aryan Books International, New Delhi, 2000.
23. For which see P.V. Kane, *op.cit.*, pp.1267-72.

* Included here from *Haryana Sahitya Akademi Journal of Indological Studies*, Vol. II - 1 & 2, Chandigarh, Spring 1987.

Chapter 17

"Root-Germinants" in the Sanskrit Language (√GHAS: √AD)

Roots have been believed to be at the basis of the formation of many words in a language; and as far as the Sanskrit language is concerned, scholars are familiar with the controversy between the Nairuktas and Śākaṭāyana on the one hand and the adherents of Gārgya on the other.[1] The former believed that all the names in a language (here in this context, Sanskrit) have their origin in a root; the latter that this is true in only a few cases. It is also an established fact that a language has adjectives formed from the roots, and are known as the participles, etc.

It is interesting to note that, in certain cases, roots give rise to new roots. This is not to point to the Causals, the Desideratives or such other forms where the original root is the same, the form only changing. What is intended to be pointed here is that, with a slight phonetic change, a new root is created; but the meaning is the same.

The Sanskrit language, like other languages, has a number of cases of similar words (i.e. phonetically similar) having different meanings. Among the roots we may point out √*dā* which means "to give" and also "to cut"; and it is indicated by the tradition by calling the latter one *dāp* and giving the appellation *ghu* to the former one.[2]

Instances of similar nature may be easily multiplied. We are not concerned with them for our present purpose; for in this case the phonemes of the two roots are the same in the actual usage.

Before we come right to the point, we may also note the system of the *ādeśa*-s. Pāṇini, at various places, points out that a particular root comes as the *ādeśa* of certain other root, as for example is the case in the aphorism *iṇo gā luṅi* which indicates that in the Aorist the forms of the root √*gā* are substituted (and not simply the sound *gā*) for the root √*i* ("to go"). This indicates that some roots already lost some of their forms, and had to be adjusted with other roots showing the remaining forms of their own.[3] The principle of *ādeśa* worked also in the sphere of the roots, the meaning being the same; but there is no doubt that the roots in these cases were quite different from one another. And there is no case of the creation of a new root.

For what we have proposed earlier as the motive of this paper, we shall take a small unit of roots as an example, which will not only explain the *ādeśa*-principle of the grammarians but also exemplify the formation of a new root from the original one. We take the roots, √*ad,* √*ghas* and √*khād*, all meaning "to eat" and recorded in the *Dhātupāṭha* ascribed to Pāṇini.

Under the *adhikāra-sūtra, ārdhadhātuke* (*Pāṇ.* 2.4.35), the *Aṣṭādhyāyī* gives the various *ādeśa*-s of the root √*ad*. Thus we have:

(i) √*ad* has the *ādeśa* √*jagdh* (*jagdhi* with *i* for pronunciation only); before the suffix *lyap*, *ti* and the one having an indicatory *k* (*Pāṇ.* 2.4.36)
(ii) The same root has √*ghas* in the Aorist and in the Desiderative (*Ibid.,* 37)
(iii) It has the form √*ghas* before the suffixes *ghañ* and *ap* (*Ibid.*, 38).
(iv) In the Vedic *mantra*-s this substitution is seen variously (*Ibid.*, 39).
(v) In a Vedic *mantra* it occurs (once) in the Perfect.

The examples of the rules mentioned above are respectively—*jagdha* or *jagdhvā, aghasat* (Aorist), *ghāsa, pra-ghasa, vi-ghasa,*[4] *ghastām or sagdhi* (which is formed from *sa* (i.e. *samānā*) and *gdhi* (from √*ghas* + the termination *ti* (*ktin*) which forms a noun), and lastly *jaghāsa,*

Out of these examples the formation of *jagdha* or *jagdhvā* and that of *sagdhi* is quite similar; for in all these the root is *ghas*; and it loses its penultimate vowel (*a*), as the following suffix begins with a consonant, i.e. the phoneme *t*, and has been provided with the indicatory sound *k* (*Pāṇ*. 6.4.96-100). Thus we have *sagdhi* — √*ghas* + *ti* > *ghs* (with *a* dropped) + *ti*; then, with the dropping of the *s* (cf.*jhalo jhali Pāṇ*. 8.2.26), we get *gh* + *ti* > *gh* + *dhi* (*Pāṇ*. 8.2.40), > g+ *dhi* = *gdhi* (Cf. *Pāṇ*. 8.4.53) *sagdhi* showing *gdhi* is peculiar to the Veda. From the aphorism (*Pāṇ*. 2.4.36) it appears that the language at Pāṇini's time had a form *jagdhi* (in *ktin*) meaning "food".

When we likewise examine the forms in the suffixes *ta* (*kta*) and *tvā (ktvā*), the question is: why is it necessary to take the *ādeśa* as *jagdh?* The answer is not far to seek. For, if *ghas* were taken to be the *ādeśa,* the forms expected would have been *ghasta* or *ghasitvā,* which the language does not warrant. The forms are *jagdha* or *jagdhvā*. It should be no great task to note that even here the root is *ghas;* but the base is a reduplicated one. Thus √*ghas* > *gha-ghas* > *ga-ghas* > *ja-ghas;* then *jaghas*+ *ta* or *tvā*; and with the process already noted *jaghas* + *ta* (*tvā*) > *jaghs* (*a* dropped) + *ta* (*tvā*) > *jagh* (*s* dropped) + *ta* (*tvā*) > *jagh* + *dha* (*dhvā*) > *jagdha* (*dhvā*).

The aphorism enjoins *jagdhiḥ* (*jagdh*), which necessitates the dropping of *dh* either of the suffix or of the *ādeśa*. Thus, *jagdh* + *ta* (*tvā*) > *jagdh*+ *dha* (*dhvā*) > *jagdha* (*dhvā*). We feel it would have been sufficient, had the beginning aphorism been *ado luṅ-sanor ghasḷ* followed by *abhyasto lyap-ti-kiti*, instead of *ado jagdhir,* etc.

If we stick to the aphorism, the better way seems

to believe that the pronunciation of the words so formed must have shown the *dh* of *jagdh* optionally in which case the word must have been pronounced as (i) *jag**dh**dha* (***dh**dhvā*), (ii) *jag**d**dha* (***d**dhvā*) and (iii) jagdha *(gdhvā)*.

The *Ṛgveda* has *akṣan* (I.82.2), *aghaḥ* (VIII.12.8), *ghasaḥ* (III.52.3), *ghāsim* (I.162.14), etc. as the forms of √*ghas*. This would show that there already existed an independent root (*ghas*), which is also noted by Bhaṭṭoji in his remark *ayaṁ na sārvatrikaḥ* (*SK* note on the root *ghas*). The independent status of √*ghas* is clear even to Pāṇini as seen from the *sūtra* (*Pāṇ*. 6.4.100),[5] where the root *ghas* does not seem to be a secondary one; and the forms *ghasaḥ* (in the *leṭ*) and *aghaḥ* (Aorist according to Sāyaṇa, while Imperfect according to GRASSMANN *Wörterbuch*, p. 422) are proof thereof. There is no room absolutely for the contention that √*ghas* is "a defective root used only to form certain tenses of √*ad*",[6] which would reflect a layman's approach to Sanskrit grammar.

Now the next interesting point is the new root, in fact, forms of the root *ghas,* obviously with a phonetic adjustment:

(i) √*jakṣ* which is the reduplicated *ghas*; and Pāṇini has noted it in his *sūtra*, *jakṣityādayaḥ ṣaṭ*. Thus, *ghas* = *ga - ghas* = *ja-ghas*> *jaks,* the change from *g*> *k* being due to the following *s* (*Pāṇ*. 8.4.55) > *jakṣ,* the change *s* > *ṣ* by *Pāṇ*. 8.3.57). (The process may be seen also in √*sthā* > √*tiṣṭhā* and √*drā* > √*daridrā* and certain other roots.)

(ii) √*kṣad* and √*khād* which are phonetically akin appear to be formed from the combination of √*ghas* and √*ad*, so closely associated in the system of the *ādesa,* as we have noted above. Thus **ghas-ad* > *ghs-ad* > *kṣ-ad* > *kṣad.*

We have in the *Ṛgveda* the form *kṣadase* (I.25.17, *hoteva kṣadase priyam*) and we may compare *akṣat* (X.11.5) which can be derived both from √*ghas* and from √*kṣad*. We have, again, the reduplicated forms in the Perfect base as *cakṣadāna* (I.116.16;117.18) and *cakṣade* (X.79.7).

From √*ghas* obtains the noun *kṣu* (√*ghas*+ *u,* the root changing *g* to *k* as noted above), and from √*kṣad* obtains *kṣadman;* we have also *kṣu-mat* ("full of food").

It is not always possible to get to the most original basis of the formation of words in a language, though it is not entirely impossible to gather the probable relationship between a root and the relative physical activity. In certain cases the original activity and the root get so closely associated that it is possible to mark the association. There can be no denying that the principle of onomatopoeia works at the back of many a root; and if we look at the root √*ad*, and also √*ghas,* from this angle, we could, probably, mark a subtle difference. √*ad* denotes simple movement of the jaws with the teeth clashing with one another and producing a sound, the lips being apart. In the case of √*ghas* the most original action does not seem to be of munching or of actual eating as such. The most original idea, probably, was that of attacking, prior to the actual devouring and, at times, even devoid of eating! The same is borne out by the root √*khād,* which is a combination of √*ghas* and √*ad*, as has been indicated above. The words *vṛtra-khāda* (*Ṛgveda* III.45.2); *amitrakhāda* (*ibid.,* X.152.1) and *ā cakhādā'vasaṁ paṇim* (*ibid.,* VI.61.1) bear testimony to what has been proposed. The form *abhikṣadam* (*abhi*+ *kṣad* + *kvip* + *am*) may be compared (VI.50.1), as also *bahu-kṣadaḥ,* having the full connotation of attacking, rather than of eating. The formation of the root *kṣad* (√*ghas* + √*ad*), we have already hinted at.

If we probe the point further, we are able to formulate a general principle for our guidance. The principle may not be too rigidly applicable; but it is, nevertheless, advantageous. The principle is this:

If, with a slight change in the constituent phonemes in a morph the meaning does not change radically,

or, in other words, if the shade of the original meaning is the same, the new morph is only a variant of the former.

We can thus say that √*kṣad*, √*khād* and √*ghas-ad* are only variants of one root, which is √*ghas;* and this root had the most original sense of attacking, prior to eating. To the same may also be added the roots √*grah* and √*gras,* both being akin to √*ghas,* all of which being coined in the hunting period. The semantic closeness of √*gras* and √*grah* can be seen from the words *grasana* or *grahaṇa* used in the context of the eclipse, which is also believed to be the act of eating or swallowing on the part of the demon who attacks. We might not be wrong in believing that the roots √*ghas*, √*ghas-ad,* √*grah* and √*gras* are from one original root, may be √*gras* > *grah/ghas;* and that original root is the germinant for the others in the unit.

NOTES AND REFERENCES

1. *Nirukta,* I.4.
2. *Pāṇ,* I.1,20, *dā-dhā ghvadāp.*
3. Cf. also *aster bhūḥ* (*Pāṇ*. II.4.52); *hano vadha luṅi* (*ibid.*, 43); *bruvo vaciḥ* (53), etc.
4. Bhaṭṭoji takes the forms *pra-ghasaḥ* and *vi-ghasaḥ* (in *ap*) to be governed by the aphorism *upasarge 'daḥ;* he gives the aphorism *ghañapoś ca* (*Pāṇ*. III.3.59 and II.4.38 respectively), indicating that only the suffix *ap* would be seen after *ghas,* which is the *ādeśa* of √*ad,* if it is preceded by an *upasarga*. But we have *pra-ghāsa* (cf. *Varuṇa-praghāsa*), indicating the suffix *ghañ*.
5. The relevant aphorisms are as follows:-
   gama-hana-khana-ghasām lopaḥ kṅity aṅi (VI.4.98) and *ghasi-bhasor hali ca* (100).
6. Apte, *Sanskrit-English Dictionary*, under √*ghas.*

* Included here from *New Indian Antiquary*, Bombay, Series III, V-1., Jan 1971.

Chapter 18

Prākritization and the Germinant of the Roots of "Vision"

Generally speaking there should be no room for any fresh discussion on the point of Prākrit and prākritization. Scholars have already marked the difference between Prākrit and prākritization. Prākrit is the name given to a group of Indo-Āryan languages; but the word in itself has no special geographical or ethnic significance. The word is understood only when applied to a variety of languages closely related to Sanskrit. On the basis of the close relationship of the Prākrit languages with Sanskrit, controversies started; and they were more of a sectarian nature than scientific. It was proposed that the original language was Sanskrit, while it was also proposed that the original language was Prākrit. This problem was given the support of etymology; and two conflicting explanations came forward—(*i*) *prakṛtiḥ sanskṛtam, tata āgatam prākṛtam;* and (*ii*) *prāk kṛtam iti prākṛtam.* The first view was held by Hemacandra Dhanika (the Commentator of the *Daśarūpakam* 2.60), Simhadevagaṇin (on *Vāgbhaṭālaṁkāra* 2.2) and Narasimha (*Prākṛta-śabdapradīpikā* p.1) and others (for these views, may be consulted Pischel, *Comparative Grammar of the Prākrit Languages,* Introduction). Narasimha clearly said that Prākrit was the "*vikṛti*" of Sanskrit. The question as to which was the original language, Sanskrit or Prakrit, was connected with sectarianism by ancient scholars like Namisādhu. More searching modern scholars, hence, left the question as of no real significance; and started studying the Prākrit tendencies right in the Vedic language (Ghatge, A.M., "Prākrit-tendencies in the Ṛgveda", *IHQ*, 21-3, pp.22-26; Ghosh, B.K., "Prākrit Samdhis in the Ṛk-samhitā", *Indian Linguistics,* Poona, 9, pp.30-57). But the old question as to the exact implication of the term *prakṛti,* whence we have the word *Prākṛta* for the languages, remained waiting.

The difference between Sanskrit and Prākrit was seen by Bharata himself when he gave the ruling that for certain characters Sanskrit was not to be used, while Prākrit was to be used for good reason — (*kāraṇam tu vyapadeśya prākṛtam samprayojayet;* and *anadhītottamānām ca saṁskṛtam naiva yojayet*). In the words "*anadhīta-uttama*" not being given the Sanskrit speech lies the indication that, at the time of Bharata education was the main criterion of the *samskāra;* and that those who learnt the texts in Sanskrit could speak the language called Sanskrit. As women did not have traditional education, they did not have the source of the Sanskrit learning; hence generally speaking they could not speak the Sanskrit tongue. The same was the case with the Vidūṣaka, who, though a brahmin by birth could not speak Sanskrit; he could not speak Sanskrit as he had stayed away from traditional learning. This will show that Sanskrit had come to be the status-language, while the general language was the local form of the Indo-Āryan speech, which was generally called Prākrit. The *bhāṣā* was designated as the Prākrit; and it denoted the regional language getting its name from that region. The languages called *vibhāṣā* were the tribal languages, though they were denoted by the name Prākrit, and were loosely included in the general term Māgadhī. The reason of this inclusion was that Māgadhī was the Easternmost phase of the Indo-Āryan; and the Eastern tongue had the tradition of being considered to be the lower type, as compared to the Northern or the North-eastern, right from the Vedic times (cf. *Kauṣītaki Br.* VII. 6 – *udañca u eva yanti vācam śikṣitum*). This would require the examination of the statement — *"prācyā vidūṣakādīnām"*. Though the *Prācyā* is said to be only a phase of the language Śaurasenī (Mārkaṇḍeya — *"prācyāḥ siddhiḥ śaurasenyāḥ*), the exact nature of the speech is not very clear. The import appears to be rather, that he speaks an "eastern tongue", and this was in continuation with the old concept of the eastern speech being a slightly corrupt speech. This is no place to go into the details of the allotment of the various Prākrits to the various characters. But the point is that Bharata's concept of Prākrit included all languages other than the status-speech, which was called the chaste speech (*saṁskṛta*). The term also included such languages as of the Śabaras or the Cāṇḍālas, that might not be strictly Indo-Āryan. In the Sanskrit drama they were denoted by the most corrupt tongue like the Māgadhī. As these tribes were also *a-saṁskṛta* (without the traditional learning and lacking in the practice of uttering the medium of the learning through the help of the then available sources of traditional learning) they were given the Prākrit language, irrespective of their own language.

What has been said above will show that at Bharata's time, Prākṛta came to indicate the speech of the common people. Among them may be the people who were the non-Sanskrit (i.e. non-educated) mass of the Āryan -speech-peoples, as also those who did not speak the Āryan tongue, but had their tribal speech, or even a foreign tongue. This will show also that the word *"prakṛti"*, in the hitherto known definitions of *Prākṛta*, does not indicate a language as such, and in the least Sanskrit. Pischel's opinion that Sanskrit could not be the source-language of the languages called Prākrit is acceptable; for, as he rightly says, Prākrit languages have many words that are not seen in Sanskrit but get directly connected with the Vedic (*op.cit.,* p.4. Ed. English Tr. 1965); and the suggestion, that all Prākrits go back to popular dialects, is also acceptable. But yet, what is the exact implication of *Prakṛti,* whence we have the name Prākṛta? We have to note that, Prākṛta is the "common people's speech", *prakṛti indicated the* "common people", and not the "original language" as Namisādhu said. The word *prakṛti* has been amply used in this sense (generally in the plural). The best definition will, hence, be—*"prakṛtayaḥ iti sādhāraṇāḥ janāḥ, tebhyaḥ āgatam prākṛtam"*. This will mean that Prākṛta was the common man's speech and also the mode of the common man's Indo-Āryan, *"prakṛtīnām bhāṣā"*. This also shows that *prākṛta,* in its original sense, indicated the fluid language that kept on changing, as against Sanskrit which was fixed. That is why even Marāṭhī was called *prākṛta* by early Marāṭhī poets. That the word *prakṛti,* which is at the base of the word Prākṛta (indicative of the language), indicated the *common uneducated (uncultured) people* is clear also from the fact that the word *prākṛta* indicated the *"idiom of the people"* also, though the actual wording of this idiom, when incorporated by the cultured people, was Sanskrit. This will be clear if we recall to our memory some of the Vedic ritual-*mantras* such as the *āhanasyāḥ* (*ṚV Khila* v 22) or the *jana-kalpāḥ* (*ibid.*, v 13; also *Atharvaveda* X. 128.6-11). Ṣaḍguruśiṣya, commenting on the *Aitareya Br.* (VI. 30 = 30.4) wherein some of these *mantra*-s are incorporated, warns that the efficacy of these *mantra*-s will be lost if more mixture of *prākṛta* was made—(*naśyed etadgato lābho bahu-prākṛta-miśraṇāt*) indicating some *prākṛta* mixture already done. Ṣaḍguruśiṣya flourished in the twelfth century A.D., which will show that the connotation of the term *prākṛta* till quite late was associated with the *prakṛtayaḥ* (the common masses). The same, obviously, was the thought of Bharata in differentiating *prākṛta* from the *Samskṛta* by which he meant to differentiate the speech of the *common man* from that of the educated. This difference is exactly maintained in the Rāmāyaṇa when it indicates that the speech of the *dvijāti*-s was chaste (*samskṛtā*—cf. *Sundara* 18, *yadi vācam pradāsyāmi dvijatīriva saṁskṛtām*). To talk in the chaste (*Saṁskṛtā*) language was the etiquette of the *dvijāti*-s, for it is they who were educated (*adhīta*); and even among them those who were not educated spoke only their natural tongue, the general Prākṛta. Saṁskṛta and Prākṛta were, thus, concurrent both being fluid. Later Sanskrit got fossilized while, as the speech of the people went on ever showing various phases of phonetic changes, the Prākṛta remained fluid, till it slanted towards more change and getting itself fossilized got differentiated from the Apabhraṁśa or the later (NIA) languages.

But though the Prākṛta language as such, thus, got to indicate a particular stage of human speech, the tendency of prākritization is seen even in the so-called status-language, and was never restricted to a particular period. Certain avowedly Prākṛta words came to be used by the people speaking the status-language obviously in the fluid stage, and thus, got to be called Saṁskṛta. Thus, the change from *bh* to *h* was a clear Prākṛta-change, indicating the retaining of the vowels and eliding the initial consonant. But, roots like *hṛ* and *gṛh–grah* came to be accepted as Sanskrit roots, their original being √*bhṛ* and √*gṛbh*. The Vedic forms are √*bhṛ* > *bharati* and √*gṛbh* > *gṛbhṇāti*, while the Sanskrit are *harati* and *gṛhṇāti*; and yet the direct nominal form √*gṛbh* is preserved both in the Vedic and Sanskrit as *garbha*. Likewise, the word *gṛha* is a prākritized form of *gṛbha*, both meaning "house"; but whereas *gṛbha* is not used in the Sanskrit language, its prākritized form *gṛha* is common. In the Vedic, however, both are to be seen (*ṚV* VII. 21.2 *gṛbhāt*, "from the house"; *gṛha* occurs at a good number of places). Further, the regular prākṛta-form *giha* > *geha* is also seen; and that too right in the Vedic (*geh-yam*, "belonging to the house" *ṚV.* III.30.7). A good number of traditional grammatical rules are useful for such a study; and in the present case the *vārtika "hṛ-gṛhor bhaś cchandasi"* (*Vār.*

4823) indicates the direction of prākritization. Comparison of the two phases of the root √*bhṛ,* or of the root √*gṛbh* shows that √*gṛh* and √*grah* are cognates. The same is true of √*bhṛ* and √*hṛ*; and though both are found as separate roots in the Vedic and the Sanskrit languages there is no doubt that the germinant was the one with the *bh*-sound. Thus,

√*gṛbh*	→ *gṛbh* / → *gṛh*	√*bhṛ*	→ *bhṛ* / → *hṛ*

Prākritization, thus, helps give root-reflexes, of which one is the germinant and all are cognates.

The present author has been studying the root-germinants for quite some time. For the present study are taken up roots indicative of "Vision" and "knowledge through Vision". The proposition, as given on the former occasion, is that apparently different roots are cognates, and are formed from the same arch-root, if with the sound-nucleus the meaning of all is conceptually the same; and secondly that the difference in the phonemes is accountable.

The Prākṛta-roots of "vision" are as follows, along with the known Sanskrit originals:—

√*cakkha*	<	*cakṣ*	√*lakkha*	<	*lakṣ*
√*ikkha*	<	*īkṣ*	√*pāsa*	<	*dṛś (paśy)*
√*pekkha*	<	*pra+ īkṣ*			

We have also the nouns *cakkhu* (> *cakṣu*); *akkhi, akkha* (*añkhi—āñkh* in NIA) from Skt. *akṣan* and *akṣi*. We do not have the nouns as **pekkhu* (√*prekṣ*, **ikkhu* (*īkṣ*) or **lakkhu* (> *lakṣ*). The *Pāiasadda-mahaṇṇao* records also *dakkhu*, obviously from √*dakkha*, and traces it to Skt. √*darś* > *dṛś*. It also connects the word "*dakkhaṇa*" with SKT "*darśana*", when we expect PKT "*daṁsaṇa*" from SKT "*darśaṇa* ! The SKT-PKT change ś > *kh* is rather uncommon, the natural being SKT ś to PKT s, as in *pāsai, dīsai,* etc., and SKT *ks* or *ṣ* to PKT *kkh,* as seen in the other roots noted above, and also at other places. If that is clearly the case, we have to presuppose a root with the *kṣl ṣ* sound for *dakkhaṇa* and it will be √*dṛkṣ—dṛṣ*. Though the root *dṛkṣ* is not seen in the Classical Sanskrit, the Vedic shows its forms (*ṚV* I.6.7 *dṛkṣase*), in spite of the fact that these forms are taken to be from √*dṛś* in the injunctive or subjunctive (with the infix *s. sip* technically). The explanation of Sāyaṇa, based on the general aphorism of Pāṇini, (*Pāṇ.* VIII.2.36;-41;-3.39;-57) as to the change of the final *ś* > *ṣ* and then *k* before the *ṣ*-sound (of the injunctive or the desiderative) only proves what we have said under the present circumstances; and Pāṇini simply helps reconstructing the *kṣ*-root, lost at his time, by a known root in *ś*. We actually have the prākritized form as *kkha* < in *dekkha-dakkhu*, and even *dekkhaṇa* > Marathi *dekhaṇā*) which expects the *kṣ* sound, rather than the *ś*-sound. Then we have the following position as regards the root *dekkha*:—

PKT— √*dekkha* < *dṛkṣ* ⇅ *dṛkṣ* / *dṛś*

In this connection, and as convincing, we may refer to the forms such as "*sariccha*" (cf. *Karpūramañjarī*—I. 19, *mahiṣī-dahiṇo sarìcchā*") which, without doubt, expect *sadṛkṣāḥ* (as the *chāyā* reveals).

The validity of the hypothesis that there was a root as *dṛkṣ* "to see", is clear in such forms as *īdṛkṣa-īdṛṣī, kīdṛkṣī* and *tādṛkṣa-tādṛkṣī* (where *s*-sound does not follow) along with the ending in the palatal sound (*ś*). Another such alternation may be seen in the roots √*aś* and/*akṣ*, both meaning primarily "to pervade", which gave the noun *akṣa-akṣi* (eye) in Sanskrit and, in the Prākrit language, *akkha-akkhi*.

A cursory glance at the roots, and the nouns from them, is apt to indicate that the common sound in all of them is SKT *kṣ*, PKT *kkh* which also indicates that √*aś*

(SKT) is a reflected root; so also is the case with √*dṛś* (SKT). The germinant is, then, with the cluster *kṣ*, whatever it originally may be. For the time being our position is that the SKT *kṣ* appears to be associated with the root-germinant of the roots of "vision". But let us probe further. We take the root √*cakṣ* (SKT), which is supposed to have given the root √*cakkha* (PKT), on the basis of the general tendency of change SKT *kṣ* > PKT *kkh*. From the very face of it, the root √*cakṣ* does not appear to be the original root; on the contrary, it is the reduplicated form of the probable root in *kṣa*; but as the Sanskrit (and the Indo-Āryan) has no roots in *a*, the probable root has to be contemplated as **kṣā*, whence we get, by the general mode of reduplication the following pattern: **kṣā~kṣā-kṣā~kṣa-kṣā~ka-kṣā~ca-kṣā*, and finally √*cakṣ*. Now, it may be asked what is the basis of this hypothesis? And here the aphorism of Pāṇini comes to our rescue—"*cakṣiṅaḥ khyāñ*" (II.4.54); and the meaning of √*cakṣ* is "to see" as also "to speak" or "to tell" (*cakṣiṅ vyaktāyām vāci ayam darsane' pi*). The same is the case with the root √*khyā*, which has the sense of "seeing" in the Vedic, along with its classical sense of "conveying" or "telling" or "relating". The point is that in certain tenses √*cakṣ* is seen (i.e., in the conjugational), while for the *same meaning* in the other (non-conjugational) tenses √*khyā* is seen. As a matter of significance it may be noted that the substitution for roots generally is divided according to the conjugational and non-conjugational tenses. The substitute is found in one arrangement (i.e., non-conjugational), while the original is found in the other. This is clear in the *adhikāra*—aphorism "*ārdha-dhātuke*" (*Pāṇ*. II.4.5). With √*khyā* the position is:

√*cakṣ* < √*cakṣ* (conjugational)
√*cakṣ* < √*khyā* (non-conjugational)

But the point is—Which is the original root—√*cakṣ*, **kṣā*, or *khyā*? The root √*cakṣ* has no claim to originality as we have seen. Now, between *√*kṣā* and √*khyā* the latter is the root, as recorded by the *Ṛkprātiśākhya,* which takes √*khyā* as the basic root, and adds that, in this root, some utter the sounds *k-ś* (palatal), and the examples given by Uvaṭa (the commentator) are *akhyat* (*ṚV.* IV.14.1). The Vedāṅga adds further that the same is done in the case of the nouns *khyāti* and the like (*Ṛkpr.* VI.55; 56). Pāṇini has maintained this position in the aphorism we have already noted (*cakṣiṅaḥ khyāñ*), and the phonetic alternation of *khy-kś* is noted by Kātyāyana and maintained by Patañjali. When Kātyāyana suggests "*śasya yo vā*" (*Vār.*1586) he admits that the original sound was *kś* (palatal), and the final *ś* changed to *y*. And Patañjali starts a regular discussion on the original sound in this root saying "*kim ayam kśādiḥ āhosvid khyādiḥ*"; and replies by suggesting a sort of emendation to Pāṇini as—"*cakṣiṅaḥ kśāñ-khyāñau*", and further, "*khaśādir va bhavati*". The position taken by these authorities is thus—

√*cakṣ* → √*cakṣ*
√*cakṣ* → √*khyā* / *kśā* / *kkhyā-khyā*

wherein they suppose √*cakṣ* to be the original root. But the older text (*Prātiśākhya*) takes √*khyā* as a separate root, pointing out the variation as √*khyā-kśā*. As the root *cākṣ* is clearly a reduplicated form, there is no doubt that the original is √*khyā-kśā*; and as both *ś* and *y* are palatal, it is quite clear that *ś* was uttered for *y* by some, or in a particular region. The most original root was, then √*khyā*, meaning "seeing" (Vedic), or "telling" both centering round the concept of cognition. It is the eye that "tells" first; hence the word for the eye came from the root of mixed connotation indicative of "telling" and "seeing" as in the case with the word "*nayana*" (√*nī* "to carry"). The root *khyā* is retained in the Prākrit language with the idea of "telling", and is also the most original as we have noted. And as the normal speech of the common people, as seen from the retention in the Prākrit language, shows the *kha* sound in the place of the *kṣ* sound, we may safely say that the roots of "vision" with the *kṣ* sound were reflected roots from the germinant √*khyā*; or at any rate from √*khyā-kśā*. The position now is as follows:

cakṣ (SKT) *cakṣu* (noun)
√*khyā-kśā* > *cakhyā-cakśā* <
→ *cakkha* (PKT) *cakkhu* (noun)

Now, as we have noted, the germinant is √*kkhyā-kśā* later retained as *khy/kś* and further normalized as *kṣ* in Sanskrit. With this we may not be wrong in supposing that the roots that have this prime element, and have the same connotation, were only reflexes of one original root, with an addition of a phoneme, or even a slight change in a single phoneme, the main sound remaining the same. We might put this in the following way:

kśā-khyā

VEDA-SKT	PKT
√*khyā* (to see, to tell)	√*khyā*
√*kṣā*	—
√(*ca*)*kṣ* (Redup)	(*ca*)*kkha* (Redup) (cf. Vedic *cakhvāṃsam*—*Ṛ*V.II.14.4)
√(*i*) *kṣ*	(*i*) *kkha*
√(a) *kṣ* (*akṣa-akṣi* "*eye*")	*√(*a*) *kkh* (*akkha*—*akkhi*)

Now we enter into a really difficult problem; but, on the basis of what has been said above, we may make another observation; but prior to that we may compare √*dṛkṣ* and *dṛś*. From what we have seen, both these roots are possible; and this has been attested by the lexicon. Comparing what has been said about *kś-kh-kṣ*, it appears that even here the original element was *kṣ* (< *kh-kś*); and *dṛ* was added later. If so, we suppose the hypothetical position will be—

(*i*) *khyā-kśā* > (*ca*)*kṣ* (*cakkha*), (*ī*)*kṣ* (*ikkha*), (*a*)*kṣu* (*akkha*)

(*ii*) (*dṛ*)-*khyā-kśā* < (*dṛ*)kṣ (> *dekkha*)
                          dṛṣ / *dṛś*

Though we do not have **drakṣu* (eye), on the analogy of *cakṣu* we have *dakkhu* (PKT).

Now there is another interesting question that crops up in this connection. We have suggested that the original root gave the other roots by addition of vowels (*ikṣ, akṣ*); but there is also a probability of the change in the initial vowel. The process of prākritization shows the initial vowel *ṛ* changing into *a* or *i*. There are any number of cases of this change. Even so, with the supply of *ṛ* the reconstructed roots will be — √(*ṛ*)*khyā*-(*ṛ*)*kśā*-(*ṛ*)*kṣ*-*rṣ*. The last one is actually a root, whence we have the word *ṛṣi*, and the last but one is seen in such nouns as *ṛkṣa*, though the traditional method is to derive it from √*ṛṣ* with the suffix *ksa*. The root √*ṛṣ* generally conveys the meaning of "going". But it is pertinent to note that when Yāska derives the noun *ṛṣi*, he connects it with √*dṛś*, "to see"— "*ṛṣir darśanāt*" (*Nir.*II.12). Yāska also shows the "going"-connotation when he says "they are *ṛṣi*-s as to them did the *brahma* approach" (*tad-yad-enāns-tapasyamānān brahma svayambhu 'abhyā-narṣat ta ṛṣayo 'bhavan'*); and yet he connects the word with "*darśana*". He could well have said "*ṛṣir arṣanāt*", meaning "from approaching" as he actually uses the expression "*abhyānarṣat*". Does it indicate then, that in Yāska's time the root *ṛṣ* had also the connotation of "seeing"? In the same family may be taken the lost √*ṛkṣ*, which gives the noun *ṛkṣa*, which, though means "bear", also means "stars" (*ṚV.*1.24.10), the idea, probably being that they "look" upon the world. In this connection we may note another word, *spaśaḥ* (plural), which means "spies" (from √*spaś*, "to see"); and Varuṇa's spies are the stars. The point to be noted is that even in the word *ṛkṣa*, the element *kṣ* is present; and we may again refer to Yāska who gives the etymology of this word as follows—"*ṛkṣā udīrṇānīva khyāyante*", (hence *ṛ*-

kyā) where the original element *khyā* is present. √*Ṛkṣā* and √*ṛṣ* are, then, cognates having the shade of "seeing", and between them √*ṛkṣ* appears to be the original root. Then the position seems to be as follows:—

*√*ṛkṣ* > √*ṣṛ*

But, then, how do we explain the addition of *ṛ* to the original *kṣ-kh* (*khyā*)? Here we may suggest that in certain cases, it has been noted, that two roots combine to form a new root. Such is, for example, the case with √*ghas* + √*ad* = √*kṣad*. (For a detailed study, see "Root-germinants" in the Sanskrit Language √GHAS: √AD in this book). In the present case we may note that the combining roots are √*ṛ* "to go" and √*khyā-kṣ*. The next stage, in the formation of certain roots of similar connotation, as we have noted above, is of the prākritization of the initial *ṛ,* which changes into *i* or *a*. Thus:

√*ṛ* "to go" + √*khyā-kṣ* = √*ṛkṣ* "to see" (or "to shine" later), where √*ṛ* is joined with the root of "vision" (*khyā-kṣ*) on the analogy of √*nī nayana* which also indicates "going". This traditional belief was already current; for Durga commenting on "*ṛṣir darśanāt*" actually quotes a maxim "*ye gatyarthās te jñānārthāḥ*". We may propose the process in this case as follows:

(1) √*ṛ* + *khyā-kṣ* = √*ṛkṣ-ṛṣ* ↗ *ṛṣi* (noun, "seer")
↘ *ṛkṣa* (noun, "stars" = seers)

The concept of the stars and the "seers" (*ṛṣi*) is mingled in the "seven seers" (*Ursa Major*). Might we propose as follows:—

(2) √*ṛkṣ* > *ikṣ* (prākritization in the initial vowel) > √*īkṣ*

(*i*) **ṛkṣ* < *īkṣ* / *īṣ* } to "see" (among other senses)

(*ii*) *ṛkṣ* < √*akṣ* (noun "*akṣi*") / √*aś* (noun "*aśī*" Avestan "evil eye")

In both, the sense of pervading is present though these roots as such have lost their original phase of "seeing". The combined base-root gives another direction of root-formation:

*√*ṛkṣ* > √*lakṣ* (Pkt/*lakkha*)

So finally—

√*ṛ*+ *khyā* = √*ṛkṣ*

* √*ikṣ-iṣ*
  - √*īkṣ-is* (SKT)
  - √*ikkh* (PKT)

(i) √*akṣ* (*akkha* PKT)

(*ii*) √*lakṣ* (*lakkha* PKT)

(*iii*) √*d-ṛkṣ* (*-d-ṛs*) by addition {dekkha / *dakkha*} PKT.

As we have noted earlier, the roots √*īkṣ*, *akṣ* or *lakṣ* have also the probability of addition (or *i*, *a* or *la* to the germinant/*khyā-kṣ*). In any case the element of change akin to prākritization is clear. Thus, the roots of "vision" show the germinant √*khyā-kśā-kṣ;* and, though in some cases the original sense of "seeing" is changed, it can be marked. Another root PKT √*pās* is not from SKT √*dṛś* as is supposed. It is:—

√*spaś* "to see" (Vedic cf. *spaśaḥ*)
= √*paś* (with the dropping of the initial *s*)
= √*pāsa* (PKT)

The change √*spaś* > *paś* being forgotten, the root, √*paś* was, probably, conduced with √*paś* "to bind" (whence we have the noun *paśu*) and the root of "vision" was seen as a substitute (*ādeśa*) of another phonetically dissimilar "vision"—root √*dṛś*, which itself was a compound root, as we have noted.

We may close by another observation, which, though does not come under strict prākritization, is interesting from the point of addition and has relation to the concept of vision. We have noted above that the roots √*akṣ* and √*aś* are cognates; that both have the meaning of "going" or "pervading"; and that both originally were reflexes of √*khyā-kś-ṣ*. Now it is to be noted, that, in certain forms √*aś* takes the addition of *n* initially and the root-base becomes √*naś* as in *ānaśe* (perfect, cf. *Pāṇ*. VII.4.72). If we extend this tendency to √*akṣ* also, we get √*nakṣ*, "to move" having the idea of pervasion, but also of "seeing" if we look to the original root*√*akṣ (akṣa-akṣi)*. This also shows the way to the etymology of the word *nakṣatra*, which has been a problem (*Vedic Index*). The meaning in the word then, is of "seeing" rather than of "moving"; and this corresponds to the word *ṛkṣa*, the formation of which we have discussed, and is so conspicuous in the *Saptarṣi*-s being the Ursa Major.

* Included here from the *Proceedings*, of the National Seminar of Prākṛta Studies, Dept. of Sanskrit, University of Bombay, Bombay, 1971.

Chapter 19

Root-Germination and Reduplicated Roots in Sanskrit

A survey of the roots in the Sanskrit language reveals that not all the roots are primary. This tendency has been noticed by scholars.[1] But a more penetrating study in the case of certain cognate roots shows that between themselves some are the germinant roots, while the others are germinated. These phonetically similar roots could be taken to be only the variant forms of one primary root; for in many cases the little change in the phoneme does not change the meaning. This phonetic change is seen in the initial, the middle or the final letter; and even in the case of the apparent change the shade of meaning is generally the same. This will be seen from the following examples, which are taken from the Pāṇinian Dhātupāṭha.

1. *Initial Change:—*

   √*kurd—khurd* "to play"; also √*gurd;* √*gṛ—ghṛ* "to sprinkle"; √*yug—jug* "to discard"; √*tev—dev* "to get disgusted"; √*kaḍ—khaḍ* "to pound"; √*kuḍ—guḍ;* also √*kuṭh—guṭh* "to cover"; √*rabh—labh* "to gain"; √*rap-lap* "to speak", etc.

2. *Final Change:*

   √*valk — valg* "to prattle"; √*nāth—nādh* "to beg",

3. *Insertion:*

√*svad-svard* "to taste"; √*īrṣy—īrkṣy* "to hate"; √*kuj—kuñj* "to coo"; √*vraj—vrañj* "to go"; √*cit—cint* "to think, comprehend", etc.

4. *The Middle Change*:

śrath—ślath "to be loose"; √*garh—galh* "to censure".

Among such new roots, germinated from the primary ones, can be listed the special "*abhyasta*" variety, where the new root retains the meaning of the primary root. And also certain roots from suffixes like the desiderative, etc. obtain. But the difference between the "*abhyasta*" and the roots noted in the list above on the one hand, and those from the desiderative, etc. on the other, is that the latter obtain with the addition of a suffix, which is not the case with the former. Others are, for example, √*muc—mokṣ;* √*śak—śikṣ,* etc. But as the sense of the desiderative is wanting in them, they are on the same status as of the "*abhyasta*" or the formerly mentioned, in as much as the principle, of meaning not being changed, remains the same. The "*s*" sound which is seen in such cases, then, may not be taken to be of the desiderative, in the strict sense of "desiring". Similar is the case of the roots such as √*bhakṣ*, √*bhikṣ*, which can be traced to √*bhaj* or √*bhas* "to partake of", or "to eat" (Whitney), where the original sense of the desiderative is absent. In such secondary roots, the requirements of the desideratives, viz. reduplication and the meaning of desiring are not seen, though they might have been present formerly. In the case of √*mokṣ, guṇa (*√*muc> mokṣ; u> 0)* is also noted, which is not usual with the desiderative forms. This fact is noted by Pāṇini (VII.7.54,57). The expected reduplication is dropped even with the sense of the desiderative in certain roots; but they have to be differentiated from these where the sense of the desiderative is absent. The term "germination" is sought to be applied in the case of those roots that do not show the change in the meaning, with a slight change in, or addition of, the phoneme to such an extent that it is entirely different. In this sense, the cases of the apparent desiderative, as noted above, have to be taken as those of the addition of the "*s*" sound, with the general phonetic similarity maintained. In the case of roots where, even with the meaning being the same, there *appears* to be no outward phonetic similarity, help is available from the aphorisms of Pāṇini. Such is, for example, the case of the roots √*ghas* and √*jakṣ*[2] or √*cakṣ* and √*khyā*.[3]

Though the guiding material for the study of roots generally notes the most common roots, there are certain roots, that are not recorded; or, they could be taken as lost in the later times; and, hence, not noticed. In the category of such roots could be placed √*ah* "to speak" (which has been noted by Whitney, *op.cit.*) which presupposes the root √*agh*, obtained in some NIA languages (cf. Hindi "*aghānā*" —"to be statisfied" or "to praise"?). The *Dhātupāṭha* takes note of the root √*ah*, "to go" or "to pervade", while the forms *āha*, etc. (perfect), or even as substituted for the present forms of the root √*brū*, presuppose √*ah* "to speak". Likewise, may be mentioned the root √*vāgh*, "to praise" (cf. *ṚV* I.3.5 *upa brahmāṇi vāghataḥ; vāghate* at I.31.14; *vāghatām* at III.3.4, etc.). The tradition (cf. Sāyaṇa), however, does not see any verbal form here; but it says that the word comes in the list of words indicating the priests (*ṛtviṅnāmasu*); or the word is rendered as "the persons that lead the sacrifice" (*Nir.*III.18.3). But the difficulty for this assumption comes when we are confronted with the expression "*punāno vāghad-vāghadbhir amartyaḥ*" (IX.103.5) in the context of Soma, where Sāyaṇa renders it as "being borne" (*uhyamānaḥ*) or, alternately, "accomplishing" (*prāpayan*). This shows that the real implication of the root was lost, nay the word was lost as a root! Similarly the root √*khud,* though occurring in the *ṚV* (X.101.12 *khudata vājasātaye*) and other texts (cf.

AV. XX.137.2) is not recorded in the *pāṭha,* though it occurs in the same sense (of digging) in the later languages. To trace the root√*khud* to √*khurd* (as Sāyaṇa does), and to take it as the Vedic form of √*khurd*, with the "*r*" sound dropped as a Vedic peculiarity (cf. *khurda krīḍāyām...rephalopaśchāndasaḥ)* does not seem sound. Especially in the face of the fact that have "*khodana*" (and not *khudana*) also as the Vedic form (*ṚV* Khila V.22.10; *AV*.XX.136.15, etc.), as also the intensive form "*kanīkhudat*" *(Taitt. Br.* noted by Whitney). One wonders if the root could not be an early prākritized variant form of √*kṣud*! Likewise the root in, *vāghat-vāghatām*, etc., is likely to have been lost even in the Vedic times, though it could be, probably, linked with such NIA forms as "*vāhavā*" (Marathi and Hindi) as we have in the expression "*vāhavā karaṇe*" (Marathi, etc.), where the probability is of "*vāh-vāh*" *(vāhavā)* being indicative of praise. Of the lost root √*vāgh*, then, the form *vāghat* appears to be the Pre. P., indicative of "praising" by means of the *mantra-s*, which is the duty of the priest. *Vāghat* being included in the list of words meaning "priest" is a further step.

The position of the two roots mentioned above, then, appears to be:

√*agh—ah* "to praise", "to speak"
√*vāgh—vāh* "to praise"

It could also be the other way round, in which case the consonant will have to be taken as being added to the simple aspirate. But this seems to be less probable. That there was a root like √*vāgh,* which germinated the root √*vāh*, with the consonant dropped, is supported by the Vedic usage. Thus, the latter root is indicated in the form "*vāhas*" (*Ṛ*V. III.30.20= —.50.4; cf.—53.3), though the tendency is to trace this word to √*vah*, and understand it to indicate the "vehicle in the form of the hymn" indicating the "praise in the *mantra*".[4]

The tendency for the germination of the roots is, thus,

clear. This tendency was hinted at by Whitney, and before him by Roth (Whitney, *op.cit.* at various roots). But it has to be remembered that this tendency is not of the type of such forms as the causal, the desiderative or the like; for in these forms the root remains the same, while the sense of the new form substantially changes. In the case of the principle of germination, however, a variant root itself is germinated, as can be seen from the examples noted above, with no substantial change in the original sense; or, we may say that in the latter case the status of the root does not change, while in the case of the causals, etc. the status undergoes a change. The forms of the causal, etc. are, if we follow the tradition, arrived at by adding suffixes to the root; while in the case of the germination, there is no suffix added; the addition, if any, could be regarded as a meaningless augment only. The change in the speech-habit changes the form of the root, with the original root-status being maintained. From this point it is interesting to examine the roots that have come down as Reduplicated Roots ("*abhyasta*").

In the Sanskrit language, the roots get reduplicated, as a general rule, when the sense is of the Desiderative, the Frequentative (Intensive) and in the case of the Perfect or a type of the Aorist. But that is not the point here; for, even there the sense gets changed. What we are examining are roots that are primarily seen as reduplicated. This will also exclude the roots of the Third Conjugation, that show reduplication in actual use, as, for example, √*dā—dadāti* (gives), etc. The roots in question are such as are treated as reduplicated in themselves, yet they are primary roots (cf. *Pāṇ.*VI.1.6). These roots are:-

√*jakṣ : jāgṛ : daridrā : cakās : dīdhī : vevī : śās.*

In all they are seven, including the root √*jakṣ*.

The purpose of their being mentioned as "reduplicated" (*abhyasta*) is seen in the fact that: (*i*) they have the initial vowel as acute, while, by the general aphorism (rule), a root has the acute accent on the final vowel (*Pāṇ*.VI. 1.162); and (*ii*) in the present participle (Pr.P.) forms these do not show the insertion of the *n* sound, as is the case with other roots (in the *parasmaipada*); thus, the forms for these roots are *jákṣat* (and not *jákṣant*), *jāgrat* (and not *jāgrant*), etc.

Apart from these indications, we expect these roots not to be further reduplicated, as they are already termed as "reduplicated". As the roots are said to be reduplicated, their primary roots have to be noted. This is not difficult in the case of the roots √*vevī,* (< √*vī,* "to enjoy"), √*dīdhī* (< *dhī*, or *dhyai*" to meditate), √*cakās* (< *kās,* really √*kāś*, "to shine"), √*daridrā* (< √*drā* "to walk defectively"). In the case of the roots √*jāgṛ* and √*jakṣ,* the primary roots, it is clear, are √*gṛ* (meaning?) and √*ghas* "to eat" (as rightly shown by Whitney). The case, as regards the form and the meaning, of the root √*jakṣ* (< *ghas*) is simple; and it is as follows:

√*ghas—ghas ghas—jaghas*

(By natural reduplication; and for the change from *gh* to *ja, Pān.* VIII.4.54).

Then, *jaghas—jagh* ()s
(loss of the penultimate *a, Pāṇ.* VI.4.98)

and *jaks—jakṣ*
(*Pāṇ.* VIII.4.55; and VIII.3.57 and later).

In the case of the root √*jāgṛ*, however, closer thought is needed. If the root is a germinated root from the primary root √*gṛ*, as it clearly seems, what could be the original implication in the root √*jāgṛ*? The root √*gṛ* has in the *Ṛgveda* the sense of singing or praising, and also of keeping awake. Might it be that the original sense was that of singing or praising, and that the sense of keeping awake or awakening came as a secondary one? Or, in other words, was keeping awake, while singing the *mantra*-s a probable plane of meaning, whence the sense of simply, keeping awake or awakening came? (We might compare such expressions as *viprāsaḥ vi-panyavaḥ jāgṛvāṁsaḥ* at *ṚV* I.22.21; and *jāgṛvadbhiḥ jaramāṇaḥ* at X.91.1, where the words *jāgṛvāṁsaḥ* and *jāgṛvadbhiḥ* do not appear to imply simply "keeping awake" or "being watchful" in view of *vipanyavaḥ* and *jaramānaḥ*, both meaning "praising".)

In the case of √*daridrā,* the original root was, obviously, √*drā* (Whitney *op.cit.,* p.79, where he also indicates that the roots √*dram* and √*dru* could have a common germinant). The sense of "to be poor" in the root √*daridrā*, obviously, was a later shade from the primary sense of "wandering" (√*drā*). The root √*daridrā* became separate in the intensive of the original √*drā*, which gave, in its original sense, the words as *kadrīcī* ("having improper gait"; Sāyaṇa "invisible gait", *adṛśyamāṇa-gamanā*), where, in addition to the root √*drā* we have also √*añc* "to go" (*kad,* + √*drā* + √*añc*), *cakadrā* (cf. *viścakadrā-karṣaḥ Nir.*II.4), and also, probably, *Kadrū* (which comes later as the name of the mother of the serpents), "of zigzag gait" (Serpentine).

Out of the roots noted above √*dīdhī* and √*vevī* occur in the Vedic language only. About the root √*śās*, its being termed as the reduplicated root is due to the fact that it does not get the expected *n* sound (*nUM*) in its Pr.p. forms (cf. *ṚV.* 1.51.8 (*śāsat;* also III.31.1). Otherwise the accent is no matter; for the acute on the initial vowel would come in its similar form as the subjunctive also. This means that its being termed as the reduplicated root is only technical. Reduplication is not actually seen.

The fact that the roots mentioned above are technically called "reduplicated" is expected to suggest also that their further reduplicated forms should not be seen. But this does not seem to be a case in actual use; for we do have such further reduplicated forms of, for example, √*śās* in the *ṚV* itself (cf. *sáśāsa* at II.29.5; III.1.2). Such is not the case with √*dīdhī*, √*vevī,* nor with the other roots, except √*jāgṛ*; but the case of the last root is not supported from the *Ṛgveda*. However, the form with further reduplications appears to have been current later.

As such, the statement of Patañjali, that in the case of the root √*jāgṛ*, reduplicated forms in the perfect (where reduplication is a general rule) are optionally seen, is puzzling in the face of the example that he gives, viz. "*yo jāgāra tam ṛcaḥ kāmayante*" and, in the same breath, "*yo jajāgāra tam ṛcaḥ kāmayante*" (*M.Bhāṣya* on *Pāṇ*. VI.1.8). Actually the passage quoted by him is *ṚV* V.44.14,abc; (cf. also *ibid.,* 15a) and the metre does not at all allow "*jajāgāra*"; and there is no variant. The puzzling question is, where does Patañjali quote it from? And could it ever be right? Or, does Patañjali quote arbitrarily? Later Bhaṭṭoji gives the reduplicated form *jajāgāra*, but does not quote the text, as it was not his method (*S.Kau.* under 2480). But the further reduplicated forms of √*śās,* as we have noted, show that this particular root was not factually a reduplicated root; but it was included in the list because of its not taking the *n* sound in the Pr.p. It was not strictly a reduplicated root, on the same status as the others.

Apart from the roots that are technically called "reduplicated", we have certain others like √*tiṣṭh*, which was later merged in √*sthā,* only to be understood as the latter's form in the formation of Verbs. In the original usage, however, √*sthā* appears as different from √*tiṣṭh*, and has forms in itself, independently of √*tiṣṭh* which represented it in conjugational forms (cf. *ṚV* I.15.2;-139.11; 108.3 and at many other places). We may also note the root √*dad* which is independent of √*dā* (cf. the forms *dadade, dadadire*, instead of *dade dadire*, noted by Bhaṭṭoji, *S.Kau* 2263). But even in this case √*dā* appears to be the original root, as √*sthā* is in the case of √*tiṣṭh*, from which germinated the reduplicated ones, as far as Sanskrit is concerned.

NOTES AND REFERENCES

1. W.D. Whitney, *The Roots, Verb-forms and primary Derivatives of the Sanskrit Language,* Leipzig 1885, Michigan;

1950; G.B.Palsule, *The Sanskrit Dhātupāṭhas,* Poona, 1961, p.161f.

2. See the Chap. "Root-germinants in the Sanskrit Language".
3. See the Chap. "Prākritization and the Germinants of the Roots of Vision".
4. Sāyana on *ṚV* III.30.20; also Geldner, *Der Rigveda,* HOS Vol. 33, London, 1951; H.D. Velankar, *Ṛgveda Maṇḍala* III, Bombay, on the passage.
5. *Mahābhāṣya* of Patañjali, New Govt. of India ed., Motilal Banarsidass, Delhi, 1967, Vol. II, p.680 on *Pāṇ*. VI.1.8.

* Included here from the *Proceedings* of the Seminar on Historical Linguistics, *Journal of the University of Bombay*, Bombay, Vol.XLI, Arts No.77, Oct.1972.

Chapter 20

Dampatī and Patnī

The word *dampatī* has been included in the representative class (*ākṛti-gaṇa*) *'rājadantādi'* (*Pāṇ*.II. 2.31), which also includes the words *bhāryāpatī, jāyā-patī, jam-patī,* etc. It will be seen that all these words have *pati* as the second member. The word *pati* gets the technical appellation *ghi* (i.e. words ending in *i* and *u*) only in a compound, i.e. as the second member of a compound (*Pāṇ*. I.4.8); but according to another aphorism the word designated as *ghi* would be placed as the first member of the dual compound (II.2.32). As the formation of the words noted above does not conform to the rule for the *ghi* (here the word in question being *pati*), they were taken to be exceptions and were placed in a separated class called *rājadantādi*, in which were accommodated such words, where the expected first position of the first member is seen as the second in actual use; for according to the principle for the *ghi*-words, the words noted above are **pati-bhārye, *pati-jāye, *pati-dam* (?) and so on. The fact that the words *dampatī* and *jampatī* are included along with the words *bhāryāpatī* and *jāyāpatī* is clearly indicative of the former two being taken to be compound words indicating the dual (*dvandva*). But, as can be seen, these two words are not on the same level of the other two. For as regards the constituents, *dam* and *jam* are not like *jāyā* and *bhāryā*.

But, as in actual usage the words *dampatī* and *jampatī* came to denote the couple (wife and the husband), they were supposed to be on par with the words *jāyāpatī* and *bhāryāpatī*; and this is the reason why Bhaṭṭoji flatly takes them as the variants of *jāyā*. But as it was difficult to account for the queer change *jāyā> dam/jam,* it was stated that it was a case of an arbitrary change (*nipāta*).[1] So to put the position taken by the grammarians in a figure,

$$\{\textit{jāyā}\}\text{— — —}\quad \left.\begin{array}{l} /\textit{jāyā} \\ /\textit{dam}/ \\ /\textit{jam}/ \end{array}\right\} + \textit{pati}$$

(cf. Bhaṭṭoji on *Pāṇ*. II.2.31, *jāyā-śabdasya jam-bhāvo dam-bhāvaś ca vā nipātyate*).

It has to be borne in mind, however, that the word *dampati* is not always in the dual. This also precludes its being *always* a compound-word indicating the *dvandva*. In the *ṚV* we have the word in the dual as also in the singular; and, in the singular it comes as the epithet of Agni and Indra. Thus,

1. *sarvāsām samānam dampatim* (I.127.8, Agni)
2. *tam tvā suśipra dampate* (V.22.4, Agni)
3. *ā tū suśipra dampate* (VIII.69 16, Indra)

Here is clearly falsified the contention that the word *dam* is a variant of *jāyā*, which is the feminine form. The form *jampati* does not occur in the Vedic literature. It is clear, however, that even this form is not a variant of *jāyā*. It is quite probable that in *jam* we have the change of the initial letter (fr. *dam> jam*), as can be noted in the following cases:- *dyut* > *jyut* (to shine); *dyutiḥ* > *jyotis;* also Greek *diamitron* and Sanskrit *jāmitra*. Moreover the change *j* > *d*, to support the contention *jāyā> dam*, is unsound. This was obvious even to those who suggested it; and it is, hence, that they said that it was by *nipāta*. It is to be noted that the inclusion of *dam-patī* (and *jam-patī)* along with *jāya-patī* and *bhāryā-patī* is not scientific. The point has to be examined.

In the *ṚV* we come across the following formations of *dam:—*

dam-su (I.134.4); *dam-sujūtaḥ* (I.122.10); *dam—supatnīḥ;* (IV.11.7) and *dam-pati* (in the singular and in the dual). The accent on *dam* in all these cases is the same, as also in the case of the word *damūnas,* which occurs quite often and is the favourite epithet of Agni. In *damūnas* the base is *dam*, the suffix being *unas.*[2] The position according to the *uṇādi* aphorism (IV.674) will be that *dam* is a root. While commenting on the word *dampati* (sing,) Sāyaṇa renders it as *gṛha-svāmin* or *gṛha-pati* taking the word as *dama,* the elision of the final *a* being, according to him, a peculiarity of the Vedic language (cf. his com. on I.127.8, *dampatim gārhapatyādi-rūpeṇa gṛhasya pālakam, dama iti gṛha-nāma.... a-kāra-lopaś chāndasaḥ*), though he is unwarrantedly influenced by the latter tradition to add at another place (VIII.84.7), that Agni is called *dam-pati* as he is a form of the husband and the wife in one (*he dampate, yadā gārhapatye vartase tadā jāyā-patisvarūpo'si*). Following the *uṇādi* aphorism, and accepting *dam* to be the root, we are quite on the path to derive the words *dam* and *dama,* meaning the 'abode', from it (the former with the zero suffix *kvin*, in conformation with the accent of the word *dam*, and the latter with *ac*). The word *dampatī* (dual*)* would, thus, indicate, primarily, the two *pati*-s of the *dam* (house). Unlike the word *dam*, the word *jāyā* has a sexual connotation, and may be compared with *jā* (in *jāmātṛ*) and with *jāḥ* (in *jās-patyam* or *jās-pati*). The following will give an idea of the formation of these words—√*jan*> *jāy-a-te;* √*jan*> *jāy*> **jāya* (Masc.) > *jāyā* √*jan+viṭ* (the zero suffix)> *jā* (*ja-n*> *ā* by *Pāṇ*.

VI.4.41, *viḍ-vanor anunāsikasya āt)*

It will be seen that in the case of *jāyā-patī*, and also in the case of *bhāryā-patī*, the compound is the dual, while in that of *dam-patī* or *dam-pati* it has to be the possessive (*ṣaṣṭhī) tatpuruṣa*. The same is the case with *jam-patī*[3] The portion *dam* (meaning "house") in these compound-words may be compared with other Aryan words such as *domain, domicile, domination, domestic,* etc.

Now we come to the word *patnī*. This word is believed to be the feminine of the word *pati* (Masc.). The word *pati*, however, has both the genders — Masc. and the Fem. Thus, the position is—

(A) *pati*
Masculine - *pati,* while Feminine <
(B) *patnī*

As an example of (A) we may cite, "*gavām patiḥ strī*" (as noted by Bhaṭṭoji on *Pāṇ*. IV. 1.34). We also come across such forms as *vṛṣala-patiḥ*/*vṛṣala-patnī* or *gṛha-pati*/ *gṛha-patnī* where alternatively *pati* (Fem.) and *patnī* are seen, which are attested by Pāṇini (IV.1.34) who says, that this is the position when the word *pati* is preceded by some other word (*vibhāṣā sapūrvasya*). While comparing ^{0}*pati and* ^{0}*patnī*, which are seen alternatively, Pāṇini observes, generally, that the latter form is seen when there is the association of sacrificial rites (*patyur no yajña-sañyoge*, cf. IV.1.33). In other words, *patnī* would indicate the wife who has the status of sitting along with her husband at the sacrificial rites. But this does not mean that the other wives of the same person, or wives of a person who has no rite for sacrificial performances (just as a *śūdra*), would not be denoted by the word *patnī*. What Pāṇini means is that *patī* (Fem.) is not seen in the setting of the sacrifice. This will show that the word *patī* (Fem.) had a restricted usage, while *patnī* had a free usage. This is exactly the case in actual usage; for it was customary to say *vṛṣalasya patnī*, as Bhaṭṭoji notes, though he gives an explanation to suggest that the wife of the *vṛṣala* can get the appellation of *patnī* on the analogy of the wife of the person who has a rite for sacrifice (cf. *vṛṣalasya patnī iti vyaste katham iti cet? patnī 'va patnī'ty'upacārāt*). The fact, however, is that any wife was called *patnī* or, alternatively, *pati* (Fem.). We have just observed that the word *patnī* was not restricted to the association of sacrifice; and that this is the real implication of the aphorism of Pāṇini, "*patyur no yajña-sañyoge*". This will be also clear from the Vedic usage. A few examples—

1. *patim na patnīr uśatīr uśantam* (*ṚV.*, I.62.11)
2. *vṛṣeva patnīr abhyeti roruvat* (*ibid.*, I.140.6)
3. *janayo na patnīḥ* (*ibid.*, I.62 10)

Examples can be multiplied; but this much is sufficient for our purpose. Among the examples cited, the first two indicate the female counterpart and have a typically sexual context. In the third example, the word does not indicate the wife; but has the connotation of the "protector" or "controller". In all the three cases there is no association of the sacrifice. And the word *patnī* is not preceded by any word.

It will be seen that the word *patnī* is not strictly connotative of the wife. As has been noted above it has the sense of "the controlling lady." This is the most original sense of the word *patnī* as can be further noted from such words as *gṛha-patnī, vāja-patnī, nṛ-patnī, viś-patnī* (which is said of the lower *araṇi*) and also *dam-supatnī*, which is indicative of the perfect control of the *dam* (house or the domain).[4]

Now about the formation of the word *patnī*. The aphorism of Pāṇini, quoted above (*patyur no,* etc.) simply says that the word *pati* gets its final vowel changed to *n* (according to the principle of *tadanta-vidhi*); but does not indicate whether the word *pati* is to be regarded as the Masculine or the Feminine. Conceptually it seems proper to understand the word to be the feminine form of *pati*, as the discussion is about feminine forms *pati*/*patnī*; but as the feminine termination *ī* (*ṅīp*) is to be added after the *n* substituted for the final vowel in *pati*, it appears that *pati* in the Masc. is intended by Pāṇini! The position that Pānini takes is:—

pati> patn + ī (ṅīp) by *Pāṇ.* - IV. 1.5 (*ṛnnebhyo ṅīp*).

It will be clear that Pāṇini takes *pati* as the base for the form *patnī,* either here or in such cases as *eka-patnī, sa-patnī*, etc. (*Pāṇ.* IV. 1.35, *nityam sa-patnyādiṣu*). But let us examine this position in the case of the word *sa-patna*. The point is—is the word *patnī* to be derived from *patn* ( ) (which is obtained from *pati*, with *n* in the place of the final (*i*) or from *patna*? In the first case the vowel (*a)* in the suffix (*na*) is to be taken only as a help to pronunciation; but in the second case the suffix is clearly *na* (with the vowel). How do we derive the word *sa-patna?* From *pati*, with *n?* In that case we have to supply the final *a* which is actually seen in the word. There is no provision for this in the aphorisms of Pāṇini. Moreover, that will be a secondary, and unnecessary (and unsound too!) step. Though the word *patnī* can be arrived at by understanding the suffix to be *n,* it poses a difficulty in the case of *sa-patna,* which anticipates the suffix as *na*. In the latter case the formation is no problem at all; for it conforms to the general rule. And we can even derive the word *patnī* from *patna* (i.e. with the suffix *na* and not *n*). Thus—

* *patna + ī (ṅīp)*
= *patn (-a) + ī*
= *patn - ( ) + ī,* the elision of *a* being common by *Pān.* VI.4 148 (*yasyeti ca)*
= *patnī*

It is, thus, better and more scientific to understand the suffix to be *with* the vowel, rather than without vowel. Now, should we take the aphorism of Pāṇini "*patyur no*", etc. to accommodate this masculine form also? In that case we would have to understand the suffix to be *na* (*with* the vowel). The position will be—

pati (Masc.) < *pati* (Masc.) / **patna* (Masc.)

But the masculine form **patna* does not obtain free from the preposition *sa* (or *a-sa*). Pāṇini does not seem to have contemplated this form; for it does not have any place in the extant aphorisms. While speaking of the substitute *patna* for *pati*, with the preposition *sa*, he only has the feminine form *patnī* in mind as is clear from his aphorism *"nityam sa-patny-'ādiṣu" (Pāṇ* IV.1.35) and this is right, as he is treating the feminine suffixes. This will make clear that in the earlier aphorism (IV.1.33 *patyur no yajña-sañyoge*) he has in mind the word *pati* in the feminine! But what about the masculine form **sa-patna*? There is absolutely no doubt, whatsoever, that the form *sa-patna*, along with its negative (*a-sapatna*) was current throughout. Thus we have in the *ṚV a-sapatnaḥ kilā'ham abhūvam* (X.171.4). We have also the plural (X.12.9; 166.2, etc). Even after the days of Pāṇini, the form was in use as we read in the *Mṛcchakaṭika*, for example, *"niḥ-sapatnaṁ bhojanam"* (*Mṛc.* I). How should we understand the position? Should we suppose that the word *sa-patna* was later suggested from the feminine form *sa-patnī?* But this is not warranted even by Pāṇini; while the normal course will be *sa-patna* > *sa-patnī* (i.e. fr. Masc. to Fem.). Pāṇini does not, again, provide explanation for the feminine form *sa-patnā,* which is presupposed in the word *a-sapatnā*. To quote an example—

a-sapatnā sa-patna-ghnī,

which occurs in the *sapatnī-nāśana*-hymn (*ṚV* X.159.4).[5] This form cannot be said to obtain from *sa-patnī.* The only way is to understand—

sa-*patna* < *sa-patna (sa-patna* + *ā* i.e. *ṭāp)* / *sa-patnī* (*sa-patna* + *ī ṅīp*)

Sapatnā in the word *sapatna-ghnī*, also reverts to the masculine form **sapatna*.

The position finally has to be that the base for the forms *sa-patnā* or *sa-patnī* is *sa-patna* (Masc.). And for *patnī* we have to postulate the form **patna*. As this form was never in use independently, Pāṇini appears to have taken the popular word *pati* as the base for *patnī*, and for other words ending in *patnī*. But the difficulty of the substitution we have already noted. This awkwardness of position can be averted if we derive the base-word **patna*, which gives the forms *patnī, sa-patnā and sa-patnī* (all Fem.), directly from a root which gives also the word *pati* (Masc. or Fem.). The word *pati* has been generally derived from √*pā* (to protect) as—

√*pā* + *ḍati* (= *ati*)

= *p* + *ati*

(the vowel *ā* of the root being elided as the suffix has an indicatory *ḍ*)

= *pati*

(on the same lines we can derive the base **patna*)

√*pā* + *ḍatna* (= *atna*)[6]

—*p*+ *atna*

(the vowel *ā* being elided due to the indicatory *ḍ* of the suffix contemplated)

= **patna*

But looking to the concept of rivalry behind the word *sa-patna* or *sa-patnī,* whose destruction forms the theme of the two hymns of the *ṚV* noted above, it does not appear plausible that the word could be derived from √*pā* (to protect) unless we also accept that this root had in itself the sense of rivalry. There is another root which seems to be more appropriate; and it is √*pat* (to rule), which is attested by the *ṚV*. Thus we have:

1. *"pṛthivīm patyamānaḥ"* (VII.18.8)
2. *agne mitro na patyase* (VI.2.1)
3. *sa havyā mānuṣāṇām iḷā kṛtāni patyate* (I.128.7)
4. *tvam (agne) viśvāni sv' anika patyase* (II.1.8)
5. *yo nāma patyate* (II.37.2)

It is not necessary to multiply instances. Sāyaṇa takes the form of this root to mean, at places, "to come" or "to fall"; but in the last two instances he renders it as *"īśvaro bhavasi"* and *"devatātvena īṣṭe"*, as at some other places (cf. VI.49.4; -22.1;-45.20; X.23.2, etc.). It is clear that later the root *pat* was lost in this sense; and its sense was submerged in the phonetically similar root *pat* (fly or to go ahead). It is interesting to note, however, that the list of roots (*dhātu-pāṭha*) ascribed to Pāṇini distinguishes between this root and the other, by mentioning the former as *pata* and the latter as *patlṛ*. Bhaṭṭoji gives √*pat* (*pata*) as a case of inversion of phonemes, in the place of √*tap* (cf. *tapa aiśvarye vā.........pata iti vyatyāsena pāṭhāntaram*). √*pat* appears to be the most appropriate root for *sa-patna*, *sa-patnī* and even for *patnī*. Thus— √*pat* + na **patna; *patna + ā > *patnā; patna + ī patnī*. The forms **patna* and **patnā* became obsolete as free forms; **patnī* remained current.

In all these forms the meaning of "control" or "lordship" remained. The word *patnī* also has the same meaning primarily; the sense of "protection" being only secondary. Even this word can be derived from √*pat*. Thus the position is this:—

√*pat* {
- *pati* (with the suffix *i*) <
  - Masc.
  - Fem.
- **patna* (with *na*) <
  - Masc. **patna*
  - Fem. **patnā / patnī*

The suffix *na* is common to many words such as *vas-*

na, praś-na, svap-na, etc. In the case of *tna* we have few cases for support. The *ṚV,* however, shows the form *cyautna*, which can be derived as √*cyu* + *tna* (with the indicatory to account for the *vṛddhi* of the initial vowel *u*> *au*), the suffix will have to be understood as *tnaṇ*, which will also conform to the accent (see *uṇādi*, 544). It is to be noted that Sāyaṇa does not give the derivation of the word *cyautna* anywhere, though it occurs ten times in the *ṚV.* It appears that the suffix gave place to *tnu* even in the Vedic time; and we have many forms in *tnu* such as *kṛtnu, drāvayitnu, hatnu, stanayitnu* and so on. Even this suffix became gradually extinct later. This is obviously the reason why Pāṇini did not think of the suffix *tna*, and even *na* in the case of the words *sapatnī,* etc.; and derived them from *pati*. The form **patna* in the word *sa-patna*, as in the word *sa-patnī* remained unnoticed.

The root *pat*, though lost later, is to be noticed in such other Aryan words as Latin-*potis, potens;* Lithuanian-*patene;* English-*potential*. We may also note the words—*pontiff* (English), *patiyāt* (Old Hindi), *pat* (Marathi and Hindi) and also *pat/pati* (Nepalese, Hindi and other Modern Indian languages) which indicate the status or the power. The compound *sa-patnī* has to be derived, hence, *not* as *samānaḥ patiḥ yasyāḥ*, but as *samanā patnī* i.e. *one who is equal in power or control,* with other wives.

Likewise

eka-patnī = *ekā eva patnī* (the only female controller)

Vīra-patnī = *vīrasya patnī* (the chief controlling wife of a brave man)

OR *vīrā patnī* (the brave chief wife).

(The word "wife" is used only as a popular word.)

In the case of the *bahuvrīhi* compound, the scientific and the most legitimate dissolution will be to show the form **patna;* but, as it never occurred without a preposition *pati* has to be shown as a *substitute*. It is not that **patna* is the substitute of *pati*.

NOTES AND REFERENCES

1. For the earliest concept of the *nipāta,* see *Nirukta*, I.2, "*uccāvaceṣu artheṣu nipatanti*", Later the term *nipāta* came to indicate a word beyond the set rules of word-formation. Generally speaking, the *nipāta* indicates a word in current usage, but not conforming to the grammatical rules.
2. Cf. *damerunasiḥ (uṇādi*, 674). It is to be noted that Sāyaṇa quotes this aphorism as *damer ūnasiḥ* (i.e. with the suffix with the long *ū*) and takes the suffix as *ūnas;* see com. on *ṚV*. 1.60.4. Amara takes the form as *damunas* (with the short *u*) "*saptārcirdamunāḥ*". Another instance where Sāyaṇa misquotes Pāṇini is *Pāṇ*. IV.4.114, where the suffix laid down is *yan* (with the indicatory *n*) to account for the accent in the words *sa-garbhya*, *sa-nutya*, etc. See *ṚV*. II.30.9. Here, in spite of the accute accent of the first vowel, which requires the indicatory *n* in the suffix *ya*, Sāyaṇa lays down the rule as having the suffix with *yat*, which would have shown the *svarita* on the final vowel in *ya*!
3. The root cannot be *jam* (to eat)! We may note another word here—*jāmi* (relation). This word has been derived by Sāyaṇa from √*jam* (cf. "*jamu adane. bāhulakāt iḥ ṚV* 1.28 16). Is the idea of partaking food together? It seems far from convincing. Yāska derives it *also* from √*jan* (to procreate), *Nir*.III.6; alternatively he suggests the root *jam;* but taking it to mean "to move". It yet remains doubtful if in *jam-pati* we can take √*jan* > *jam*, in spite of the following *p* in *pati*.
4. The word is interesting. The whole expression refers to the "*staryo daṁsupatnīḥ*" (IV.19.7, the word occurs nowhere else), *milked* by Indra. As Geldner rightly remarks, they are the cloud-cows (cf. *staryo na gāvah* at VII.23.4). The cloud-cows being called *dam-supatnīḥ* indicates their control over the earthly domain, to fertilize which is their power. Indra helps. Geldner's hint that the word is an inversion for *su-daṁpatnīḥ* is perfect.
5. The verse is the same at the *sapatnī-nāśana* and the royal advance, the only difference being of the gender in *a-sapatna*, suitable to the context.

6. For the authority in suggesting this suffix, cf. *"kāryād vidyād anūbandham"* *(bhāṣya)* and *"kecid avihitā apy'ūhyāḥ"*.

* Included here from *Vidarbha Samshodhana Mandal, Annual No.*, Nagpur, 1968 (pub. in 1969).

Chapter 21

Kanyā and Kānīna

The word *kanyā* has been explained by Yāska in the following way:

i. *kanyā kamanīyā bhavati* (fr. √*kam,* "to desire")
ii. *kamanena ānīyate iti vā* (fr. √*kam* + *ā* + √*nī,* "to desire" and "to carry") (brought by one who desires)
iii. *kva iyam netavyā iti vā* (fr. *kva* + √*nī*) (where is she to be carried?)
iv. *kanatervā syāt kānti-karmaṇaḥ* (fr. √*kan* "to shine")

Yāska's comment on the word *kanyā* comes, as he quotes the following passage from the *ṚV* (IV.32. 23):

kanīnakeva vidraghe nave drupade,
babhrū yāmeṣu śobhete

and glosses on the word *kanīnakeva* (*kanīnaka+ iva* acc. to *Pada-pāṭha* while *kanīnake (*dual) *iva* according to Yāska and Sāyaṇa), as *kanyake.*

Out of the etymologies noted above, two give the root as √*kam*, while one gives it as √*kan;* and in two it is connected with √*nī.*

It is to be noted that Yāska does not give any etymology of the word *kanī* (also meaning the same as *kanyā*), though he quotes it in another context (*Nir.*X.21 on *ṚV* I.66.4. *jāraḥ kanīnām,* etc.). Actually Yāska could have found support from *kva+* √*nī* (see above iii) which would straight away connect with *kanī,* instead of with *kanyā,* on the basis of his method (cf. *Nir.*II.i *artha-nityaḥ* parī*kṣeta* and *akṣara-varṇa-sāmānyān nirbrūyāt*). It will be seen that *kanyā* or *kanī* does not get clear support from √*kam;* it is rather easy with √*kan.* Śākaṭāyana derived *kanyā* from √*kan* (with *yā*) and not from √*kam* (*Uṇādi,* IV.111). Apart from these words there are other words that have the same sense; and we shall do well to place them all side by side. Thus:—

kanā (*ṚV* X. 61.5; -10; -11; -21; only in the Gen.Sing.)
kanī (*ibid.,* I.66.4 and other places, total six; all Gen.Pl.)
kanyā (*ibid.,* at various places).
kanyanā (*ibid.,* VIII.35.5).

Sāyaṇa, at all places, derives the word *kanī* as only a form of *kanyā* by *samprasāraṇa,* which he explains as a Vedic peculiarity; but in doing so he is not uniform. We give below the derivations of *kanī* according to Sāyaṇa:

ṚV I. 66.4		*kanī* < *kanyā* by *samprasāraṇa* (*kanyā*< *kanī-ā kanī*) quotes *Pāṇ.* "*bahulam chandasi.*"
ṚV I. 116.10	fr.	*kanyā;* same explanation; but quotes "*rayer matau bahulam*" (*Vār.* 3473).
ṚV I. 152.4 — (i)	fr.	√*kan+ iÑ + ṄīṢ* (*kṛdikārād-aktinaḥ*). √*kan+ iN* (variant comm. "*iN sarvadhātubhyaḥ*"?)
OR (ii)	fr.	*kanyā* by *samprasāraṇa; Pāṇ.* not quoted.
ṚV I. 163.8	fr.	*kanyā* (*kanīnām kanyānām strīṇām*); no further comment.
ṚV II. 15.7; V.3.2	fr.	*kanyakā* (*kanīnām kanyakā-nām*); no further comment.

For *kanā* he has "*kamanīyā stutiḥ*" at three places; but at one (X.61.5) where the word is with *duhitṛ* (*kanāyā duhituḥ*) he renders it as *kāntā*. Thus he sees the root to be √*kam*. This he does also in the case of *kanyā*, following Yāska. For *kanyānām* (VIII.35.5) he has "*kanyānām āhvānam*", which shows that he understands the word as an abstract noun, meaning "invocation of the *kanyās*."

The facts noted above indicate that the words *kanā*, *kanyanā* and *kanī* pose a problem, though *kanyā* appears to be fairly derived, being rather familiar. The case for √*kam* is clearly quite weak; for the change from *m* to *n* in *kanyā* is difficult to be accounted. This is exactly why Yāska takes the help of the root √*nī* (to carry) which has *n* initially. Likewise √*kan* (to shine) also does not offer good help, in view of a clear contrast in *janī* and *kanī* (*ṚV* I.66.4 *jāraḥ kanīnām patir janīnām*, said of the Sun). Here *kanī* indicates a "younger unmarried woman" as against *janī* who is with husband and is "apt to produce" (*janī* < √*jan*). This also seems to be true with the other words that are cognates of *kanī*, such as *kanyā*, *kanā* and *kanyanā*. All these words are, most certainly, indicative of "miniature", rather than 'formal beauty' (*kānti* < √*kam*) or 'desire' (√*kāma*). In fact, the very source of this discussion, as quoted by Yāska, has this very connotation, though Yāska misses this point completely, and Sāyaṇa meekly follows him. The expression is descriptive of Indra's well-formed horses that are compared with two *kanīnakā*-s, which are tiny wooden female figurines fixed on a wooden stand (Sāyaṇa and Yāska). The passage is interesting also from the social point, as it indicates the practice of displaying tiny figurines at special occasions — here, at the sacrifices (*yāmeṣu-Sāyaṇa*).

We have indicated the probability of the words examined above indicating "miniature", or the connotation of being younger. In all these words the common part is *kan*. But it does not appear to be indicative of a root, in spite of Yāska and Sāyaṇa. This will be clear if we examine another set of words. The words we have examined are in the feminine. If we reconstruct their masculine forms, the pattern will be as follows:-

Fem.	**Masculine**	**Fem.**
kanā		*kanyanā*
} →	**kana*; **kanyana* ←	{
kanī		**kanyanī*

We have seen that *kanīnakā* was a form used by the *ṚV* (IV. 32.23 quoted above); the masculine form would be *kanīnaka*. Thus:-

Fem.	**Masc.**
kanīnakā	*kanīnaka*

Now the forms * *kana* and * *kanyana* are not found; probably they went out of use even at the time of the *Ṛgveda*. But the form *kanīnaka* was in use, as will be seen from the following quotation:

janiṣṭa yoṣā patayat kanīnakaḥ (ṚV X.40.9)

Sāyaṇa takes it to mean "*kanyā-kāmaḥ patiḥ*", thus making it dependent on *kanyā*. But there is no doubt that this is an independent form. For this we have only to compare another form—*kanīnaḥ* (I.117.18; III.48.1; VIII.69.14; X.99.10). There is, hence, no doubt that the word *kanīnaka* is only another form of *kanīna*, with *ka* added in the same sense *(svārthe)*. This also supports the feminine word *kanīnikā (*eye-ball; or, really, eye-'doll'). Thus:

kanīnaka < *kanīna (*Masc.) { *kanīnakā* (like *pāvaka,* cf. *Vār.*4527)
{ *kanīnikā (Pāṇ.* VII. 3.44)

Now the word *kanīnaka* or *kanīna* (both Masc.) not only has the sense of "miniature", but also that of, comparatively, young age, as is clear from the passage cited above; and this sense is inherent in the part *kan*, as is quite obvious. This point is supported by Pāṇini himself, who observes that *kan* is the substitute for *yuvan* and *alpa* in certain passages (V.3.64 *yuvālpayoḥ kan-anyatarasyām*). This would show that the nucleus *kan* in all these forms (including *kanyā*, *kanā, kanī* and *kanyanā*) does not indicate any root as such. Though Pāṇini teaches this *kan*-substitute in the case of such formations as are in *īyas* and *iṣṭha* (*kanīyas-kaniṣṭha*), there is no doubt that it could extend to the forms we have noted, which will save us from the fantastic etymologies; or, if a root is to be seen it could not be having the sense of "shining" or "desiring" so much as of "diminution." It may well be √*kaṇ* (*nimīlane*)—originally * √*kan*—.

We have seen how the form *kanīna-kanīnaka* gave the forms *kanīnakā* and *kanīnikā*. But there is another point to be noted *viz.* the form *kanīna* (Masc.) could also give the form (Fem.). *kanīnā*. Pāniṇi indicates it already (*Pāṇ*. IV.1.116); but he uses the form *kanīna (kanyāyāḥ kanīna ca)* without the mention of its gender; and yet the expected form is *kanī+nā (...kanīnā ca)*, in view of the gender of *kanyā*. His difficulty appears to be that the form *kanīnā* was out of use at his time. May be it was never in use! But the word *kānīna* presupposes the word *kanīnā*; and, hence, there is reason to believe that it was in use sometime but was lost! The proper explanation of the word *kānīna* would then be "*kanīnāyāḥ apatyam pumān*" and if *kanyā* is preferred in view of its current use (and which is only proper), Pāṇini's aphorism has to be read (correctly) as "*kanyāyāḥ kanīnā ca.*" Thus:

kanyā > *kanīnā* + aṆ
kānīnā (by *vṛddhi* of the initial vowel, *Pāṇ*. VII.2.117)
kānīnā+ *a* (*aṆ*) = *kānīn* + *a* (final *ā* dropped, *Pāṇ*. VI. 4.148) = *kānīna*

Here we may compare the Prākrit word *kāṇelī* (cf. *kāṇeli-mātṛ* used often by Bhāsa), which resembles *kanī* or *kanīnā*.

In fine we may note that the words *kanā, kanī, kanyā, kanyanā* (fem.), and their counterparts *kanīna-kanīnaka*, have the sense of "diminution" as is indicated by *kan (*may be √*kan*↘*kaṇ*, which also gives *kaṇa* or, *kaṇikā*), and have to be seen in respect of *kanīyas* or *kaniṣṭha*. They also had the sense of the vigour of fresh youth, later getting the general sense of "unmarried person." *Kanīna* was the youthful male; **kanīnā* was the young maiden; and *kānīna* (masc.) was the one born of a "*kanīnā.*" As the other words went out of use, leaving *kanyā, kānīna* on the stage of current usage, they were associated with one another, *kānīna* being said to be the son of the *kanyā*. Accentually *kanyā* appears to be only another form of *kanī* with an addition of *ā*; and it is not that *kanī* is from *kanyā* as Sāyaṇa remarks.

kanī↘*kanī-ā*↘*kanyā,* with the accent-shift to *svarita* of the *jātya-type*.

* Included here from *Vidarbha Samshodhana Mandal, Annual No.*, Nagpur, 1971 (pub. in 1972).

Chapter 22

Vowel-Shortening and the Sanskrit-Sandhi

As a general rule, in the Sanskrit language, two similar simple vowels[1] coming after each other get assimilated and changed into a long vowel of the same category. This has been noted by Pāṇini in his aphorism, *akaḥ savarṇe dīrghaḥ* (VI.1.101). Pāṇini's *Aṣṭādhyāyī* gives also rules for cases where a dissimilar vowel follows a vowel. According to the arrangement of Pāṇini, a vowel stands for all its types, whether long or prolated, unless specifically mentioned to the contrary (cf. I.1.9; I.1.70). Now the change of a short simple vowel into its longer type, in the case of assimilation is a feature well marked by Pāṇini. What seems to be less marked is the fact that a long simple vowel gets shortened in the condition of its being followed by a dissimilar vowel. The tendency has, however, been indicated in two aphorisms, viz. "*iko' savarṇe śākalyasya rhasvaśca*" and "*ṛty' akaḥ*" (VI.1.127 and 128). Out of these, the first is taken as indicating an option as it has been authorised by Śakalya, and the second suggests that the shortening will take place only when the following vowel is *ṛ*.

It has to be, however, observed that the tendency of the preceding long simple vowel getting shortened, when followed by a dissimilar vowel, is a general one in actual practice; and it can be marked at various stages. Thus —

In the case of the *sandhi*-s known as the *guṇa* and the *vṛddhi* the position is as follows:

ramā + *īśa* = *rameśa*
rāma + *īśa* = *rāmeśa*

This will show that the difference between the short and long preceding vowels (here *a* and *ā* respectively) goes; and in both cases the resultant vowel is the compound vowel *e* (*sandhy'akṣara* of the *Prātiśākhyas*). As the compound vowel is the combination of two vowels, it will have two moras; and it will be long.

The same observation holds good in the *Vṛddhi-saṇdhi*. Thus,

gaṅgā + *ogha* = *gaṅgaugha*
and *kapittha* + *oṣadhi* = *kapitthauṣadhi*

In combination both *a* and *ā* get similarly changed; and it is to be particularly marked that *ā* changes to the shorter vowel, as is also testified by actual hearing. We do not hear *gaṅgāugha*.

On the other hand, the short vowel following *a* or *ā* shows length after assimilation; but the normal length is only two moras. This is the case even if a long vowel follows, which indicates shortening of the following vowel.

Let us now examine the case of vowels other than *a* or *ā* followed by a dissimilar vowel. Thus, in the case of *sudhī* + *upāsyaḥ* the final long vowel of the first word will show *y* (acc. to the *yaṇ sandhi*) and the new combination will be *sudhy'upāsyaḥ* (barring the variant forms showing reduplication), and *ati* + *uttama* will show the new combination as *aty 'uttama,* thus the difference between the long and the short vowel at the end of the first word is nullified.

In the case of *sādhu ahita* and *vadhū ahita*, the final vowels (*u* and *ū*) will both show *v*, the form being, *sadhv 'ahita* and *vadhv 'ahita*, thus nullifying the difference between the long and the short preceding vowel.

From what has been stated above, it is easy to postulate a stage where, *prior to the actual combination*, the final long vowel of the first word gets shortened. The assimilation is a subsequent stage. And it is quite possible that at times there was no assimilation at all, the position being simply as—

sudhī + *upāsyaḥ* =	i.	*sudhi upāsyaḥ* (shortening)
	ii.	*sudhy 'upāsyaḥ* (change to semi-v.)
vadhū + *ahita* =	i.	*vadhu 'ahita* (shortening)
	ii.	*vadhv 'ahita* (change to semi-v.)

This would also indicate that it was never a strong and general rule that the *sandhi* must show the required *antaḥsthā* (semi-vowel) at the end of the first word. This is exactly what has been implied in the observation of Śākalya noted earlier. Bhaṭṭoji's comment quoted from the *Bhāṣya* on it that there is no further *sandhi* due to the shortening of the earlier vowel has to be taken with care. If misunderstood, it will open up comparison with such cases where there is no further *sandhi* after one formation has already taken place. Thus, for example, in *devāḥ* + *iha* changed to *devā iha* with the *visarga* (aspiration) dropped, will not have a further *sandhi* into showing *deveha* (which will be a wrong usage in general, except for a few cases of material necessity).

The case in hand is slightly different. While there is no further combination in *devā iha*, in this case the combination does appear; for the forms after *sandhi* are both *sudhi upāsyaḥ* (Śākalya) and *sudhy'upāsyaḥ*. Likewise *cakrī* (nom. sing. of *cakrin*) + *atra* will show both *cakri atra* (with the gap called the *vivṛtti*), and also *cakry'atra*. Now what guarantee is there to suggest that the latter form was not a result of a further combination of original shortening?

It has to be noted that Pāṇini's note of Śākalya as regards the shortening of the vowel in question holds good in all such cases, without reservations whatsoever; and it is only Kātyāyana who makes a difference between cases of compounds (like *sudhī-upāsyaḥ)* and mere *sandhi*-s where there is no compound, which shows a later phase of utterences (cf. Kātyāyana "*na samāse*").

We can say, thus, that the shortening of the long final vowel of the first word was a marked tendency in some parts, probably where Śākalya lived, while in certain other parts this tendency had gone a further change by which the resulting semi-vowel took the place of both, i.e. the preceding long and short vowels. The new position can best be described as—stage i., Shortening of the vowel; and the gap (*vivṛtti*); and stage ii. Loss of the vowel; and replacement by the semi-vowel. The case of *a* and *ā* was not so clearly marked.

What we have observed about the first step in utterance, in the case of the *sandhi*, being the shortening of the final long vowel before a dissimilar vowel, can be attested from other examples. It has been noted by Pāṇini that certain words ending in long *ī* or long *ū* the final is changed to *iy* or *uv*, while in certain other cases the change is to simple *y* to *v*. Here is an interesting case then. Thus we have *strī* + *am* changing to *striyam* where the *ī* gets shortened and, in addition, takes *y*. Though it may be objected that this is a case of an internal *sandhi* between a word and its suffix the tendency cannot be overlooked. In the Vedic language it is well marked. Thus optional forms like *vibhvam*/*vibhuvam*, *tanvam*/ *tanuvam*, *sudhy'ah*/*sudhiyaḥ* obtain, where the long *ī* and *ū* get changed into *y* or *v* respectively; and optionally, also show the shortened vowel with the respective semi-vowel. That the tendency is observed in certain word-formations, and not in others, only shows that in the others it became obsolete. It may well be said that in the Vedic *mantra*-s (*chandasi*) this was due to the necessity of the metre. But cases of *iy* and *uv* in the classical language, with the observation of Śākalya, should leave no doubt about the stage of vowel shortening, and the adjustment of the respective semi-vowel, prior to the latter's finally usurping the place of the former. In short the line of change is as follows.[2]

Long vowel > shortened v; > /short v.> semi-v. The forms showing the shortening, without a further *sandhi*, as noted by Śākalya, and also those showing the combined shortened v. and the semi-v (i.e. *iy* and *uv)* are then steps which have to be admitted. Though they were lost, and appear to be lost orthographically, in the general nature of the Sanskrit language described by Pāṇini, the tendency has prevailed in the MIA and NIA, where *sandhi* is not so acute as in the Sanskrit language. This is a matter of experience even in the modern speech. The final long vowel of the preceding word, as a rule, gets shortened before the next vowel, unless it is retained with special care! In the examples of the Sanskrit usage, as can be seen *iy* or *uv* is retained in the internal *sandhi*; for there a break (after shortening) was not advisable between the word and the suffix. In the case of the external *sandhi* (*pada-vivṛtti*) break was admissible. In the internal *sandhi,* the shortened vowel had *at once* to adjust with the next one, itself taking the semi-v as a balancing element. Where this was not done, the final of the word retaining its vowel, the following vowel (of the case-suffix) was lost. This was the case for the internal *pūrva-rūpa sandhi* (cf. *ami pūrvaḥ, Pāṇ.* VI.1.107; also VI.1.102).

	(1)	(2)	(3)
Thus	*strī + am =*	*striy + am =*	*striyam*
but,	*nadī + am =*	*nadī + ( ) m =*	*nadī*

Mark *strī + au = striy + au = striyau*

again, *nadī + au = (*nadiy + au) = nad ( ) y + au = nadyau*

and *strī + aḥ* (nominative) = *striy + ah = striyaḥ*

nadī + aḥ (=do=) = (*nadiy + aḥ = nad ( ) y + aḥ = nadyaḥ*

but *strī + aḥ* (accusative) = *strī = ( ) h = strīḥ*

also *nadī + + aḥ* (=do=) = *nadī + ( ) ḥ = nadīḥ*

And likewise with *bhrū* and *vadhū*

NOTES AND REFERENCES

1. Simple vowels, i.e. the *samānākṣarāṇi* of the *Prātiśākhya,* as against the *sandhy'akṣarāṇi* which are compound vowels such as *e (a/ā + i/ī), ai* (*a/ā + e*), 0 *(a/ā = u/ ū*), and *au* (*a/ā* + 0).
2. For a detailed discussion on this topic, see, Sadashiv A. Dange, "Vowel-shortening in Sanskrit", *Vidyā-vratin* (Prof. A.M. Ghatge Fel. Vol.), Sri Satguru Publications (A Division of Indian Books Centre), Delhi, 1992, pp.95-100; also by the same author, "Sandhi, Śākalya, Pāṇini VI.1.127-128 And the Vedic Evidence", *Traividyam* (Vedic Studies in Memory of Durgamohan Bhattacharyya), Subarnarekha Pubn., Kolkata, 2001, pp.63-77.

* Included here from *Vidarbha Samshodhana Mandal, Annual No.,* Nagpur, 1969 (pub. in 1970).

Chapter 23

Some Peculiarities of the Eastern Dialect according to Pāṇini

In his *Aṣṭādhyāyī* Pāṇini refers to various places or regions pointing out their speech peculiarities. Thus we have reference to the Madras, the Udīcyas, the Prācya-Bharatas and so on. The main distinction seems to be between the Udīcyas and the Prācyas. It has to be noted that this distinction prevailed in times anterior and posterior to Pāṇini. The Udīcya (or the Northern) region was supposed to be the norm for all perfection including the language, while the language of the Easterners was supposed to be sliding away from this norm. Thus the *Kauṣītaki Br.*, clearly says that people went to the Udīcyas for learning the language (VII.6 – *udañca u eva yanti vācam śikṣitum*), while in the sphere of the Prakrit language it was always the case that the language of the Easterners showed the deviation. In this case while the Śaurasenī was supposed to be the norm of Prakrits, being nearest to Sanskrit, that of the Magadhas showed a distinct decay, changing the original *r* to *l* to mention the most distinct of its peculiarities; and though the province of the Avantīs marked a commingling of the Śaurasenī and its Southern variety—called the Dākṣiṇātyā by Bharata and the Māhārāṣṭrī by Daṇḍin—there arose what was then called the *Prācyā*, which traditionally became the language of the Vidūṣaka in Sanskrit dramas (cf. *Nāṭyaśāstra*, XVII.48; *Kāvyādarśa*, I.33; also *prācyāḥ siddhih śaurasenyāḥ*, and *prācyā vidūṣakādīnām*). The distinction between the Eastern and the Northern tongue is maintained in the *Ṛk-prātiśākhya*, which mentions the Prācya and the Pāñcāla way in the *samdhi* called the *udgrāha* and the *vivṛtta* (II.33;68). This will make clear that in the Sanskrit, as well as in the Prakrit sphere, the Eastern people showed a slight distinction in the usage of the same forms. From this point it will be interesting to note the information Pāṇini gives. The distinction between the Northern and the Eastern usage of Sanskrit, as seen from Pāṇini, appears to be mainly concerning the Taddhitas and the Strī-suffixes. We shall examine the places one by one.

PLACE-NAMES

Speaking about the suffix *īya* (technically *ch*) Pāṇini says that it is seen after the nouns in the sense of 'belonging to'; but the nouns in this case are seen to start with *ā* or *ai* or *au* (which are technically called the *vṛddha* vowels, I.1.73; IV.2.114). So the forms that were in use were *mālīya* (from *mālā*), *śālīya*' (from *śālā*), etc. in both cases the original word starting with a *vṛddha* vowel (*ā*). We may imagine other forms like these, where the original word starts with *ai* or *au*. Seeing the forms *tadīya*, *yadīya* and the like, Pāṇini included them in special aphorism (I.1.74); for they cannot be strictly said to be *vṛddha,* as they do not have the initial vowel a *vṛddha* one; because they start with *tad*, *yad* (see also *madīya*, *tvadīya*, *asmadīya*, *yuṣmadīya* and so on). Now in the Eastern region a name denoting a place or region, and having *e* or *o* as the initial vowel (which are not technically the *vṛddha*) will show the suffix *īya (Pāṇ.* I.1.75, *eṅ prācām deśe*). Thus from *gonarda, Bhojakaṭa* and *eṇīpacana* the forms in the Eastern region were, as Bhaṭṭoji points out, *Gonardīya, Bhojakaṭīya* and *eṇīpacanīya;* while in the

Udīcya (or safer, in the non-Eastern region influenced by the Northern) we could possibly hear persons belonging to the places mentioned above being indicated as *Gaunardaḥ, Bhaujakaṭaḥ*, and *Aiṇīpacanaḥ*, which do not show the suffix *īya* but the usual *aṆ* (the indicatory *Ṇ* accounting for the *vṛddhi* in the initial vowel). Gonarda,* etc. were Eastern places.

A point has to be noted in this connection. When Bhaṭṭoji says that the optional forms will be Aiṇīpacanaḥ, Gaunardaḥ and Bhaujakaṭaḥ *(pakṣe*, etc.), it does not necessarily indicate that both the types of forms were in use side by side. In fact, option does not indicate sameness of region at all in the origin. The variance in forms conforms to different regions in the origin; and when there is a fusion of people from these different regions in one region, all the varieties may be seen in usage in that particular region of fusion. But it has to be remembered that the varieties pertained to different regions originally. In the present case it appears certain that Pāṇini indicates the usage of two different regions, and nothing beyond that. Hence persons belonging to the places mentioned above called themselves Gonardīya, etc. (with the *īya* suffix), which was a peculiarity of the Eastern dialect. It does not necessarily mean, however, that the Northern people used the other forms, when indicating the same persons (i.e. from the Eastern region). What it means is that place-names from the Eastern region gave adjectives in *īya* while those in the non-Eastern (or the Northern) gave epithets in *aṆ*. In the fusion of the regional influences if one is heard to introduce himself or somebody with the *īya* suffix, it indicated the Eastern influence. Thus modern surnames as Māthur show the Northern influence carried over the years, though Mathurā is actually in the Eastern region.

It is interesting to note that the Eastern tendency prevailed, and is to be widely marked even today, as can

---

* Patañjali was called Gonardīya.

be seen from some of the surnames. Thus—

Sisod > *Sisodīya > Sisodiyā (from Sisodiyāḥ Plural)
Kāṅker > *Kāṅkerīya > Kāṅkeriyā " "
Pāṭod > *Paṭodīya > Pāṭodiyā " "
Baḍjāt > *Baḍjātīya > Baḍjātiyā " "
Mālava > *Mālavīya > Mālaviyā (?) " "

These are the names from Rajasthan; but we may also compare some Maharashtriyan names formed from places. Thus:

Āpṭā > Āpṭīya > * Āpṭiyā > Āpṭe
Purandara > Purandarīya > * Purandariyā > Purandare
Karhāḍ > Karhāḍīya > * Karhāḍiyā > Karhāḍe
Varhāḍ > Varhāḍīya > * Varhāḍiyā > Varhāḍe

It can be marked that the plural forms in the Rajasthani and the Maharashtriyan names, as noted above, show a correspondence. The plural form in *īya* does not show a considerable change in the Rajasthani, simply losing the plural aspirate (*visarga*) while in the Maharashtriyan names it changed to *e*, corresponding to the general tendency of the plural in the Marathi language (cf. āmbā > āmbe; sasā > sase). The singular in the *īya* base in the Rajasthani will be *īya* > *iyo,* as *o* indicates the singular in certain cases as is the case with the Śaurasenī language.* In the Marathi language, in an older phase the singular was indicated by the suffix *yā* or *ā*, both having the same status, thus, Śirkā/Śirkyā; Āpṭā/Āpṭyā. The suffix *yā* later on got the tinge of disrespect. Concerned as we are with the place-names, it has to be noted that in the Marathi language *yā,* indicative of place, did not originally have the tinge of disrespect. The *yā* in the Marathi language is the same as the *iyo* of the Rajasthani noted above. So the position

* Rāmaḥ > Rāmo; Śivaḥ > Śivo gao.

now is:

īya (singular)	*iyo* > ( ) *yo*	Rajasthani
	īya > ( ) *yā*	Marathi

To illustrate:

Singular — Karhāḍ > Karhāḍīya > Karhādyā
Karhāḍa...Marathi
" Kāṅker > Kāṅkarīya > Kāṅkariyo Rajasthani

As there is a tendency to elide the initial *ī* of the suffix *īya* which gets shortened in the process, in the Marathi Singular forms, so is there the same in such Rajasthani forms as Baḍjātyā (Baḍjāt [i] tyā).

In the forms noted above it could be marked that in the plural, the suffix shows the shortening of the initial vowel. Thus:

Singular *Plural*
Varhāḍīya > * Varhāḍīya > Varhāḍyā > Varhāḍe
Kāṅkerīya > * Kāṅkeriya > Kāṅkeriyo > Kāṅkeriya

On minutely seeing, it is clear that, if the vowel following *y* in the original suffix *īya* gains length, the initial *i* gets shortened; but if the vowel that follows *y* is a short one (and in this case the original *a*) the initial length is retained in actual practice. More clearly now, the position of the vowel in the place-suffix is as follows:—

īya (*CH*)	*īya*	(if short v. after *y*)
	īyā	(if long v. after *y*)
	( )*yā*	(" " " ") = loss of initial v.

The names among the Maharashtriyans obviously showed *y* with the loss of the initial vowel of the suffix and the position was this—

Singular *Plural*
Āpṭā > * Āpṭiyā > Āpt ( ) yā Āpṭye Āpṭ(y)e Āpṭe

It will be clear that Pāṇini's observation of the place-indicative suffix CH (*īya*) has far-reaching strides. In his times it was found to be present after names having a long initial vowel in the Northern region (*Pāṇ*. IV. 2.114). In the Eastern region it was seen added to *place-names* to form adjectives. In yet later times, reaching the modern, also it is seen in place-names. But while at his times it was seen after Eastern names denoting a region, having *e* or *o* initially, later it is found without this restriction. We may say, in line with Pāṇini, that the scope of the term *vṛddha* has to be made much wider to include many other names. This was noted long back by Kātyāyana in his *vārtika "vā nāmadheyasya"*, adjuncted to the aphorisms I.1.73 and I.1.74.

Another suffix indicative of the place of origin is *ika* (*THAÑ*, see *Pāṇ*. IV.2.119) which changes to *ka* after stems ending in *is, us, u* (short or long), *ṛ* (short or long) (*Pāṇ*.VII.3.51). Pāṇini observes that this suffix was seen after nouns indicating place, but ending in *u* (short or long) and the forms, as shown by the tradition would be — Niṣādakarṣū > Naiṣādakarṣuka *(Pāṇ*. IV.2.119; VII.3.51, and VII.4.13). This unrestricted suffixation of *ka* (< *ika*) to the stems ending in *u* or *ū,* was not to be seen, however, in the Eastern region, where the suffix in question was seen after only those stems ending in *u* (short or long) which initially had a *vṛddha* vowel *(Pāṇ*. IV.2.120). Thus:—

Eastern—Āḍhakajambū < Āḍhakajambukaḥ (THAÑ = *ika* > *ka)*

but, Mallavāstu Māllavāstavaḥ (with *aṆ*)

Had Niṣādakarṣū been in the Eastern region, the form indicating a person belonging to that place would have been simply—Naiṣādakarṣavaḥ, and not Naiṣādakarṣukaḥ in both the cases the indicatory *Ṇ* and *Ñ*, causing initial *vṛddhi*.

We have noted the peculiar use of the suffix *īya*. While denoting the region this suffix was also seen after words ending in the word *garta*, thus showing Vṛkagartīya, Trigartīya, etc. (*Pāṇ*. IV.2.137). In the

Eastern region, however, this suffix was seen after words having *kaṭa* as the first member (IV. 2.139), as can be seen from such forms as Kaṭanagarīya, Kaṭaghoṣīya, etc.

Another peculiarity of the Easterners was to use the suffix *aka (VUÑ)* to indicate place-formed-names or adjectives where the name of the place showed *r* at the penultimate and had a *vṛddha* vowel initially as in—

Pāṭaliputra > Pāṭaliputraka

and where the place-name ended in ī (long), as in

Kākandī > Kākandaka

both being Eastern cities *(Pāṇ.* IV.2.123). Had the cities been in the Northern region, we would have expected the forms to be Pāṭaliputrīya and Kākandīya by *Vṛddhāccaḥ.*

In the sense of "hailing from that place", the Easterners were in the speech-habit of causing the *vṛddhi* of the initial vowel of the second member of a word, of which the first indicated a quarter (*Pāṇ.* VII.3.14, *prācām grāmanagarāṇām*).

1. Pūrva-iṣukāmaśamī > Pūrva-aiṣukāmaśama
= Pūrvaiṣukāmaśama (wih *aṆ*)
2. Pūrva Pāṭaliputra > Pūrva Pāṭaliputraka
(with *VUÑ*)

In the second example, the initial vowel *ū* is not changed as in 1; the *vṛddhi* in the second part is not seen due to *ā* which itself is *vṛddha.* In the non-Eastern region these forms would have been,

Paurveṣukāmaśama and
Paurvapāṭaliputraka.

If a place-name had *nagara* as the second part, the word indicating a person hailing from that place, showed *vṛddhi* in the initial vowel of both parts *(Pāṇ.* VII.4.124).

KINSHIP

In forms suggestive of blood-relation, the following points are noteworthy. The general suffix indicative of 'issue', seen after a word ending in *a* is *i* (*iÑ*) causing *vṛddhi* in the initial vowel. Thus Dakṣa's son will be Dākṣi (*Pāṇ.* IV.1.95 and the general aphorism for the *vṛddhi*- VII.2.117). But in the stems having an initial *vṛddha* vowel, the following were the usages in the Northern and the Eastern regions respectively:—

Āmragupta	Āmraguptāyani (with *PHiÑ*) Northern
	Āmragaupti (with *iÑ*) Eastern or non-Northern (*Pāṇ.* IV.1.157)

But whereas in the Northern region from a word ending in *a* and not having a *vṛddha* vowel initially, the form will be only in *i*, in the Eastern region it will show also *āyani*. Thus,

Dakṣa		Dākṣi	(*iÑ*)	Northern
	i.	Dākṣi	(*iÑ*)	Eastern
	ii.	Dakṣāyaṇi	(PHiÑ)	

It may be noted, however, that the Dakṣas were a Northern family. Pāṇini is himself said to be Dākṣīpūtra. Another example—

Glucuka		Glaucuki	(iÑ)	Northern
	i.	Glaucuki	(iÑ)	Eastern
	ii.	Glucukāyani	(PHiÑ)	(*Pāṇ.* IV.1. 157; 169).

A similar difference is to be marked in the case of words ending in *sena*, the word *lakṣaṇa*, and those indicating craft (*Pāṇ.* IV.1.152). Thus:—

Non-Northern—Hariṣeṇa> Hāriṣeṇya
or
Eastern - Lakṣaṇa > Lākṣaṇya
Tantuvāya > Tāntuvāyya
Nāpita > Nāpiti
or Nāpitya
(Pāṇ. IV.1.157)
(initial *vṛddha*)
} *Ṇya (Pāṇ.* IV.1.152)

Northern - Hariṣeṇa Hāriṣeṇi
Lakṣaṇa Lākṣaṇi
Tantuvāya Tāntuvāyi
} *iÑ*
Nāpita Nāpitāyani — *PHiÑ* *(Pāṇ.* IV.1.157)

In the case of the suffix indicative of the living *fourth in the line*, when the higher in the family-line is alive *(Pāṇ.* IV.1.163), the Easterners had a distinction. The suffix so indicative is technically called "*yuva-pratyaya*", while the person indicated thereby is the "*yuvan*" or *yuvāpatya*. Now this suffix is seen only after the usual suffix indicative of the "issue" or the "*gotra*" for which there is the same suffix *generally*. Thus:—

Dakṣa (1) > Dākṣi (*iÑ*) = Dakṣa's son (2) / Dakṣa's son's son (3)
Dākṣi > Dākṣāyaṇa (*PHAK*) *(Pāṇ.* IV.1.101; VII.1.2) (4)

It will be clear that here the suffix *PHAK* (*āyan*) comes after *iÑ*, which has been already fixed. With the addition of the suffix *PHIÑ* the new form indicates Dakṣa's son's son, i.e. the *fourth* from Dakṣa. But in the Eastern region, the fourth was indicated without the addition of the suffix indicative of the "fourth" in the line. Or, in technical language, the "*yuva-pratyaya*" was elided. The position in the Eastern region would be—

Dakṣa (1) > Dākṣi (*iÑ*) = (2)/(3)
Dākṣi (elision of *PHIÑ*) = Dākṣi (4)

It is interesting to note that two different forms are given by Bhaṭṭoji to indicate the difference. Thus:—

Eastern = Pannāgāra (1) Pānnāgāri (*iÑ*) (2) (3) (4)
Northern = Dakṣa (1) > Dākṣi (*iÑ*) (2) (3)
Dākṣāyaṇa (*PHAK*) (4)

It may be safe to believe that the family of the Dakṣas hailed from the North, as we have noted earlier and that of the Pannāgāras hailed from the Eastern region.

FEMININE FORMS

In the case of the feminine terminations, the following peculiarity was seen. Where the usual termination was *ī*, there was difference when it was seen after the suffix *ya* (*yaÑ*). In the non-Eastern region, the feminine *ī* would be seen, eliding the *y* of the previous suffix (*Pāṇ*. VI.4.150), while in the Eastern, before the feminine *ī*, another suffix was also seen; this was *āyan* (*ṢPHA, Pāṇ*. IV.1.17). Thus:—

Garga > Gārgya {
Gārgī (Fem.) non-Eastern/Eastern
Gārgyāyaṇī (Fem.) - Eastern.

This tendency seems to have influenced other non-Eastern usages in the case of Lohita, Kata, etc. whose feminine forms in *ī*, without *āyan* (*ṢPHA)*, went out of use, (*Pāṇ*. IV.I.18). Thus:—

Lohita > Lauhitya {
(*Lauhitī) - non-Eastern
Lauhityāyanī - Everywhere.

Kata > Kātya {
(*Kātī) - non-Eastern
Kātyāyanī - Everywhere

Such other forms were Kauravyāyaṇī (*Kauravī), Māṇḍūkāyanī (*Māṇḍūkī), and Kātyāyana adds Āsurāyaṇī (*vā.* 24.33). We have observed that such Eastern names drove out of use the names without *āyan*, which was a peculiarity of the Eastern usage. It is more probable that all such names were in origin only Eastern imported into the non-Eastern region.

Another interesting peculiarity to be noted is about the feminine suffixes after words indicating adjectives. We are told that the normal suffix *ī* was found among the Easterners, while its another variety *ā* was in use in other regions, as far as the word *śoṇa* was concerned *(Pāṇ.* IV.1.43 and Bhaṭṭoji). Pāṇini notes eleven adjectives, having two forms each, mutually differing in meaning; but in the case of *śoṇa* the meaning is the same. It is likely that one form (*Śoṇī*) was used in the Eastern region and the other (*śoṇā*) in the Northern. Now, the very next aphorism says that there were optional forms of the adjectives ending in short *u*, but does not mention the particular region in which they were in vogue. There is no doubt that the forms in the feminine *ī* and *ā*, which underline the option, were not prevalent in the same region originally. As such, before being used in the same locality (if we are to believe so giving the prop to the idea of option) one form must have been used in the Eastern region and the other in the non-Eastern. And, the Northern speech was supposed to be the norm, the non-Eastern indicated the Northern. The aphorism which teaches that the feminine suffix *ī* was used for *śoṇa* in the Eastern region (*Pāṇ.* IV.1.43, *śoṇāt prācām)* obviously tells something special about the Eastern usage, as far as the word *śoṇa* is concerned. It tells only that the word *śoṇa* had the feminine *ī* suffix, in the Eastern region. But we are not sure if the feminine form of this word in the Northern region was *śoṇā*, though it is mentioned as such (see Bhaṭṭoji). The probability is that the form *śoṇā* went out of use in the Eastern region, being completely eclipsed by the Northern trend of *śoṇī*. It is pertinent to note that the very next aphorism teaches that, the feminine forms of words indicative of a quality and ending in *u* (short) were ending optionally—i.e., in *ī* or the original *u*, and no special region is mentioned (*Pāṇ*. IV.1.44, *vā-uto guṇavacanāt*). If we understand the *anuvṛtti* of "*prācām*" from the earlier aphorism, we are safe in supposing that *ā* was not a *special* (but normal) feminine ending in the Eastern region, while *ī* was; and the option taught in the latter aphorism was in view of the feminine forms used in the Eastern region for bases in short *u*. Even if the *anuvṛtti* is not taken, the comparison of the two aphorisms leads us to the surmise that Pāṇini's period showed *śoṇī* in the Eastern region, while in the other case *ī-u* forms were used without any special restriction, to any region. So was the case with the words in the class "*bahu*", etc. (*Pāṇ*. IV. 1.45). So, the position, following the aphorisms of Pāṇini, is as follows:—

śoṇa	*śoṇī*	— Eastern
	śoṇā	?
mṛdu	*mṛdvī*	
	mṛdu	
bahu	*bahvī*	
	bahu	

Now the *Gaṇa-sūtra* tradition adds to this list of optional feminine forms of words ending in *i* (short), which are different from those formed by the *kṛt* suffix K*tiN (Gaṇa* 50, *kṛd-ikārād-aktinaḥ*) - i.e. not words like *bhakti* (√*bhaj* + *ti* < *Ktin*), *dhṛti* (√*dhṛ* + *ti* < *KtiN*); but such words as *rātri* (√*ra*+ *tri* < *trip)*. And according to others, the original feminine *i*-ending need not be of a *kṛt* suffix; only it should not be the *kṛt KtiN* (*sarvato-aktinn-arthād-ity-eke*). So:—

śakaṭī - *śakaṭi* -	(small cart)

Now it has to be marked that the Vedic usage, especially the *mantra*, showed the *ī* in the feminine invariable without exception *(Pāṇ.* IV.1.46, *nityam chandasi*). There is no doubt, hence, that in the case of the forms noted above the most original feminine suffix was *ī,* which was also the suffix in the normative Northern tongue; and in the Eastern region, except for *śoṇa,* the similar suffix was *ā*. In the case of *śoṇa* there are two possibilities— (i) either the Northern *ī* completely drove out of use the normal Eastern *ā* suffix; or, more likely, (ii) the word *śoṇi* was a loan-word from the North. What Pāṇini has noted about (the invariability of) the feminine suffix *ī* in *Chandas* (IV.1.46) is corroborated from textual data. We may now see the position:—

śoṇa	*śoṇī* (Eastern < Northern-loan *śoṇā* (out of use in the Eastern; Northern doubtful)	
mṛdu	*mṛdvī* (Northern) *mṛdu* (Eastern)	later mixed use in both regions
bahu	*bahvī* (Northern) - *ṚV* (I.188 5; X 97.18, etc. *bahu* (Eastern)	later mixed use
śakaṭa	*śakaṭī* (Northern) - *ṚV* (X. 146 3) *śakaṭi* (Eastern)	" "
.. ..	*rātrī* (Northern) - *ṚV* (I.35.1, etc.) *rātri* (Eastern)	" "

It is, now, safe to believe that in the case of words indicating a quality (*guṇa-vacana*) the Northern usage added *ī* to form the feminine, while the original Eastern usage was to retain them as they were, if they ended in short *u*. Though at a later stage of a mixed usage it was difficult to sift the original influences, it is not altogether impossible. It will be interesting to trace the influence in some of the modern words (new Indo-Aryan).

kaḍu { *kaduvī* (Hindi) > *kaḍuī*
kaḍu (Marathi), etc.

OTHER STYLISTIC PECULIARITIES

Another stylistic peculiarity of the Easterners was to use *tvā* with *alam* and *khalu* in denoting forbiddance (*Pāṇ.*III.4.18, *alam khalvoḥ pratiṣedhayoḥ prācām Ktvā*). Thus:—

alam datvā ← Do not give → *datvā khalu*
alam kṛtvā ← Do not perform → *kṛtvā khalu*

otherwise *mā kuru* = Do not perform, etc. (Northern).

Here the remark that the mention of the Easterners is to show respect (to them?) — (*prācām grahaṇam pūjārtham*, see Bhaṭṭoji) is rather difficult to reconcile with. Though it may be granted that it is not a case for option unlike the view of the *Kāśikā*, the mention of the Easterners has to be understood as a mode of speech, as different from that of the Northerners, as is indicated by the next aphorism (*udīcām māṅo vyatīhāre*).

The forms in *atara* and *atama* (*ḌataraC* and *ḌatamaC*) were normally used, to indicate a definite person, after *kim* (who, which), *yat* (who, which, what) and *tat* (that); but in the Eastern region, along with these forms, the forms *ekatara* and *ekatama* were in use, where the said suffixes were seen after *eka*. Thus:—

kataraḥ / katamaḥ
yataraḥ / yatamaḥ } Northern and Eastern
tataraḥ / tatamaḥ

ekataraḥ / ekatamaḥ Eastern

We close our observations with yet another interesting peculiarity. Pāṇini notes certain suffixes to denote pity (pitiable condition), suitability for admonition, etc. These are:— *ka*, if the word has two vowels; *ika* (*THAC*) if the word denotes the name of a person and has three or more vowels in it. In the later case two more suffixes are also noted viz. *iya* (*GHAN*) and *ila* (*ilaC*) - (*Pāṇ*. V.3. 76;-77;-78;-79). Another aphorism teaches that in such cases, the suffix is seen after the second vowel; and all that follows this second vowel is dropped (*Pāṇ*. V.3.83). Thus:—

Pitiable Devadatta = Deva + suffix (datta)
Deva + suffix (... ...)

The forms will be:

Devi*ka*, Devi*ya*, Devi*la*

In all these, the second part of the original word has been dropped. In the case of the first member also the final vowel is elided before the following suffix (*Pāṇ*. VI.4.148).

In the case of the suffix *ka*, however, there is no such change, and it is seen at the end of the word. Thus:— Devadattaka.

In later times, the change was manifold as is seen from the *Vārtikas;* and we are not concerned with it in this study.

In the Eastern region, however, in the case of a word denoting a human and having *upa* as its first member, two more suffixes were seen viz. *aḍa* (*aḍaC*) and *aka* (*VUC*) and the formation was the same way. Thus:—

Pitiable Upadatta = Upa + suffix

Non-Eastern:— Upiya, Upika, Upila and Upadattaka Eastern:—All the above forms PLUS- Upaḍa Upaka	} The second part in the original word (datta) being lost.

This will give a general idea of the changes in certain words in the Eastern region as known to Pāṇini. There are also a few accentual peculiarities; but being minor may not be included in this study.

* Included here from *Vidarbha Samshodhana Mandal, Annual No.,* Nagpur, 1970 (pub. in 1971).

Bibliography

SANSKRIT TEXTS (WITH ABBREVIATIONS)

SAṀHITĀS

(*AV*) Atharvaveda-Saṁhitā; Ed. S.D. Satawalekar, Pardi, 1957.

(*Mait.Sam.*). Maitrāyaṇī-saṁhitā; Ed. Leopald von Shroeder, 1923; S.D. Satawalekar, Vik. Saṁvat 1998.

(*ṚV*) Ṛgveda-saṁhitā; Ed. Vaidik Samshodhan Mandal, Pune, 1933-1951.

(*Taitt.Sam.*) Taittirīya-saṁhitā; S.D. Satawalekar, New Print, Saṁvat 2039; Anandashram, Pune, 1948.

BRĀHMAṆA-TEXTS

(*Ait/Ai. Br.*) Aitareya-brāhmaṇa; Anandashram, Pune, Part-I 1930, Part II 1970.

(*Jai. Br.*) Jaiminīya-brāhmaṇa; Eds. Raghuvira and Lokesh Chandra, Nagpur, 1954; reprint, Motilal Banarsidass, Delhi, 1986.

(*Jai .Up. Br.*) Jaiminīya Upaniṣad-Brāhmaṇa; Hans Ortel, American Oriental Society.

(*Kauṣītaki Br.*) Kauṣītaki-brāhmaṇa (= Śāṅkhāyana-brāhmaṇa), Anandashram, Pune 1911.

Pañcaviṁśa-brāhmaṇa (= Tāṇḍya Mahābrāhmaṇa) Kashi Sanskrit Series, Chawkhamba, Benares, 1936.

(*Śat.Br.*) Śatapatha-brāhmaṇa (Mādhyandina), Kashi Sanskrit Series, 2nd print, Varanasi, Chawkhamba, V. Saṁvat 1997; (Kāṇva) Raghuvir and Caland, 1939
(*Taitt.Br.*) Taittirīya-brāhmaṇa, Anandashram, 3rd Ed., Pune, 1979.

UPANIṢAD-TEXTS

(*Bṛhad.Up.*) Bṛhadāraṇyaka-upaniṣad, Gita Press, Gorakhpur.
Chāndogya-upaniṣad, Gita Press, Gorakhpur.
(*Kaṭha Up.*) Kaṭha-upaniṣad, Gita Press, Gorakhpur.
Kauṣītakibrāhmaṇa-upaniṣad

SŪTRA-TEXTS

(*Āśv. / Āśvalāyana G.S*) Āśvalāyana Gṛhyasūtra, ed. with Marathi tr. by Shivram Shastri Shintre, Mumbai, 1938.
(*Baudh.Dh.S.*) Baudhāyana Dharmasūtra, ed. by A. Chinnaswami Shastri, pub.in Kashi Sanskrit Series, Benares, 1934.
(*Bau.P.S.*) Baudhāyana - pitṛmedha - sūtra.
(*Gaut.Dh.S.*) Gautama Dharmasūtra, ed. by I. Srinivas-acharya, Mysore, 1917.
(*K.Ś.S.*) Kātyāyana Śrautasūtra, Chowkhamba Sanskrit Series, Benares, 1933.
Kauśika Sūtra (of Atharvaveda), ed. by M. Bloomfield, Motilal Banarsidass, Delhi, Reprint 1972 (1889 Journal *JAOS*).
Vaikhānasa-smārta-sūtra, ed. by Caland in B.I. Series with Eng.tr. (1927 text, 1929).
(*Vas.Dh.S.*) Vasiṣṭha Dharmasūtra, ed. by A.A. Führer, in Bombay Sanskrit Series, 3rd ed., Poona, 1930.
Viṣṇu Dharmasūtra, ed. by J. Jolly, Calcutta, 1881.

EPICS

(*Ram.*) Rāmāyaṇa, ed. Chinnaswami Shastri/ Subrahmanya Shastri, 2nd ed., Mylapore, Madras, 1958.

(*Mb.*) Mahābhārata, ed. (with the commentary of Nīlakaṇṭha), Chitrashala Press, Pune; Crit. Ed., BORI, Pune; and Gita Press, Gorakhpur.

SMṚTI-TEXTS

(*Manu S./Sm.*) Manusmṛti (with Kullūka's comm.), Nirnayasagara, Bombay, 1946.
(*Yāj. S./Sm.*) Yājñavalkyasmṛti (with the comm. Mitākṣarā), Nirnayasagara, Bombay, 1937.

PURĀṆA-TEXTS

(*Agni P.*) Agni Purāṇa, ed. Anandashram, Poona, 1900.
(*Bhāgavata P.*) Bhāgavata Purāṇa, ed. Gita Press, Gorakhpur.
(*Brahmāṇḍa P.*) Brahmāṇḍa Purāṇa, ed. Venkateshwar Press, Bombay, 1912.
(*Brahmavaivarta P.*) Brahmavaivarta Purāṇa, ed. Anandashram, Poona, 1935.
(*Garuḍa P.*) Garuḍa Purāṇa, ed. Chawkhamba, Varanasi, 1964.
(*Matsya P.*) Matsya Purāṇa, ed. Jivananda Vidyasagar, Calcutta, 1879.
(*Padma P.*) Padma Purāṇa, ed. Anandashram, Poona, 1893-1894.
(*Śiva P.*) Śiva Purāṇa, ed. Venkateshwar Press, Bombay.
(*Skanda P.*) Skanda Purāṇa, ed. Venkateshwar Press, Bombay.
(*Varāha P.*) Varāha Purāṇa, ed. Hrishikesh Shastri, Calcutta, 1893.
Viṣṇudharmottra Purāṇa, Gaikwad, Oriental Series III.

OTHER TEXTS

Arthasaṅgraha, ed. S.M. Paranjape, Bombay, 1927.
(*Artha.*) Arthaśāstra, ed. R.P. Kangle, University of Bombay, Bombay, Part I, 2nd ed. 1969, Part II, 2nd ed. 1972.
Aṣṭādhyāyī of Paṇini

Bhagavadgītā, with Śaṅkara's com., Ashtekar and Company, 2nd ed., Poona, 1929.

Bṛhaddevatā, ed. with Eng. tr. by A.A. Macdonell, in Harvard Oriental Series, Vols. 5 & 6, Cambridge, Massachusetts, 1904.

Bṛhatsaṁhitā, with Eng. tr. by V. Subrahmanya Sastri and M. Ramakrishna Bhat, 2 vols., Bangalore, 1947.

Chullavagga

Daśarūpakam of Dhanañjaya, with Dhanika's com., ed. and tr. in Hindi by Ramji Upadhyaya, Bharatiya Samskriti Samsthana, Allahabad, Vikram Sam. 2036.

Dūtavākyam, in *Bhāsanāṭakacakram,* Crit.ed. C.R. Deodhar, 2nd ed., Poona, 1951.

Harṣacarita, ed. by P.V. Kane, Nirnayasagar, 1st ed., Bombay, 1918.

Karakaṇḍacariu, ed. with Eng. and Hindi tr., Hiralal Jain, 2nd ed., Calcutta, 1964.

Karpūramañjarī, 4th ed., Nirnayasagar, Mumbai, 1949.

Kāvyādarśa of Daṇḍin, with the com. of Pt. Rangacharya Raddi Shastri, BORI, Poona, 1938.

Kāvyaprakāśa with Bālabodhinī, BORI, 7th ed., Poona, 1965.

Kāvyālaṅkāra of Rudraṭa, ed. in the Kāvyamālā Series, Bombay.

Kumārasambhava, with the com. of Mallinatha, 12th ed., Nirnayasagar, Bombay, 1935.

Laṅkāvatāra, pub. by Buddhist Text Society, Calcutta, 1902.

Mahābhāṣya of Patañjali, Vol.II, Motilal Banarsidass, Delhi, 1967.

Mahāparinirvāṇa-sūtra (Mahāparinibbāna-Sutta), ed. Bhikshu Kittima, Benares, Vikram Saṁvat 1998 (= A.D. 1941).

Meghadūta, ed. with Eng. tr. and notes by M.R. Kale, 3rd ed., Gopal Narayan & Co., Bombay, 1934.

Nāṭyaśāstra of Bharata, pub. in Kashi Sanskrit Series, 1929.

(*Nir.*) Nirukta, ed. Nirnayasagar, Bombay, 1930.

Pratijñāyaugandharāyaṇa, in *Bhāsanāṭakacakram*, Crit. ed. C.R. Deodhar, Oriental Book Agency, 2nd ed., Poona, 1951.

Pūrvamīmāṁsāsūtra of Jaimini, Anandashram, Poona.

Uttarajjhayaṇa-sūtra (=Uttarādhyayana-sūtra), Nirnayasagar, Bombay, 1937.

Uttararāmacarita of Bhavabhūti, ed. P.V. Kane, 1st ed., Nirnayasagar, Bombay,1915.

Vāgbhaṭālaṅkāra of Vāgbhaṭa, pub. in Kāvya Mālā Series.

Vyaktiviveka of Mahimabhaṭṭa, pub. in Trivandrum Series, 1909.

OTHERS

Ali, Muzafer S., 1973 (1966): *The Geography of the Purāṇas,* People's Publishing House, 2nd ed., New Delhi, Ahmedabad, Bombay.

Banerji, R.D., 1950 (1914): *Prehistoric Ancient and Hindu India,* Blackie and Son (India) Ltd., Bombay, Calcutta and Madras.

Barnett, L.D., 1922: *Hindu Gods and Heroes,* London.

Betty Sue Flowers, 1988: *The Power of* Myth (Ed. Interview of Joseph Campbell with Bill Moyers), Doubleday, New York.

Cavendish, Richard, 1974: *Legends of the World*, Barnes and Nobles, New York.

Chambers Twentieth Century Dictionary.

Charpentier, J., 1920: *Die Suparṇasage*, Uppsala.

Claude Lévi–Strauss, 1980: *Myth and Meaning*, Routledge and Kegan Paul, London.

Clement, C.J. Webb, 1937 (1910): *A History of Philosophy,* Thornton Butterworth Ltd., London.

Colebrooke, 1837: *Miscellaneous Essays*, Vol.I, Madras.

Crawford, S. Cromwell, 1982 (1974), *The Evolution of Hindu Ethical Ideas,* Hawaii.

Dange, Sadashiv A., 1969: *Legends in the Mahābhārata*, Motilal Banarsidass, Delhi.

——, 1971: *Vedic Concept of 'Field' and the Divine Fructification*, University of Bombay, Bombay.

Dange, Sadashiv A., 1979: *Sexual Symbolism from the Vedic Ritual,* Ajanta Publications, Delhi.
——, 1986-1990: *Encyclopaedia of Puranic Beliefs and Practices*, Navrang, New Delhi (Vols. I-V).
——, 1992: *Divine Hymns and Ancient Thought,* Vol.I (Ṛgveda Hymns and Ancient Thought), Navrang, New Delhi.
——, 1994: *Purākathāncā Artha — Vāda āṇi Vivecana* (Marathi), Continental Prakashan, Pune.
——, 1995: *Divine Hymns and Ancient Thought*, Vol.II (Ritual and the Quest for Truth), Navrang, New Delhi.
——, 1996: *Towards Understanding Hindu Myths,* Aryan Books International, New Delhi.
——, 1997: *Myths from the Mahābhārata,* Vol.1, *Quest for Immortality,* Aryan Books International, New Delhi.
——, 2000: *Images from Vedic Hymns and Rituals,* Aryan Books International, New Delhi.
——, 2000: *Vedic Sacrifices — Early Nature*, Vols. I & II, Aryan Books International, New Delhi.
——, 2001: *Myths from the Mahābhārata,* Vol. 2, *Study in Patterns and Symbols,* Aryan Books International, New Delhi.
——, 2001: *Myths from the Mahābhārata,* Vol. 3, *Probe in Early Dim History and Folklore*, Aryan Books International, New Delhi.
Dange, (Mrs.) Sindhu S., 1980: *Bauddha Dharma āṇi Tattvajñāna* (Marathi), Continental Prakashan, Pune.
——, 1980: *Jaina Dharma āṇi Tattvajñāna* (Marathi), Continental Prakashan, Pune.
——, 1989: *Puranic Etymologies and Flexible Forms*, Viveka Publications, Aligarh.
——, 1996: *Aspects of Speech in Vedic Ritual*, Aryan Books International, New Delhi.
Darmesteter, James, 1988 (1887): *The Zend-Avesta,*Part I, SBE Vol.4, Motilal Banarsidass, Delhi.

Darmesteter, James, 1988 (1882): *The Zend-Avesta,* Part II, SBE Vol.23, Motilal Banarsidass, Delhi.

——, 1988 (1887): *The Zend-Avesta,* Part III, SBE Vol.31, Motilal Banarsidass, Delhi.

Dasgupta, S.N. (Editor), 1947: *A History of Sanskrit Literature* — Classical Period, Vol.I, University of Calcutta, Calcutta.

Davies, H.A., 1950 (1928): *An Outline History of the World,* Oxford University Press, London.

Faraday, Anna, (no year mentioned): *The Dream Game*, Harper and Row, New York.

Fergusson, J., 1967: *History of Indian and Eastern Architecture*, Vol.I, Delhi.

Freud, Sigmund, 1925: *Collected Papers*, London.

——, 1952: *On Dream*, Norton, New York.

——, 1953 (1900): *The Interpretation of Dreams,* Basic Books, New York.

Geldner, K.F., 1978 (1951): *Der Rig-Veda,* Vols.I-III, HOS Vols.33-35, Cambridge-London.

1957: Vol.IV Index, HOS Vol.36, Harvard University, Cambridge.

Good News Bible, 1988 (1970), Delhi.

Gonda, J., 1959: *Epithets in the Ṛgveda*, Mouton and Co., Gravenhage.

Green, Peter, 1991: *Alexander of Macedon,* University of California Press, Los Angeles, Oxford.

Halls, Calvin S., *The Meaning of Dreams.*

Hamilton, Edith, 1942: *Mythology,* Little Brown and Co., Boston.

Hastings, J., *Encyclopaedia of Religion and Ethics,* Vol.IX.

Held, C.J., 1935: *The Mahābhārata,* London, Amsterdam.

Hopkins, E.W., 1901: *The Great Epic of India,* New York.

——, 1986 (1915): *Epic Mythology,* Motilal Banarsidass, Delhi.

Kane, P.V., 1951: *The History of Sanskrit Poetics* in his ed. of *Sahityadarpaṇa*, 3rd ed., Bombay.

——, 1968: *History of Dharmaśāstra*, Vol.I, pt.I, 2nd ed., BORI, Poona.

Kane, P.V., 1974: Vol.II, pt.I, 2nd ed., BORI, Poona.
——, 1974: Vol.II, pt.II, 2nd ed., BORI, Poona.
——, 1973; Vol.IV, 2nd ed., BORI, Poona.
——, 1977, Vol.V, pt.II, 2nd ed., BORI, Poona.
Karl, Abraham, 1909: *Dreams and Myths*.
Kolangade, R.G., 1946: *Tyāgarāja Bhagavān Gotama Buddha* (Marathi), pub. by himself, Mumbai.
Kramer, S.N., 1944: *Sumerian Mythology*, American Philosophical Society, Philadelphia.
Kulkarni, V.M. (Ed.), 1994: *A Treasury of Jain Tales,* Sharadaben Chimanbhai Educational Research Centre, Ahmedabad.
Lang, Andrew, 1913 (1887): *Myth, Ritual and Religion,* Vol.I, London.
Macdonell, A.A., 1961 (1898): *Vedic Mythology*, (Hindi tr.), Chowkhamba, Varanasi; 1995: Motilal Banarsidass, Delhi.
Mackenzie, Donald (no year mentioned): *Myths of Babylonia and Assyria*, Gresham, London.
—— (no year mentioned): *Egyptian Myth and Legend*, Gresham, London.
—— (no year mentioned): *Myths of Crete and Pre-Hellenic Europe*, Gresham, London
—— (no year mentioned): *Myths of China and Japan*, Gresham, London.
Mainkar, T.G., 1961: *Mysticism in the Ṛgveda*, Popular Book Depot, Bombay.
——, 1966: *Some Poetical Aspects of Ṛgvedic Repetitions,* University of Poona, Poona.
Meyer, J.J., 1952: *Sexual Life in Ancient India*, Calcutta.
Miller, Hugh, 1835: *Scenes and Legends*, London.
Mistree, Khojeste, 1982: *Zoroastrianism - An Ethnic Perspective*, Bombay.
Mitra, Rajendralal, 1981 (1882): *Sanskrit Buddhist Literature of Nepal*, Cosmo Publication, Delhi.
Nakamura, Hajime, 1992 (1975): *A Comparative History of Ideas*, Motilal Banarsidass, Delhi.

O'Flaherty, Wendy Doniger, 1981: *Anthology from the Ṛgveda,* Penguin.

Palsule, G.B., 1961: *The Sanskrit Dhātupāṭhas,* Poona.

Pischel, R., 1965 (Eng.tr.): *Comparative Grammar of the Prakrit Languages.*

Pusalkar, A.D., 1968 (1940): *Bhāsa—A Study,* Munshiram Manoharlal, 2nd ed., Delhi.

Ramakein (Thai Rāmāyaṇa).

Rao, S.R., 1982: *The Decipherment of the Indus Script,* Asia Publishing House, Bombay (Calcutta, New Delhi, Lucknow).

Robertson, William, 1997: *History of America.*

R.T. Rundle Clark, 1959: *Myth and Symbol in Ancient Egypt,* Thames and Hudson, London.

Sen, Asis, *Animal Motifs in Ancient Indian Art,* Firma K.L. Mukhopadhyay, Calcutta.

Stall, Frits, 1983: *Agni* (The Vedic Ritual of the Fire-altar), Vols.I & II Motilal Banarsidass, Delhi.

Suzuki David and Kundston Peter, (no year mentioned): *Wisdom of the Elders,* Bantam Books, New York.

Vats, Madho Sarup, 1940: *Excavations at Harappa,* Vol.I, Calcutta.

Velankar, H.D. 1962: *Ṛgveda Maṇḍala* VII, University of Bombay, Bombay.

——, 1968, *Ṛgveda Maṇḍala* III, University of Bombay, Bombay.

Whitney, W.D., 1950 (Leipzig, 1885): *The Roots, Verb-forms and Primary Derivatives of the Sanskrit Language,* Edwards Brothers, Inc., Michigan.

PAPERS

Agrawal, R.C., "Agni in Early Indian Art", *Journal of Indian History,* Trivandrum, April, 1965.

Bodewitz, H.W., "What did Indra do with the Yatis?", *Amṛtadhārā* (Prof. R.N. Dandekar Fel. Vol.), Delhi, 1984.

Dange, Sadashiv A., "Religious Suicide in the Vedic Period (?)", *Indologia Tauriensia,* 8-9 (1980-81), Torino, Italy.

——, "Presidential Address" of the Vedic Section, *Proceedings* of the All India Oriental Conference, XXX Session (Vishva Bharati University, Santiniketan), 1980, pub. by BORI, Poona, 1982.

——, "Ritual Variations and the Principle of Sampad", *Brahmavidyā* (Golden Jubilee Vol.), Madras, 1986.

——, "Vowel-shortening in Sanskrit", *Vidyā-vratin* (Prof. A.M. Ghatge Fel. Vol.), Sri Satguru Publications (A Division of Indian Books Centre), Delhi.

——, "Sanskrit Poetics and Semiotics", *Journal of the Asiatic Society of Bombay,* Bombay, Vol.71 (for 1996), 1997.

——, "Vāstupuruṣa", *Purāṇa-Itihāsa-Vimarśa* (Essays in honour of Prof. S.G. Kantawala), Bharatiya Vidya Prakashan, Delhi, 1998.

——, "Dream, Myth and the Hindu Context", *Annals* of BORI, Vol.LXXIX (1998), Pune, 1999.

——, "Kumāra, Kārttikeya and the Peacock", *Journal of the Asiatic Society of Bombay,* Bombay, Vol.74 (for 1999) (New Series), 2000.

——, "Sandhi, Śākalya, Pāṇini VI.127-128 and the Vedic Evidence", *Traividyam* (Vedic Studies in Memory of Durgamohan Bhattacharyya), Subarnarekha Publication, Kolkata, 2001.

Dange, (Mrs.) Sindhu S., "Autovertism in the Ṛgveda", *Vishveshvaranand Indological Journal,* Panjab University, Hoshiarpur, Vol.XIV, pt.I, March 1976.

——, "The Stage of Bharata: Some Symbolic Rites", *Ṛtam* (Baburam Saksena Fel.Vol.), Lucknow, 1983.

——, "Sūta — The Paurāṇika", *Purāṇa,* All India Kashiraj Trust, Varanasi, Vol.XL, No.2, July 1998.

Desai, Devangana, "Hayagrīva in the Vaikuṇtha Pantheon of Khajuraho", *Colloquium on Viṣṇu*, Birla Archaeological and Cultural Research Institute, Hyderabad, 1993.

Desai, Devangana, "An Unpublished Viśvarūpa Sculpture in the Khajuraho Museum", *Journal of the Asiatic Society of Bombay,* Bombay, Vol.72, 1997 (New Series).

De Souza, J. Patrocinio, "The Symbol of the Double-headed Eagle: Its Origin, Diffusion and Significance", *Journal of the University of Bombay, Bombay,* Oct. 1969, No.74, Vol.XXXVIII.

Ghatge, A.M., "Prākrit-tendencies in the Ṛgveda", *Indian Historical Quarterly,* 21-3.

Ghosh, B.K., "Prākrit Samdhis in the Ṛksamhitā", *Indian Linguistics,* Poona, 9.

Handa, Devendra, "Vaikuṇṭha Images from Panjab", *Ajaya-Śrī*-Recent Studies in Indology (Prof. Ajaya Mitra Shastri Fel.Vol.), Sundeep Prakashan, Delhi, 1989.

Jung, C.G., "The Archetypes and Collective Subconscious", in the *Collected Works of C.G. Jung,* Vol.IX, pt.1 (tr. in Eng. by R.F.C. Hull), Bollingen Series, XX, Princeton University Press, Princeton, 1990 (1968).

Krishna Deva, "Images of Hayagrīva as Vaikuṇṭha", *Viśvambharā* (Prof. V.S. Pathak Fel. Vol.), Harman Publications, New Delhi, 1995.

Mehendale, M.A., "Presidential Address" of the Vedic Section *Proceedings* of the AIOC XVII Session (Kurukshetra), 1974, published by BORI, Poona, 1976.

——, "Satī — Kahīn Pracīna Sandarbha", *Navabhārata,* Wai, Jan. 1988.

——, "The Custom of Sahagamana, some early references", *Proceedings* of the National Seminar on Living Customs and their Ancient Indian Sources, CASS, University of Poona, Poona, 1991.

Parpola, Asko, "The Metamorphosis of Mahiṣa Asura and Prajāpati", in: *Ritual, State and History in South India* (Essays in honour of J.C. Heesterman), E.J. Brill, Leiden, 1992.

Ramachandran, T.N., "A Brief Survey of Buddhistic Art", in *2500 Years of Buddhism,* Govt. of India Publication, New Delhi, 1976 (1959).

Ram Gopal, "Vedic Vāstu and its Derivatives", *Bhāratīya Vidyā,* Vols. XLV-XLVII (Mm.Prof. J.H. Dave Fel. Vol.), Bombay, 1987.

Talim, Meena V., "Origin of the Chabbaggiyas", *Proceedings* of the Prakrit Seminar, University of Bombay, Bombay, 1971.

Velankar, H.D., "Kavi and Kāvya in the Ṛgveda", *Proceedings* of AIOC, XXIII Session (Aligarh 1966), BORI, Poona, 1969.

Vidyabhusana, J., "Persian Affinities of the Licchavis", *Indian Antiquary,* Vol.37, 1908.

Wordsworth, W., "Poetry and Poetic Diction", Preface to the 2nd ed. of *Lyrical Ballads*, 1800.

Abbreviations of Modern Titles

ABORI	:	Annals of the Bhandarkar Oriental Research Institute
AIOC	:	All India Oriental Conference
B.I.	:	Bibliotheca Indica
BORI	:	Bhandarkar Oriental Research Institute
CASS	:	Centre of Advanced Study in Sanskrit
Ency. P.B. & P.	:	Encyclopaedia of Puranic Beliefs and Practices
Hist. of Dh.S	:	History of Dharmaśāstra
HOS	:	Harward Oriental Series
IHQ	:	Indian Historical Quarterly
JASB	:	Journal of the Asiatic Society of Bombay
MIA	:	Middle Indo-Aryan
NIA	:	New Indo-Aryan
SK	:	Siddhānta-Kaumudī of Bhaṭṭoji
VIJ	:	Vishveshvaranand Indological Journal
VSM	:	Vidarbha Samshodhan Mandal
VVBIS & IS	:	Vishveshvaranand Vishva Bandhu Institute of Sanskrit and Indological Studies
VVRI	:	Vishveshvaranand Vedic Research Institute

Part - II

1. A Short Biographical Sketch of Dr. Sadashiv Ambadas Dange
2. Bibliography of the Writings of Dr. Sadashiv Ambadas Dange

A Short Biographical Sketch of Dr. Sadashiv A. Dange

Name: **Sadashiv Ambadas Dange**

Academic qualifications: M.A. (Sanskrit); M.A. (Hindi); Sahityaratna (Hindi); Diploma in Linguistics; Ph.D. (Sanskrit); D.Litt. (Sanskrit).

BIOGRAPHICAL DETAILS

Span of life: August 23, 1922 to October 25, 1999

EDUCATION:

B.A. 1942	:	Nagpur University, Nagpur, Maharashtra, India
	:	Dedicated eight years of life to social work
M.A. (Sanskrit) 1952	:	Bombay University, Bombay, Maharashtra, India
Sahityaratna (Hindi) 1955	:	Prayag, Uttar Pradesh, India
M.A. (Hindi) 1957	:	Nagpur University, Nagpur, Maharashtra, India
Ph.D. (Sanskrit) 1960	:	Nagpur University, Nagpur, Maharashtra, India

Diploma in Linguistics 1966	:	Deccan College, Poona, Maharashtra, India
D. Litt. (Sanskrit) 1969	:	Nagpur University, Nagpur, Maharashtra, India

POSTS HELD

1. Head (1954-1962): Department of Sanskrit, G.S. College, Khamgaon, Maharashtra
2. Lecturer in Sanskrit (1962-1969): Department of Post-graduate Studies, Nagpur University, Nagpur, Maharashtra
3. Reader in Sanskrit (1969-1979): Department of Sanskrit, University of Bombay, Bombay, Maharashtra
4. R.G. Bhandarkar Professor of Sanskrit and Head (1979-1982; until retirement): Department of Sanskrit, University of Bombay, Bombay, Maharashtra

BRANCHES OF SPECIALIZATION

Veda-literature and Rituals; Hindu Mythology (Epics and Purāṇas) in comparison with other mythologies in the world; Dharmashastra and Grammar.

HONOURS AND AWARDS (*Selected ones*)

1. Three awards for the book *Hindu Dharma āṇi Tattvajñāna* (1973): (i) State Govt. of Maharashtra, for the best book in Marathi (1974-1975); (ii) Chiplunkar prize, Poona University (1974); (iii) Prize of the Kesari - Maratha Trust, Poona (1974).
2. Award from the State Govt. of Maharashtra for the book *Aśvatthācī Pāne* (1975-1976).
3. Silver Medal from the Asiatic Society of Bombay, for outstanding contribution to the study of Indology (1983; for the year 1980).
4. Vishishta Puraskāra from the Uttar Pradesh Sanskrit Academy (1989; for the year 1987).

5. Honoured by the State Govt. of Maharashtra for his service and contribution to Sanskrit and its study, 1990.
6. Honoured by the President of India with the Certificate of Merit for his contribution to Sanskrit study, 1993.
7. Award from the State Govt. of Maharashtra for the book *Purākathāncā Artha-Vāda-āṇi Vivecana (Meaning of Myth - Theories, Discussion and Evaluation)* in Marathi, (1994-1995).

* Honorary Membership and Awards conferred, by many academic and cultural institutions in Maharashtra.

EDITORIAL AND OTHER RESPONSIBILITIES

1. Editor (Hon.) for the Indian Section, *Journal of Ultimate Reality and Meaning,* Regis College, Ontario, Canada (1970-1980).
2. Consulting member of the Editorial Board for the *Encyclopaedia of Human Ideas on Ultimate Reality and Meaning* (Regis College, Ontario, Canada.)
3. President of the Vedic Section of the All India Oriental Conference (Santiniketan 1980 and Ahmedabad 1985) XXX and XXXII Sessions.
4. Consultant for the television series "Discovery of India", directed by Shyam Benegal, sponsored by Govt. of India (1988).

THESIS AND COURSE RESPONSIBILITIES

1. A Ph.D. guide for twelve students.
2. Instrumental in starting the Certificate and Diploma Courses in Sanskrit in Department of Sanskrit, Bombay University, Bombay.

INVITED LECTURES *(A partial list of more than 100)*

1. Bhau Vishnu Ashtekar Lecture Series (Vedic) — 5 lectures, University of Poona, Poona, 1968.
2. Murgudkar Shastri Lecture Series - 2 lectures, Poona, 1969.

3. Pathak Shastri Lecture Series - 3 lectures, Dhule, 1978.
4. National Lecturer of Sanskrit: Selected by the University Grants Commission, New Delhi and delivered several lectures in various universities (1980-1981).
5. Vishvabandhu Memorial Lectures — 3 lectures, University of Panjab (two at Chandigarh and one at Hoshiarpur), 1981.
6. Inaugurated the National level School of Vedic Interpretation, Bangalore University, Bangalore, twelve lectures in the Lecture Series on "Modern Interpretation of the Veda and Vedic Topics", 1982
7. Fifteen lectures in the Lecture Series, "Hindu Myths", International Institute of Semiotics and Structural Studies, Central Institute of Languages, Mysore University, Mysore, December 1984-January 1985
8. National Centre for Performing Arts lecture series (7 lectures), "Indian Myths and Symbols", Bombay, 1988 (a part of a month-long course for actors, directors and performing artists).
9. Invited lecture on the Seventy-second Death Anniversary of Dr. R.G. Bhandarkar, "Dream, Myth and the Hindu Context", Bhandarkar Oriental Research Institute, Poona, Sept. 1997.

* On invitation, National Seminars attended, sessions chaired and papers presented: 40.
* Sessions attended of the All India Oriental Conference and papers presented: 20

Bibliography of Dr. Dange's Writings

BOOKS: (A total of 27 including revised editions and book volumes)

1. S.A. Dange and (Mrs.) S.S. Dange, *Critiques on Sanskrit Dramas,* Darshan Printers, Moradabad, 1963. Second revised edition, Aryan Books International, New Delhi, 1994.
2. S.A. Dange, *Legends in the Mahābhārata,* Motilal Banarsidass, New Delhi, 1969. Second revised edition, *Myths from the Mahābhārata: Quest for Immortality,* Vol.1, Aryan Books International, New Delhi, 1997.
3. S.A. Dange, *Pastoral Symbolism from the Ṛgveda*, University of Poona, Poona, 1970.
4. S.A. Dange, *Vedic Concept of 'Field' and the Divine Fructification,* University of Bombay, Bombay, 1971
5. S.A. Dange, *Hindu Dharma āṇi Tattvajñāna* (in Marathi), Shri Lekhan-Vacan Bhandar, Poona, 1973.
6. S.A. Dange, *Aśvatthācī Pāne* (in Marathi), Hindu Dharma Sanskriti Mandir, Nagpur, 1974.
7. S.A. Dange, *Cultural Sources from the Veda*, Bharatiya Vidya Bhavan, Bombay, 1977.
8. S.A. Dange, *Sexual Symbolism from the Vedic Ritual*, Ajanta Publications, New Delhi, 1979.

9. S.A. Dange, *Vedic Myths in Social Perspective,* VVRI, Hoshiarpur, 1982
10. S.A. Dange, *Puranic Myth and Culture,* Ajanta Publications, New Delhi, 1987
11. S.A. Dange, *Encyclopaedia of Puranic Beliefs and Practices,* Navrang, New Delhi Vol.1: 1986, Vol.II:1987, Vol.III:1987, Vol.IV.1989, Vol.V:1990
12. S.A. Dange, *Divine Hymns and Ancient Thought,* Navrang, New Delhi, Vol.I: *Ṛgveda Hymns and Ancient Thought*, 1992. Vol.II: *Ritual and the Quest for Truth*: 1995
13. S.A. Dange, *Purākathāncā Artha-Vāda āṇi Vivecana (Meaning of Myth - Theories, Discussion and Evaluation)* (in Marathi), Continental Prakashan, Poona, 1994
14. S.A. Dange, *Towards Understanding Hindu Myths*, Aryan Books International, New Delhi, 1996.
15. S.A. Dange, *Images from Vedic Hymns and Rituals,* Aryan Books International, New Delhi, 2000.
16. S.A. Dange, *Vedic Sacrifices—Early Nature,* Vols. I & II, Aryan Books International, New Delhi, 2000.
17. S.A. Dange, *Myths from the Mahābhārata: Study in Patterns and Symbols*, Vol.2, Aryan Books International, New Delhi, 2001.
18. S.A. Dange, *Myths from the Mahābhārata: Probe in Early Dim History and Folklore*, Vol.3, Aryan Books International, New Delhi, 2001.
19. (Mrs.) S.S. Dange (Ed.), *Gleanings from Vedic to Puranic Age* (Collected Papers of Dr. Sadashiv A. Dange), Aryan Books International, New Delhi, 2002.

RESEARCH PAPERS (More than 260)

1. Journal articles; articles in Proceedings and articles contributed to Encyclopaedic Projects: 226.
2. Invited articles: 5 (in press).
3. Review articles: > 33.

PUBLISHED RESEARCH PAPERS OF DR. S.A. DANGE

VEDA

1. "Kadrū-Vinatā and the Wager", *Purāṇa*, All India Kashiraj Trust, Varanasi, Vol.III-2, July 1961, pp.203-214.
2. "About the words *garut* and *garutmān* in the Ṛgveda", *Indian Historical Quarterly*, Calcutta, Vol.XXXIX-1 & 2, Mar.-June 1963 (pub.1967), pp.134-137.
3. "Prajāpati and his Daughter", *Purāṇa*, All India Kashiraj Trust, Varanasi, Vol.V-1, Jan. 1963, pp. 39-46.
4. "Sāvitrī and the Banyan", *Purāṇa*, All India Kashiraj Trust, Varanasi, Vol.V-2, July 1963, pp.258-266
5. "Indra āṇi Dyāvāpṛthivī" (Marathi), *Vidarbha Samshodhan Mandal* (VSM), Nagpur, *Annual No.*, 1963 (pub.1964), pp.71-79.
6. "Three Stages of the Advent of Soma", *Journal* (*Jnl.*) *of the Oriental Institute*, M.S. University of Baroda, Baroda, Vol.XIV-1, Aug.1964, pp.62-69.
7. "Ketu or the War-banner in the Ṛgveda", *Journal of Indian History,* Trivandrum, Vol.XLII-2, Aug. 1964, pp.377-379.
8. "Parvata in the Ṛgveda", *VSM,* Nagpur, *Annual No.,* 1964 (pub.1965) pp.47-60.
9. "Ṛgvedātīla yātu āṇi Yātudhāna" (Marathi), *Navabhārata*, Wai, 17 (10), July 1964, pp.12-16.
10. "'Survivals' in the Ṛgvedic Indra-Myth", *Nagpur University Journal*, Nagpur, Vol.XV-2, Apr. 1965, pp.166-188.
11. "The Ritual of Soma and the Theory of Kāvya-rasa", *VSM*, Nagpur, *Annual No.*, 1965 (pub.1966), pp.93-108.
12. "The Birth of Vasiṣṭha", *Journal of the Mythic Society*, Bangalore, Vol. LV-3 & 4, Oct. 1964-Jan.1965, pp.83-91.

13. "Adornment as a Protective Measure in the Vedic Ritual", *Dr. Mirashi Fel. Vol.,* Vidarbha Samshodhan Mandal, Nagpur, 1965, pp.87-103
14. "Aspects of War from the Ṛgveda", *Journal of Indian History*, Trivandrum, Vol.XLIV-1, Apr. 1966, pp.125-138.
15. "A Virility Charm from the Ṛgveda", *Nagpur University Journal,* Nagpur, Vol.XVI-2, Apr. 1966, pp.127-145.
16. "Ṛgvedātīla Sūkti (mhaṇī) āṇi Lokanīti" (Marathi), *Navabhārata*, Wai, 19(12), Sept.1966, pp.19-28.
17. "Mahānagnī and Apālā", *VSM*, Nagpur, *Annual No.,* 1966 (pub.1967), pp.186-210.
18. "Vasiṣṭha āṇi Sudās-kula" (Marathi), *Navabhārata*, Wai, 20 (3), Nov.-Dec.1966, pp.12-21.
19. "A Folk-custom in the Aśvamedha", *Journal of the Oriental Institute*, M.S. University of Baroda, Baroda, Vol.XVI-4, June 1967, pp.323-335.
20. "Virgin and the Divine Seed-layer", *Journal of Indian History,* Trivandrum, Vol.XLV-2, Aug.1967, pp.369-398.
21. "Sasarparī and the Horse of Sudās", *Vishveshvaranand Indological Journal* (*VIJ*), Panjab University, Hoshiarpur, Vol.V-1, Mar.1967, pp.25-32.
22. "The Field and the Plough-share (A Ritual at Ṛgveda X.101)", *Nagpur University Journal,* Nagpur, Vol.XVII-2, Apr.1967, pp.158-178.
23. "The Gaviṣṭi (Go-iṣṭi) and the Mehanā in the Ṛgveda", *Nagpur University Journal,* Nagpur, Vol.XVIII-2, Oct. 1967, pp.78-108.
24. "Sūryajala" (Marathi), *Navabhārata*, Wai, 21(2), Nov.1967, pp.32-39.
25. "The Bull of Mudgala", *VSM*, Nagpur, *Annual No.,* 1967 (pub.1968), pp.43-62.
26. "The Bull and the Fiery Fluid from the Ṛgveda", *Journal of the Oriental Institute,* M.S. University of Baroda, Baroda, Vol.XVII-3, Mar.1968, pp.209-229.
27. "On the Vedic Word *vāṇa*", *Journal of Indian History*, Trivandrum, Vol.XLVI-2, Aug.1968, pp.271-280.

28. "'Field' and the 'Ritual-husband' (from the Vedic Tradition)", *Nagpur University Journal,* Nagpur, Vol.XIX-1 & 2, July-Oct.1968, pp.1-28.
29. "Holāṣṭakopaniṣad" (Marathi), *Navabhārata*, Wai, Nov.1968, pp.67-69.
30. "Cyavana—Eka Vegale Darśana" (Marathi), *Navabhārata*, Wai, May 1969, pp.15-19.
31. "Aspects of the Great Roar in the Ṛgveda", *Journal of the University of Bombay,* Bombay, Vol.XXXVIII, Arts No.74, Oct. 1969, pp.11-18.
32. "Try'ambaka (the genesis of the concept)", *Journal of the Oriental Institute,* M.S. University of Baroda, Baroda, Vol. XIX-3, Mar.1970, pp.223-227.
33. "Admasad", *VIJ*, Panjab University, Hoshiarpur, Vol.VIII-1 & 2, Mar.-Sept. 1970, pp.35-37.
34. "Cosmic Foetus and the Symbolism of Rain from the Ṛgveda", *Journal of the University of Bombay,* Bombay, Vol.XXXIX, Arts No.75, Oct. 1970, pp.1-5.
35. "Śiprin and Śipiviṣṭa", *Umesh Mishra Comm. Vol.,* Ganganath Jha Research Institute, Allahabad, 1970, pp.501-510.
36. "Maṇḍūka-Brāhmaṇa āṇi Lokaviśvāsa" (Marathi), *Samskṛtisugandha (V.T Shete Fel.Vol.),* Joshi-Lokhande Prakashan, Poona, 1970, pp.37-50.
37. "The Vision of Vasukra", *Journal of the University of Bombay*, Bombay, Vol.XL, Arts No.76, Oct.1971, pp.1-26.
38. "Āmā meṅ Pakva" (Hindi), Veda Spl. Issue, *Viśvajyoti,* 21 (3-4), Hoshiarpur, May 1972, pp.115-117.
39. "The Thunder-cow and the Asya-Vāmīya", *Journal of the University of Bombay,* Bombay, Vol.XLI, Arts No.77, Oct. 1972, pp.28-51.
40. "Upaniṣadoṅ meṅ Suparṇa aur Aśvattha kā Vivecana" (Hindi), *Viśvajyoti*, 22 (1-2), Hoshiarpur, May 1973, pp.82-84.
41. "The Ṛgvedic Seer and the Fire-Water Complex", *Journal of the University of Bombay,* Bombay, Vol. XLII, Arts No.78, Oct.1973, pp.18-42.

42. "Indrāṇī-karma", *Journal of the Ganganath Jha Research Institute,* Allahabad, Vol. XXIX—1 to 4, 1973, pp.221-228.
43. "Godāna āṇi Govikarta" (Marathi), *VSM,* Nagpur, *Annual No.,* 1973 (pub.1974), pp.29-42.
44. "Vāmadeva and the Dog's Entrails (Ṛgveda IV.18.12-13)", *VIJ,* Hoshiarpur, Vol.XII-1 & 2, Mar.-Sept. 1974, pp.76-88.
45. "Cosmo-sexualism in the Vedic Ritual", *Charudeva Shastri Fel.Vol.,* Charudeva Shastri Fel. Committee, Delhi, 1974, pp.23-44.
46. "Patnī āṇi Yajñīya Mithuna-saṅketa" (Marathi), *VSM,* Nagpur, *Annual No.,* 1974 (pub.1975), pp. 8-22.
47. "Metempsychosis and the Ṛgveda" *Journal of the University of Bombay,* Bombay, Vol.XLIII, Arts No.79, Oct. 1974, pp.1-12.
48. "Urvaśī — The Water-Belle (A fresh interpretation of *ṚV* X.95)", *Journal of the Oriental Institute,* M.S. University of Baroda, Baroda, Vol.XXV-1, Sept. 1975, pp.17-46.
49. "The Mithuna and the Vedic Ritual", *Journal of the University of Bombay,* Bombay, Vol.XLIV-XLV, Arts Nos. 80-81, Oct. 1975-76, pp-1-6.
50. "Patnī-saṁyāja āṇi Mithuna-saṅketa" (Marathi), *VSM,* Nagpur, *Annual No.,* 1975 (pub.1976), pp.18-24.
51. "The Vedic Mithuna — Concept and Practice", *Journal of the Oriental Institute,* M.S. University of Baroda (Silver Jubilee Vol.), Baroda, Vol.XXV-3-4, Mar.-June 1976, pp.197-212+chart.
52. "Menā-eka Mithuna-saṅketa" (Marathi), *VSM,* Nagpur, *Annual No.,* 1976 (pub. 1977), pp.21-29.
53. "Yama-Yamī, the cosmic Twins", *Some Aspects of Indo-Iranian Literary and Cultural Traditions (V.G Paranjpe Comm.Vol.),* Ajanta Publications, Delhi, 1977, pp.24-37.

54. "The 'wife' and the Divine Mates", *Journal of the University of Bombay*, Bombay, Vol.XLVI, Arts No.82, Oct. 1977, pp.1-10.
55. "Sex in Stone and the Vedic Mithuna", *Annals of the Bhandarkar Oriental Research Institute (ABORI)*, Diamond Jubilee Vol., Poona, May 1978, pp.543-560.
56. "Dīrghatamas — The Vedic Philosopher", *Prabuddha Bhārata*, Mayavati, 83, Aug.1978, pp.543-548.
57. "The Marriage of Heaven and Earth in the Vedic Ritual", *Prof. Kundanlal Sharma Fel. Vol.*, Merath Vishwavidyalaya Sanskrit Adhyapak Parishat, Merath (Meerut), Mar. 1977, pp.1-6; also pub. in the *Proceedings*, All India Oriental Conference (XXVIII Session, Dharwar, 1976), Poona, 1978, pp.213-218.
58. "Aspects of Ultimate Reality from the Ṛgveda", *Jnl. Ultimate Reality and Meaning*, Ontario, Canada, Vol.1, No.2, 1978, pp.71-99.
59. "Vedic Dvibarhas — A Wonder-working Priest", *VIJ*, Panjab University, Hoshiarpur, Vol.XVII, 1979, pp.5-8.
60. "Rain and Sex-pairing", *Journal of the Asiatic Society of Bombay*, Bombay, Vols.49-51, 1979, pp.61-71.
61. "Garta and Garta-āruk in the Ṛgveda", *Ludwick Sternbach Fel.Vol.*, Part One, Akhil Bharatiya Sanskrit Parishad, Lucknow, 1979, pp.83-87.
62. "Purūravas — Vādagrasta Yājñika" (Marathi), *VSM*, Nagpur, *Annual No.*, 1979 (pub. 1980), pp.13-22.
63. "Ajāmitā and Speech-coupling", *Journal of the Ganganath Jha Research Institute*, Allahabad, Vol.XXXVI — 1 to 4, January-Dec. 1980 (pub.1983), pp.77-85.
64. "Śiśnadeva and the Vedic Cult of the Nude", *Bhāratībhāṇam* (Light of Indology) (*Dr. K.V. Sarma Fel. Vol.*), Panjab University, Indological Series-26, Panjab University, Hoshiarpur, Dec.1980, pp.22-25.

65. "Purūravas — A Research for Identity", *A Corpus of Indian Studies (Gaurinath Shastri Fel. Vol.)*, Sanskrit Pustak Bhandar, Calcutta, 1980, pp.52-60.
66. "Religious Suicide in the Vedic Period (?)", *Indologica Taurinensia (Ludwick Sternbach Comm.Vol.)*, Vols. VIII-IX, Torino (Italy), 1980-81, pp.113-121.
67. "Veda aur Tāntrika Tattva" (Hindi), *Sanmārga*, (Veda Spl. Issue for the 75th Year), Varanasi, Aug.1981, pp.83-87.
68. "Kṛṣṇamṛga Yajñīya Paśu" (Marathi), *VSM*, Nagpur, *Annual No.*, 1981, (pub.1982), pp.14-22.
69. "Ritual-coupling and Speech-symbolism in the Veda", *Journal of the Oriental Institute,* M.S. University of Baroda, Baroda, Vol.XXXI-3, Mar. 1982, pp.225-237.
70. "The Son-husband in the Vedic Concept", *Journal of the University of Bombay,* Bombay, 125 year Vol. (Arts, Humanities and Social Sciences), 1982, pp.88-93.
71. "The Crying Worlds (*krandasī*)", *Prof. Jagannath Agrawal Fel.Vol.,* Ajanta Publications, Delhi, 1982, pp.9-16.
72. "Presidential Address" — Vedic Section, *Proceedings* of the All India Oriental Conference (XXX Session, Santiniketan 1980), *BORI,* Poona, 1982, pp.23-34.
73. "The Riddle of the Black Antelope", *Abhinandanabhāratī (Prof. K.K. Handiqui Fel. Vol.),* Kamarupa Anusandhana Samiti, Gauhati, 1982, pp.27-33.
74. "Veda and the Śramaṇa Culture", *Āmbhṛṇīyam (Acharya R.C. Shukla Fel.Vol.),* Acharya Ramesh Chandra Shukla Fel. Committee, Aligarh, 1983, pt.V, pp.1-8.
75. "Indus Civilization and the Vedic Culture — Reexamination of the Problem", *Journal of the Mythic Society,* Bangalore, Vol.LXXIV-1, Jan-Mar. 1983, pp.49-82.
76. "The Eye of Prajāpati", *Journal of the Asiatic Society*

of Bombay, Bombay, Vols.54-55 (1979-80), 1983, pp.27-30.

77. "The Kuntāpa-hymns and the Śilpa", *Amṛtadhārā (Prof. R.N. Dandekar Fel. Vol.)*, Ajanta Pubns., Delhi, 1984, pp.85-93.
78. "The Upaniṣads and the Ultimate Real One", *Journal Ultimate Reality and Meaning,* Vol.7, No.4, Ontario, Canada, 1984, pp.252-269.
79. "Some Ritual-Variations from the Aitareya Brāhmaṇa", *Aligarh Journal of Oriental Studies* , Aligarh *(R.S. Tripathi Comm. Vol)*, Vol.II-1 & 2, 1985, pp.45-52.
80. "The Yatis and the Uttaravedi", *Haryana Sahitya Akademi Journal of Indological Studies*, Vol.I-1, Chandigarh, Spring 1986, pp.66-71.
81. "Altars and Platforms in Ancient India (with special reference to the Samarāṅgaṇasūtradhāra)", *Journal of the Asiatic Society of Bombay*, Bombay *(Bhagawanlal Indraji Comm.Vol.)*, Vols. 56-59 (1981-84), 1986, pp.122-135.
82. "Vaidika Mithunoṅ meṅ Yauna-saṅketa" (Hindi), *Vikrama* (Spl. Issue on Myths), Vikram University, Ujjain, Vol. 2-4, May-Nov. 1986, pp.223-232.
83. "Ritual Variations from the Brāhmaṇas (Agniṣṭoma)", *Ṛtambharā (Udayavira Shastri Fel.Vol.),* Society for Indic Studies, Ghaziabad, 1986, pp.3-6.
84. "Ritual Variations and the Principle of Sampad", *Brahmavidyā* (Golden Jubilee Vol.), Adyar Library Bulletin 50, Adyar, Madras, 1986, pp.498-511
85. "Pradakṣiṇā" (Marathi), *VSM,* Nagpur, *Annual No.,* 1986 (pub.1987), pp.13-24.
86. "Woman's Share and the Mīmāṁsā Rule: Dvayoḥ Praṇayanti", *Bhāratīya Vidyā,* Bombay, Vol.XLV-XLVII, 1 to 4 (*J.H. Dave Fel. Vol.*), 1987, pp.59-64.
87. "The Prāyaṇīya and the Udayanīya Iṣṭis (A study in variation and evolution), *Journal of the Dept. of Sanskrit,* University of Calcutta, Calcutta, 1987, pp.27-37.

88. "The Double Altar", *Annals of the Bhandarkar Oriental Research Institute* (*ABORI*), Poona, (*R.G. Bhandarkar 150th Birth-Anniversary Vol.*), Vol.XLVIII, 1987, pp.349-358.

89. "Ukhā, Variations from the Śatapatha Brāhmaṇa", *Proceedings* of the All India Oriental Conference (XXXII Session, Ahmedabad, 1985), Poona, 1987, pp.151-157.

90. "Features of Tantrism and the Veda", *The Journal of Oriental Research* (The Kuppuswamy Sastri Research Institute), Madras, Vols. XLII-XLVI (1972-1977), 1987, pp.78-88.

91. "Mother-goddess on the Vedic Scene", *Vāṇījyotiḥ* (Journal of the Dept. of Sanskrit, Utkal University), Vol.II, Bhubaneswar, 1987, pp.1-6.

92. "Moral Value and the Pūrvamīmāṁsā", *Haryana Sahitya Akademi Journal of Indological Studies*, Chandigarh, Vol.II-1 & 2, Spring 1987, pp.59-67.

93. "The Audgrabhaṇa Offerings", *Aligarh Journal of Oriental Studies,* Aligarh, Vol.V-1 & 2, 1988, pp.57-65.

94. "Sabardughā and Kāmadhenu", *Svarṇa-Bhāratī* (Souvenir of the Golden Jubilee 1938-88), Nalbari Sanskrit College, Nalbari (Assam), 1988, pp.74-80.

95. "Vāruḷa-prācīna saṅketa" (Marathi), *VSM*, Nagpur, *Annual No.,* 1988 (pub.1989), pp.1-7.

96. "Soma and the Ritual-Waters", *Studies in Indology — Prof. R.V. Joshi. Fel.Vol.*, Shree Publishing House, New Delhi, 1989, pp.73-83.

97. "Yūpa — Its Nature and Evolution", *Bhāratī* (*R.C. Mujumdar Comm. Vol.*), Vol.16 (for 1985-87), Banaras Hindu University, Varanasi, 1989, pp.1-10.

98. "Vedic Symbolism", *New Horizons of Research in Indology,* Centre of Advanced Study in Sanskrit (CASS), Poona University, 1989, pp.10-16.

99. "The Havirdhāna-maṇḍapa", *Glory of Knowledge* (*Ram Murti Sharma Fel. Vol.*), Eastern Book Linkers, Delhi, 1990, pp.88-92.

100. "Malamāsa āṇi Deva-malimluca" (Marathi), *VSM*, Nagpur, *Annu*al *No.*, 1990 (pub.1991), pp.25-35.
101. "Ultimate in the Ritual of Soma", *Ultimate in Ancient Indian Thought and Discipline* (*Proceedings* of the National Seminar, Dept. of Sanskrit), University of Bombay (Mumbai), 1991, pp.197-206.
102. "Mahāvedīce Saṅketa" (Marathi), *Vedaprabhā (Yajñeśvara Shastri Kasture Fel. Vol.)*, Savita Prakashan, Aurangabad, 1991, pp.37-45.
103. "Vedic Sexual Symbolism", *Dravidian Encyclopaedia,* Vol.I, International School of Dravidian Linguistics, Trivandrum, 1991, pp.643-644.
104. "Yūpa — Images and Evolution", *VIJ,* Panjab University, Hoshiarpur, Vol.XXV-i & ii (June-Dec. 1987), pub.1991, pp.12-19.
105. "The Bones of Dadhīci", *Samāmnāya, Journal of the Maharshi Veda-Vijñāna Academy,* Ahmedabad, Vol.I-i, 1992, pp.63-69.
106. "The Aryan Culture as reflected in the Veda", *The Aryan Problem,* Bharata Itihāsa Sankalana Samiti, Pune, 1993, pp.183-191.
107. "The Attire of the Vedic Sacrificial Post", *Studies in Indology and Musicology (Dr. P.N. Kawthekar Fel. Vol.)*, Pratibha Prakashan, Delhi, 1993, pp.77-80.
108. "Urvaśī — The Weaver of the Web of Life", *Śrījagannāthajyotiḥ, Jagannath University Journal of Indology*, Puri, Vol.6, pp.63-67.
109. "The Principle of Continuity in the Vedic Ritual", *Centenary Vol.,* Chawkhamba Sanskrit Series office, Varanasi, 1993, pp.236-241.
110. "Manu āṇi Iḍā" (Marathi), *VSM,* Nagpur, *Annual No.,* 1993 (pub.1994), pp.9-20.
111. "Varuṇapraghāsa and the Wife", *Śruticintāmaṇiḥ (C.G. Kashikar Fel.Vol.)*, Tilak Maharashtra Vidyapeeth, Pune, 1994, pp.29-35.
112. "Antarvedi-Bahirvedi", *Cultura Indica (Dr. Asoke*

Chatterjee Tributes Vol.), Sharada Publishing House, Delhi, 1994, pp.31-33.

113. "Hotṛvūrya", *VIJ*, Panjab University, Hoshiarpur, Vol.XXVII-1 & 2, 1994 (for June-Dec. 1989), pp.1-4.

114. "Dakṣiṇa-Āhavanīya", *Samāmnāya, Journal of the Maharshi Veda-Vijñāna Academy,* Ahmedabad, Vol.III, 1994, pp.9-12

115. "Vāgdevī - Puṁścalī" (Marathi), *VSM,* Nagpur, *Annual No.,* 1994 (pub.1995), pp.8-23.

116. "The Principle of Double Value in Vedic Ritual", *Indian Heritage,* Burdwan, Vol.I, Issue 6, Sep.1995, pp.22-24.

117. "Perspiration of the Creator", *Śrījñānāmṛtam (Prof. Shrinivas Shastri Smṛtigranth,* Kurukshetra), Parimal Pubns., Delhi, 1996, pp.1-5.

118. "Visions in the Poetry of the Ṛgveda", *Journal of the Oriental Institute,* M.S. University of Baroda, Baroda, Vol.XLV, Nos. 3-4, Mar.-June 1996, pp.136-147.

119. "Ṛgveda and the Buffalo Sacrifice?", *Oriental Journal,* Sri Venkateswara University, Tirupati, Vol. XXXIV, pts. 1 & 2, 1996, pp.53-59.

120. "Vīṇāgāthin āṇi Dhṛtihoma" (Marathi), *VSM,* Nagpur, *Annual No.*, 1996 (pub.1997), pp.13-29.

121. "Speech — Divine and Puṁścalī", *Bhārata Vidyā Saurabham (Biswanarayana Shastri Fel.Vol.*), Manorama Prakashan, Guwahati, 1997, pp.49-53.

122. "Dream (svapna) in the Vedic Context", *VIJ,* Panjab University, Hoshiarpur, Vol.XXX, pts. i-ii, (June-Dec. 1992), 1997, pp.1-6.

123. "Stūpa — Vedic and Buddhistic", *Oriental Journal,* Sri Venkateswara University, Tirupati, Vol. XXXVII, pts. 1 & 2 (Jan.-Dec.1994), 1997, pp.1-8.

124. "Veda and Indian Mythology", *Lokaprajñā, Journal of Indological Studies*, jointly pub. by SARASVATI (Puri) and Dept. of Sanskrit, Hari Singh Gour Vishwavidyalaya, Sagar (*Pt. Vasudeva Dvivedi Shastri Fel.Vol.*), Vol.III, 1997, pp.1-9.

125. "Araru āṇi Nārmara" (Marathi), *VSM*, Nagpur, *Annual No.*, 1997, pp. 1-20.
126. "Metaphors in the Aśvamedha", *Metaphors in Vedic Literature (Proceedings* of the National Seminar), CASS, University of Poona, Pune, 1998, pp.1-15.
127. "Manūcyā Patnīcī Purākathā" (Marathi), *VSM,* Nagpur, *Annual No.*, 1998 (pub.1999), pp.17-34.
128. "Vāstoṣpati, Rudra and Cyavana", *Oriental Journal,* Sri Venkateswara University, Tirupati, Vol. XLII, pts. 1 & 2, 1999, pp.13-22.
129. "Vaidika Yajñīya Vedi-Vikāsa āṇi Saṅketa" (Marathi), *Dr. Devisingh Chauhan Fel. Vol.,* Marathawada Samshodhan Mandal, Latur, 1999, pp.45-61.
130. "Vedic Gods - Classification and Evolution", VIJ, Panjab University, Hoshiarpur, Vols. XXXIII - XXXIV pts. i-iv (June-Dec. 1995-96), 2000, pp.29-48.
131. "The Relevance of Vedic Studies in the Modern World", *Brahmarshi Daivarāta's Chando-Darshana — A Critical Study* (A Collection of Research Papers), Samskrita Shodha Samsthana (SAMSHODHANA), Sirsi, Jan. 2001, pp.57-71.
132. "Veda and Indian Mythology", *Vedic Foundations of Indian Śāstric Traditions,* ed. by Radha Vallabh Tripathi, Pratibha Prakashan, Delhi, 2001, pp.1-11.

PUBLICATIONS IN PERIODICALS

VEDA

1. "Vṛtra-eka Sṛṣṭitattva" (Marathi), *Jīvana-vikāsa,* Ramakrishna-ashram, Nagpur, Jan.1964, pp.587-591.
2. "Aśvamedhātīla Aśva-Rāṇī — Sambandha" (Marathi), *Lokasatta,* Bombay, *Dīpāvalī Spl. Issue,* 1971.
3. "Indrālā Vīryaśālī Karaṇārā Vṛṣākapi Koṇa?" (Marathi) (On the real nature of Vṛṣākapi), *Lokasatta,* Bombay, *Dīpāvalī Spl. Issue,* 1976, pp.120-124.

4. "Vedāntīla Kṛṣi āṇi Utpādana" (Marathi), *Dharmabhāskara,* Bombay, *Dīpāvalī Spl. Issue,* 1976.
5. "Mithuna-Śilpāncī Paramparā āṇi Pārśvabhūmi" (Marathi), *Lokasatta,* Bombay, *Dīpāvalī Spl. Issue,* Nov. 1977.
6. "Indra: eka pratīkātmaka netṛtva" (Marathi), *Dharmabhāskara,* Bombay, 6(12), 1977, pp.7-8.
7. "Vedavāṅmayam kiñca janaviśvāsaḥ"? (Sanskrit), *Saṁskṛta-Bhavitavyam,* Nagpur, 1978, 8.4, pp.3-4.
8. "Ātmatattvācā prathama draṣṭā Vaidika ṛṣi Dīrghatamas (Marathi), *Dharmabhāskara*, Bombay, 8(11), 1979, pp.46-48, 54.

EPICS AND PURĀṆAS

1. "The Pāṇḍava Riddle", *Journal of the University of Bombay*, Bombay, Vol. XXVI-2, Arts No.32, Sep. 1957, pp.159-176.
2. "Gajendra-Mokṣa", *Journal of the Mythic Society,* Bangalore, Vol.LI-2, July 1960, pp.55-66.
3. "The Garuḍas", *Indian Historical Quarterly,* Calcutta, Vol.XXXVII-2 & 3, June-Sept. 1961, pp.165–176.
4. "Rāmaṇīyaka, the Island of the Nāgas", *Purāṇa*, All India Kashiraj Trust, Varanasi, Vol.III-1, Jan. 1961, pp.64-71.
5. "Mahābhārata men Garta" (Hindi), *Viśvajyoti,* Vishveshvaranand Vedic Research Society, Hoshiarpur, May 1970 (Mahābhārata Spl. Issue), pp.27-29.
6. "Śayyā-Śilpa āṇi Dāna" (Marathi), *VSM,* Nagpur, *Annual No.,* 1977 (pub.1978), pp.45-55.
7. "Dīpāvalī - The Festival of Lights", *Yuvabhāratī,* Madras, (Dīpāvalī Spl. Issue), Nov. 1977, pp.6-12.
8. "The Jar in Belief and Custom", *Prabuddha Bhārata*, 83, Mayavati, Dec. 1978, pp.501-506.
9. "Nadyāncyā Janmakathā" (Marathi), *VSM,* Nagpur, *Annual No.,* 1978 (pub. 1979), pp.40-53.

10. "The Puranic Motif of the River-cow", *Indica* (*Fr. A. Esteller Fel.Vol.*), Bombay, 16-1, March 1979, pp.41-45.
11. "Dānava-kathā āṇi Bhaugolika Satya" (Marathi), *VSM*, Nagpur, *Annual No.,* 1980 (pub.1981), pp.21-27.
12. "The Gift of the Bed", *Brahmavidyā* (Adyar Library Bulletin) *(K.K. Raja Fel. Vol.)*, Madras, Vols. 44-45, 1980-81, pp.333-343.
13. "The Birth of Gaṇapati", *Aruṇabhāratī (A.N. Jani Fel.Vol.)*, Prof. A. N. Jani Fel. Committee, Oriental Institute, Baroda, 1983, pp.1-7.
14. "Two Wives of the Sun-God", *Ṛtam*, Journal of Akhila Bharatiya Sanskrit Parishad, Lucknow, Vols.XI-XV (1979-1983) (*Baburam Saksena Abhinandana Viśeṣāṅka–Fel. Vol.*) 1983, pp.109-118.
15. "Reṇukā" (Marathi), *VSM,* Nagpur, *Annual No.,* 1983 (pub. 1984), pp.8-17.
16. "The Fifth Face of Brahmā", *Śrījagannāthajyotiḥ — Jagannatha University Journal of Indology*, Puri, Vol. 1-1, Mar. 1984, pp.31-38.
17. "Ghaṭa āṇi Hiraṇyagarbha" (Marathi), *VSM,* Nagpur, *Annual No.,* 1984 (pub.1985), pp.1-6.
18. "Śiva-mūrti āṇi Rudra-śīrṣa" (Marathi), *VSM,* Nagpur, *Annual No.,* 1985 (pub.1986), pp.24-30.
19. "The Indian Gem-Culture (Puranic Records)", *Śrījagannāthajyotiḥ-Jagannatha University Journal of Indology,* Puri, Vol.III, pp.88-93.
20. "Purāṇa and the Paurāṇika", *Jñānāmṛtam* (*A.C. Swain Fel. Vol.*), P.G. Dept. of Sanskrit, Utkal University, Bhubaneswar, 1985, pp.125-128.
21. "Devālaya āṇi Viṣṇūce Śīrṣa" (Marathi), *VSM,* Nagpur, *Annual No.,* 1987 (pub.1988), pp.10-19.
22. "Pāṇḍu, Mādrī and their Bodies", *Bhāratī (Bulletin of the College of Indology,* Benaras Hindu University), Varanasi, Vol.17, 1987, pp.1-6.
23. "The Horse-faced Goddess", *Amalā Prajñā (P.V. Bapat, Fel.Vol.),* Sri Satguru Pubns. (A Division of

Indian Books Centre), Delhi, 1989, pp.531-536.

24. "Vāmana, Baṭu āṇi Khujā" (Marathi), *VSM,* Nagpur, *Annual No.,* 1989 (pub.1990), pp.9-18.
25. "Śiva-liṅga", *Kalyāṇa-Kalpataru* (*Śiva Spl. Issue*), Gorakhpur, Vol. XXXVI, No.1, Oct. 1990, pp.47-51.
26. "Tanks and Trees", *Environmental Awareness reflected in Sanskrit Literature* (*Proceedings* of the National Seminar), *CASS*, Poona University, Poona, 1991, pp.191-199.
27. "Meḍhī and Toraṇa", *Living Customs and their Ancient Indian Sources (Proceedings* of the National Seminar), CASS, Poona University, Pune, 1991, pp.187-191.
28. "Aṣṭama" (Marathi), *VSM*, Nagpur, *Annual No.,* 1991 (pub.1992), pp.13-23.
29. "Triśaṅku āṇi Svargārohaṇa" (Marathi), *VSM*, Nagpur, *Annual No.,* 1992 (pub.1993), pp.9-20.
30. "The Abduction of Sītā", *Journal of the Asiatic Society of Bombay*, Bombay, Vols.64-66 (for 1989-91), 1993, pp.24-28.
31. "Satī, Mādrī āṇi Mahābhārata" (Marathi), *Navabhārata*, Wai, 1993, Apr.-June, pp.157-164.
32. "Beliefs about Trees from the Purāṇas", *Sasigauravāmṛtam (Śaśidhara Śarmā Fel. Vol.)*, being pt.5 of *Horizons of Indic Studies*, Shri Sahitya Sudha Sadanam, Chandigarh, 1994, pp.68-72.
33. "The Myth of Dhundhu", *Modern Evaluation of the Mahābhārata (Prof. R.K. Sharma Fel. Vol.)*, Nag Publishers, Delhi, 1995, pp.132-137.
34. "Naūcī Navalāī" (Marathi), *VSM,* Nagpur, *Annual No.,* 1995 (pub.1996), pp.39-51.
35. "Purāṇa and Śāstra", *Purāṇa,* All India Kashiraj Trust, Varanasi, Vol.XL, No.2, July 1998, pp.92-101.
36. "Durvāsas — A Pattern", *Purāṇa,* All India Kashiraj Trust, Varanasi, Vol.XLI, No.1, Jan.1999, pp.39-47.
37. "Kumāra, Kārttikeya and the Peacock", *Journal of the Asiatic Society of Bombay*, Mumbai, Vol.74 (for 1999) (New Series), 2000, pp.39-53.

MYTHOLOGY AND FOLKLORE

1. "Lokakathāntīla Rākṣasa" (Marathi), *Sarvodaya (Folklore Spl.Issue)*, State Govt. of Maharashtra, Bombay, May 1961.
2. "Death and Rebirth in Initiation Ceremonies", *Indian Antiquary*, Bombay, III Series, Vol.I-2, Apr.1964, pp.104-109.
3. "Purāvṛtta āṇi Itihāsa-Saṅketa" (Marathi), *Navabhārata*, Wai, 23(1), Oct.1969, pp.60-67.
4. "Purāvṛtta āni Vidhi-saṅketa" (Marathi), *Navabhārata,* Wai, 23(3), Dec.1969, pp.43-50.
5. "Indrālā Lāj Vāṭāvī Mhaṇūn" (Marathi), *Marathawada Samshodhan Mandal,* Sirur Tajband, *Annual No.,* 1970, pp.66-73.
6. "Sexual Symbology and the Hindu Myths", *Proceedings* of the Seminar on Indian Symbology, Industrial Design Centre, Indian Institute of Technology, Bombay, 1987, pp.11-20.
7. "Tribal and Other Accounts of Creation", *Myths of Creation (Proceedings* of the Seminar), Dept. of Sanskrit, University of Bombay, Bombay, 1987, pp.60-68.
8. "Sacrifice and the Cult of the Mother-goddess", *Sacrifice in India — Concept and Evolution (Proceedings* of the National Seminar, Dept. of Sanskrit, University of Bombay), Viveka Pubns., Aligarh, 1987, pp.165-176.
9. "Beast-Heads and Human Bodies", *Benudhar Sharma Comm. Vol.,* Kamarupa Anusandhana Samiti, Guwahati, 1987, pp.13-21.
10. "Proto-Philosophy in Myths", *Journal of the Indian Musicological Society*, Spl. Issue on: Music and Mythology, Book 2, Vol.18, No.2, Indian Musicological Society, Baroda, Dec. 1987, pp.30-37.
11. "Meaning of Myth and the Vedic Context", *Annals* of the Bhandarkar Oriental Research Institute, Poona, (Amṛtamahotsava Vol.), Vol. LXXII-LXXIII, 1991-1992, pp.171-180.

12. "Simha-Āsana", *Spectrum of Indian Culture (Prof. S.B. Deo Fel. Vol.* — I & II), Agam Kala Prakashan, Delhi, 1996, Vol.II, pp.469-478.
13. "Therianthropomorphism and Multiple-Head Motifs in Ancient India and the Middle East", *Journal of the Asiatic Society of Bombay,* Mumbai, Vol.73 (for 1998), (New Series), 1998 pp.8-23.
14. "Dream, Myth and the Hindu Context", *Annals* of the Bhandarkar Oriental Research Institute, Pune, Vol.LXXIX-1998), 1999, pp.61-82.

PUBLICATION IN PERIODICAL

15. "Jīvātmā āṇi Jana-viśvāsa" (Marathi), *Jīvana-vikāsa*, Ramakrishna-ashram, Nagpur, June 1978, pp.208-214.

SANSKRIT DRAMAS

1. "The Order of the 'Duryodhana' — Plays of Bhāsa", *Journal of the University of Bombay*, Bombay, Vol.XXIII-2, Arts No.29, Sept.1954, pp.49-59.
2. "Vipralambha in the Uttararāmacarita", *Journal of the University of Bombay*, Bombay, Vol.XXV-2, Arts No.31, Sep.1956, pp 67-81.
3. "Śarvilaka not a resident of Ujjayinī", *Journal of the Ganganath Jha Research Institute,* Allahabad, Vol.XVI — 1 & 2, Nov.-Feb. 1958-59, pp.39-48.
4. "Suggestion in Sanskrit Dramas", *Journal of the Mythic Society,* Bangalore, Vol.XLIX-4, Jan.1959, pp.238-251.
5. "Genesis of the Story of Jīmūtavāhana", *Journal of the Asiatic Society of Bombay*, Bombay, Vols. 34-35 (for 1958-60), 1962, pp.68-74.
6. "The Mendicant of the Mṛcchakaṭika-Once More", *Journal of the Asiatic Society of Bombay*, Bombay, Vols.52-53, 1981, pp.76-92.
7. "Candra-Rohiṇī Mithuna āṇi Khaṇḍamodaka Candra" (Marathi), *VSM*, Nagpur, *Annual No.*, 1982, pp.6-16.

8. "The Priyānuprasādana Vrata (*Vikramorvaśīyam*)" *Anupama-Kālidāsaḥ (Prof. A.G. Bhatta Comm. Vol.)*, Sanskrit Sahitya Academy, Gandhigram, 2001, pp.457-463.

PUBLICATION IN PERIODICAL

9. "Bhavabhūtīcyā Nāṭakāntīla Kālapriyānāth" (Marathi), *Jīvana-vikāsa*, Ramakrishna-ashram, Nagpur, Aug.1962, pp.320-326.

POETICS

1. "Rasa-pratīti āṇi Vyaktimattva" (Marathi), *Navabhārata,* Wai, Nov. 1970, pp.51-61.
2. "Sanskrit Poetics and 'Semiotics", *Journal of the Asiatic Society of Bombay,* Bombay, Vol.71 (for 1996), 1997, pp.47-56.

DHARMAŚĀSTRA

1. "Godāna — The Hair-ritual", *P.V. Kane Comm. Vol.*, University of Bombay, Bombay, 1974, pp.26-35.
2. "Kane's History of Dharmaśāstra (Need for a Real Edition)", *Haryana Sahitya Akademi Journal of Indological Studies,* Chandigarh, Vol.III-1&2, Spring 1988 (pub.1990), pp.61-67.
3. "Heir-Apparent and Putrikāputra", *Ajaya-Śrī*—Recent Studies in Indology *(Prof. Ajay Mitra Shastri Fel. Vol.* I & II), Sundeep Prakashan, Delhi, 1989, Vol. II, pp.597-602.
4. "Hindu Dharma āṇi Dharma-nirapekṣatā" (Marathi), *Marathawada* (Spl.Issue), Aurangabad, 1989, pp.159-160.

PUBLICATIONS IN PERIODICAL

5. "Ṛṇa-Kalpanā" (Marathi), *Dharmabhāskara*, Bombay, Apr. 1978.
6. "Samāja-dhāraṇa, Puruṣārtha āṇi Āśramavyavasthā" (Marathi), *Dharmabhāskara,* Oct. 1978.

SANSKRIT GRAMMAR

1. "Dampatī and Patnī", *VSM*, Nagpur, *Annual No.*,1968 (pub.1969), pp.158-171.
2. "Vowel-shortening and the Sanskrit Sandhi", *VSM,* Nagpur, *Annual No.,* 1969, (pub.1970), pp.211-217.
3. "Root-germinants in the Sanskrit Language (√GHAS: √AD)", *New Indian Antiquary*, Bombay, Series III, V-1, Jan.1971, pp.1-5.
4. "Some Peculiarities of the Eastern Dialect according to Pāṇini", *VSM,* Nagpur, *Annual No.,* 1970 (pub. 1971), pp.174-191.
5. "Kanyā and Kānīna", *VSM,* Nagpur, *Annual No.*, 1971 (pub.1972), pp.179-185.
6. "Prākritization and the Germinants of the Roots of Vision", *Proceedings* of the National Seminar on Prākṛta Studies, Dept. of Sanskrit, University of Bombay, Bombay, 1971, pp.67-75.
7. "Root-germination and Reduplicated Roots in Sanskrit", *Proceedings* of the Seminar on Historical Linguistics, *Journal of the University of Bombay*, Bombay, Vol.XLI, Arts No.77, Oct. 1972, pp.208-214.
8. "Ad > ghas āṇi Dhātvādeśa-vivecana" (Marathi), *VSM,* Nagpur, *Annual No.,* 1972 (pub.1973), pp.95-110.
9. "Sphoṭa — A Reappraisal", *Proceedings* of the Seminar on Ancient Indian Theories on Sentence-meaning", University of Poona (1979), CASS, Poona, 1980, pp.69-78.
10. "Vowel-shortening in Sandhi", *Vidyā-vratin (*Prof. A.M. Ghatge Fel. Vol.), Sri Satguru Publications (A Division of Indian Books Centre), Delhi, 1992, pp.95-99.
11. "Sandhi, Śākalya, Pāṇini VI.1.127-128 and the Vedic Evidence", *Traividyam* (Vedic Studies in Memory of Durgamohan Bhattacharyya), Subarnarekha Pubn., Kolkata, 2001, pp.63-77.

MISCELLANEOUS

1. "Bhakti-Kalpanā āṇi Jñāneśvarī" (Marathi), *Jīvana-vikāsa*, Ramakrishna-ashram, Nagpur, May 1962, pp.169-171.

2. "Jaina Dharma āṇi Bhāratīya Samskṛti" (Marathi), *Bharata Itihāsa Samshodhana Patrikā* (Quarterly Journal of the Bharata Itihasa Samshodhaka Mandal), Pune, 1979, Year 58, Nos. 1-4, pp. 1-44.
3. "Mudrāeṅ" (On the various signs of palms) (Hindi), *Varivasyā*, Tripureśvarī Śakti–pīṭha, Lucknow, Vol. I-1, Aug. 1984.
4. "Cooling Devices in Ancient India", *Viśvambharā: Probings in Orientology (Prof. V.S. Pathak Festschrift*–I & II), Harman Publishing House, New Delhi, 1995, Vol. II, pp.496-497.

CONTRIBUTION TO RESEARCH PROJECTS

1. Article on "Purāṇa" as also on
2. "Aśvamedha Yajña — In Legends and History", in the *Encyclopaedia of Hinduism,* a Project of India Heritage Research Foundation for the Third Millennium (IHRF), University of South Carolina, Columbia, U.S.A., under the (Chief) Editorship of Prof. K.L. Seshagiri Rao.
3. "Resolution of Conflicts — Vedic Reflection", in the Project *Veda-Vedanta and Conflict Resolution*, Dharam Hinduja International Centre for Indic Research, Delhi, under the Chairmanship of Prof. Ram Murti Sharma.

REVIEW ARTICLES OF DR. S.A. DANGE

1. *The Concept of Beauty in Poetics* (by Dr. G.T. Deshpande). *Nagpur University Jou*rnal, Nagpur, Vol.XV-1, Oct. 1964, pp.143-146.
2. *Rashtrīya Utthānāta Sāhityāce Sthāna (The Place of Literature in National Uplift)* (by Dr. G.T. Deshpande), *Nagpur University Journal*, Nagpur, Vol.XVI-2, Apr.1966, pp.255-257.
3. *A Survey of the Śrauta-sūtras* (by Dr. C.G. Kashikar), *Vishveshvaranand Indological Journal,* Panjab University, Hoshiarpur, Vol.VII— I & II, 1969, pp.175-178.

4. *Gaṇeśa-Kośa* (by Shri Prabhudesai), *Jīvana-vikāsa*, Nagpur, March 1969.
5. *Devi-Kośa* (by Shri Prabhudesai), *Jīvana-vikāsa*, Nagpur, March 1969.
6. *India as seen in the Bṛhatsa=mhitā of Varāhamihira* (by Dr. A.M. Shastri), *Journal of the University of Bombay,* Bombay, Arts No. XL, No. 76 (New Series), Oct. 1971, pp. 248-252.
7. *Puruṣārthopadeśa* of Bhartṛhari (ed. by Dr. K.V. Sarma), *Vishveshvaranand Indological Journal*, Panjab University, Hoshiarpur, Vol. VIII—i-ii, March & Sept. 1970, pp. 272-273.
8. *Praśastikāśikā* of Bālakṛṣna Tripathin (ed. by Dr. K.V. Sarma), *Vishveshvaranand Indological Journal*, Panjab University, Hoshiarpur, Vol.VIII—i-ii, Mar. & Sept.1970, pp.285-286.
9. *R.N. Dandekar Fel. Vol. (Indian Antiquary* III Series, Nos.1-4, ed. by Dr. G.V. Devasthali), *Journal of the University of Bombay,* Vol.XXXIX, Arts No., Oct.1970, pp.362-365.
10. *Anubhavānandalaharī* of Keśavānanda Yati (by Dr. K.V. Sarma), *Vishveshvaranand Indological Journal,* Panjab University, Hoshiarpur, Vol.VIII-i-ii, Mar. & Sep. 1970, pp.315-316
11. *Evolution of the Sanskrit Language* (by Dr. S.D. Laddu), *Journal of the University of Bombay,* Bombay, Vols. XLIV & XLV, Nos.80-81, 1975-76 (Arts No.), pp.440-444.
12. Marāṭhawāḍa Sa=mśodhana Maṇḍala, *Annual No. Journal of the Oriental Institute,* M.S. University of Baroda, Baroda, Vol.XXVI, No.2, Dec. 1976, pp.207-210.
13. *Ṣaḍvi=mśa Brāhmaṇam (*ed. by B.R. Sharma), *Journal of the Asiatic Society of Bombay,* Bombay, 1977, pp.176-178.
14. Nārāyaṇa Bhaṭṭa's *Prakriyāsarvasva* (by S. Venkatasubramonia Iyer), *Journal of the Asiatic Society of Bombay*, Bombay, 1977, pp.178-180.
15. *Śrauta-dharmācī Svarūpa-cikitsā* (Marathi) (by C.G.

Kashikar), *Journal of the Asiatic Society of Bombay*, Bombay, Vols. 49-50-51/1974-75-76 (New Series), pub. in 1979, pp.247-250.

16. *Introduction to Pāṇini-I* (by P.B. Junnarkar), *Journal of the Asiatic Society of Bombay*, Bombay, Vols.49-50-51/1974-75-76 (New Series), pub. in 1979, pp.231-232.
17. *Aśvinā in the Ṛgveda and Other Indological Essays* (by Dr. G.C. Jhala), *Indica*, Journal of the Heras Institute of Indian History and Culture, Bombay, Vol.17, 1980, pp.79-81.
18. *Studies in Pāṇini* (by Hari Prapanna Dwivedi), *Journal of the Asiatic Society of Bombay*, Bombay, Vols.52-53 (1977-78, New Series), pub. in 1981, pp.387-389.
19. *Meaning of Tenses and Moods* (by Dr. Jayashree Gune), *Journal of the Asiatic Society of Bombay*, Bombay, Vols.52-53 (1977-78, New Series), pub. in 1981, pp.389-390.
20. *Verses Attributed to Murari* (by Ludwik Sternbach), *The Indian Historical Review*, Delhi, Vol.VII-1 & 2, July 1980–Jan.1981, pp.251-252.
21. *Unknown Verses Attributed to Kṣemendra* (by Ludwik Sternbach), *The Indian Historical Review*, Delhi, Vol.VII — 1 & 2, July 1980-Jan.1981, pp.252-253.
22. *Abhinavagupta and his Works* (by Dr. V. Raghavan), *Journal of the University of Bombay*, Bombay, Post-Centennial Silver Jubilee Year Commemorative Vol. (1982), pp.61-62.
23. *India as seen in the Kuṭṭanīmata of Damodaragupta* (by Dr. A.M. Shastri), *Journal of the University of Bombay*, Bombay, Post-Centennial Silver Jubilee Year Commemorative Vol.(1982), pp.307-309.
24. *Indian Society, Religion and Mythology* (by Dr. A.J. Rawal), *Journal of the Oriental Institute*, M.S. University of Baroda, Baroda, Vol.XXXII, Nos.3 & 4, March-June 1983, pp.338-340.
25. *Vaidika Vāṅmayātīl Praśnottare* (Marathi) (by Dr.

M.A. Mehendale), *Journal of the Asiatic Society of Bombay*, Bombay, Vols. 54-55, (1979-80 combined), pub. in 1983, pp.235-239.

26. *Sexual Metaphors and Animal Symbols in Indian Mythology* (by Wendy Doniger O'Flaherty), *The Indian Historical Review,* New Delhi, Vol.XI-1 & 2, 1984-85, pp.189-191.
27. *Bhāratīya Mithyāncā Māgovā* (Marathi) (by Vishwanath Khaire), *Bhāṣā āṇi Jīvana,* Marathi Abhyāsa Pariṣada Patrikā, Pune, Vol.V-2, (Summer Issue), 1987, pp.38-50.
28. *Vedic Tantrism* (by Dr. M.S. Bhat), *Journal of the Asiatic Society of Bombay*, Bombay, Vol.60-61, (New Series for 1985-86), pub. in 1991, pp.133-137.
29. *Vāstusūtropaniṣad* (by Alice Boner, Sadaśiva Rath Śarma and Bettina B¥aumer), *Journal of the Asiatic Society of Bombay,* Bombay, Vol.60-61 (New Series for 1985-86), pub.in 1991, pp.126-130.
30. *Oaths and Ordeals in Dharmaśāstra* (by S.N. Pendse), *Journal of the Asiatic Society of Bombay,* Bombay, Vol. 60-61 (New Series for 1985-86), pub. in 1991, pp.131-132.
31. *A Comparative History of Ideas* (by Hazime Nakamura), *Journal of the Asiatic Society of Bombay*, Bombay, Vols.67-68 (combined for 1992-93-94), pp.368-372.
32. *An Essay on the Myth of the Ṛbhus* (by Félix Néve, tr. from French into English by G.V. Davane), *Journal of the Asiatic Society of Bombay,* Bombay, Vol.70 (for 1995), pp.169-171.
33. *The Ṛgveda as Oral Literature* (by Nilanjana Sikdar Datta), *Journal of the Asiatic Society of Bombay,* Mumbai, Vol.74 (for 1999), New Series, pub. in 2000, pp.264-267.
34. Ṛgveda and the Indus Script (by Egbert Richter—Ushanas), *Journal of the Oriental Institute, M.S. University of Baroda*, Baroda, Vol. XLIX (in press, to be published shortly).

Index

(Figures in the bracket indicate numbers in the notes)